Glucolipotoxicity and the Heart

Guest Editors

PETER P. TOTH, MD, PhD
VASUDEVAN A. RAGHAVAN, MBBS, MD, MRCP (UK)

HEART FAILURE CLINICS

www.heartfailure.theclinics.com

Consulting Editors
RAGAVENDRA R. BALIGA, MD, MBA
JAMES B. YOUNG, MD

Founding Editor
JAGAT NARULA, MD, PhD

October 2012 • Volume 8 • Number 4

SAUNDERS an imprint of ELSEVIER, Inc.

W.B. SAUNDERS COMPANY
A Division of Elsevier Inc.

1600 John F. Kennedy Boulevard • Suite 1800 • Philadelphia, Pennsylvania 19103-2899

http://www.theclinics.com

HEART FAILURE CLINICS Volume 8, Number 4
October 2012 ISSN 1551-7136, ISBN-13: 978-1-4557-4892-1

Editor: Barbara Cohen-Kligerman
Developmental Editor: Teia Stone

Heart Failure Clinics (ISSN 1551-7136) is published quarterly by Elsevier Inc., 360 Park Avenue South, New York, NY 10010-1710. Months of publication are January, April, July, and October. Business and editorial offices: 1600 John F. Kennedy Boulevard, Suite 1800, Philadelphia, PA 19103-2899. Periodicals postage paid at New York, NY, and additional mailing offices. Subscription prices are USD 224.00 per year for US individuals, USD 347.00 per year for US institutions, USD 76.00 per year for US students and residents, USD 268.00 per year for Canadian individuals, USD 398.00 per year for Canadian institutions, USD 285.00 per year for international individuals, USD 398.00 per year for international institutions, and USD 96.00 per year for Canadian and foreign students/residents. To receive student and resident rate, orders must be accompanied by name of affiliated institution, date of term, and the *signature* of program/residency coordinator on institution letterhead. Orders will be billed at individual rate until proof of status is received. Foreign air speed delivery is included in all *Clinics* subscription prices. All prices are subject to change without notice. **POSTMASTER:** Send address changes to *Heart Failure Clinics*, Elsevier Health Sciences Division, Subscription Customer Service, 3251 Riverport Lane, Maryland Heights, MO 63043. **Customer Service: 1-800-654-2452 (US and Canada). From outside of the US and Canada, call 314-447-8871. Fax: 314-447-8029. For print support, e-mail: JournalsCustomerService-usa@elsevier.com. For online support, e-mail: JournalsOnlineSupport-usa@elsevier.com.**

Reprints. For copies of 100 or more of articles in this publication, please contact the Commercial Reprints Department, Elsevier Inc., 360 Park Avenue South, New York, NY 10010-1710. Tel.: 212-633-3812; Fax: 212-462-1935; E-mail: reprints@elsevier.com.

Heart Failure Clinics is covered in *MEDLINE/PubMed (Index Medicus)*.

Cover artwork courtesy of Umberto M. Jezek.

Printed and bound by CPI Group (UK) Ltd, Croydon, CR0 4YY

Transferred to Digital Print 2012

Contributors

CONSULTING EDITORS

RAGAVENDRA R. BALIGA, MD, MBA
Vice Chief, Division of Cardiovascular
Medicine, Professor of Internal Medicine,
Ohio State University Medical Center,
Columbus, Ohio

JAMES B. YOUNG, MD
Professor of Medicine and Executive Dean,
Cleveland Clinic Lerner College of Medicine,
George and Linda Kaufman Chair, Cleveland
Clinic, Cleveland, Ohio

GUEST EDITORS

**PETER P. TOTH, MD, PhD, FAAFP, FNLA,
FCCP, FAHA, FACC**
Professor of Clinical Family and Community
Medicine, University of Illinois College of
Medicine, Peoria, Illinois; Director of Preventive
Cardiology, CGH Medical Center,
Sterling, Illinois

**VASUDEVAN A. RAGHAVAN, MBBS, MD,
MRCP (UK)**
Associate Professor, Division of Diabetes,
Endocrinology & Metabolism, Department of
Internal Medicine, Texas A&M Health Sciences
Center and College of Medicine; Director,
Cardiometabolic, Lipid Clinic and Medical
Weight Management Services, Scott and
White, Temple, Texas

AUTHORS

ANNAYYA R. AROOR, MD, PhD
Research Assistant Professor, Department
of Internal Medicine; Diabetes and
Cardiovascular Research Center, University
of Missouri School of Medicine, Columbia,
Missouri

NICHOLAS A. AVITABILE, MD
Chief Fellow, Section of Endocrinology,
Tulane University Health Sciences Center,
New Orleans, Louisiana

AJAZ BANKA, MD
Fellow, Section of Endocrinology, Tulane
University Health Sciences Center,
New Orleans, Louisiana

CHRISTOPH BODE, MD
Department of Cardiology and Angiology,
University Hospital of Freiburg, Freiburg,
Germany

DAVID N. BRINDLEY, PhD, DSc, FRSC
Signal Transduction Research Group,
Department of Biochemistry, School of
Translational Medicine, University of Alberta,
Edmonton, Alberta, Canada

HEIKO BUGGER, MD
Department of Cardiology and Angiology,
University Hospital of Freiburg, Freiburg,
Germany

ELISABETTA BUGIANESI, MD, PhD
Division of Gastro-Hepatology, Department
of Internal Medicine, San Giovanni Battista
Hospital, University of Turin, Turin, Italy

SRUTI CHANDRASEKRAN, MD
Department of Medicine, Division of
Endocrinology, Diabetes and Nutrition,
University of Maryland, Baltimore,
Maryland

ANNA MARIA J. CHOY, MD, FRCP, FACC
Division of Cardiovascular and Diabetes
Medicine, Medical Research Institute,
Ninewells Hospital and Medical School,
University of Dundee, Dundee, United Kingdom

KATHLEEN DUNGAN, MD
Division of Endocrinology, Diabetes and
Metabolism, Department of Internal Medicine,
The Ohio State University, Columbus, Ohio

VIVIAN A. FONSECA, MD
Professor of Medicine and Pharmacology;
Chief, Section of Endocrinology, Tullis-Tulane
Alumni Chair in Diabetes, Tulane University
Health Sciences Center, New Orleans,
Louisiana

ALAN J. GARBER, MD, PhD, FACE
Professor, Division of Diabetes, Endocrinology
and Metabolism, Department of Medicine,
Baylor College of Medicine, Houston, Texas

AMALIA GASTALDELLI, PhD
Institute of Clinical Physiology, National
Research Council, Pisa, Italy

IRA J. GOLDBERG, MD
Professor, Division of Preventive Medicine
and Nutrition, Columbia University, New York,
New York

JEONG-A KIM, PhD
Assistant Professor of Medicine, Division of
Endocrinology, Diabetes, and Metabolism,
Department of Medicine, UAB Comprehensive
Diabetes Center; Department of Cell Biology,
University of Alabama at Birmingham,
Birmingham, Alabama

BERNARD P.C. KOK, PhD
Signal Transduction Research Group,
Department of Biochemistry, School of
Translational Medicine, University of Alberta,
Edmonton, Alberta, Canada

ALEXANDRA KÖNIG, BS
Department of Cardiology and Angiology,
University Hospital of Freiburg, Freiburg,
Germany

CHIM C. LANG, MD, FRCP, FACC
Division of Cardiovascular and Diabetes
Medicine, Medical Research Institute,
Ninewells Hospital and Medical School,
University of Dundee, Dundee, United Kingdom

CHIRAG H. MANDAVIA, MD
Post-Doctoral Fellow, Department of Internal
Medicine, Diabetes and Cardiovascular
Research Center, University of Missouri School
of Medicine, Columbia, Missouri

DOUGLAS L. MANN, MD
Lewin Professor and Chief, Center for
Cardiovascular Research, Division of
Cardiology, Department of Medicine,
Washington University School of Medicine,
St Louis, Missouri

MONICA MONTAGNANI, MD, PhD
Department of Biomedical Sciences and
Human Oncology, Pharmacology Section,
University Aldo Moro at Bari, Policlinico,
Bari, Italy

JARED MOORE, MD
Department of Internal Medicine, The Ohio
State University, Columbus, Ohio

TAE-SIK PARK, PhD
Associate Professor, Department of Life
Science, Gachon University, Seongnam,
Gyunggi-do, South Korea

SAMPATH PARTHASARATHY, MSc, PhD
Florida Hospital Chair in Cardiovascular
Science and Professor of Medicine, Burnett
School of Biomedical Sciences, University
of Central Florida, Orlando, Florida

MICHAEL J. QUON, MD, PhD
Professor of Medicine, Professor of
Physiology, Division of Endocrinology,
Diabetes & Nutrition, Department of Medicine,
University of Maryland, Baltimore, Maryland

**VASUDEVAN A. RAGHAVAN, MBBS, MD,
MRCP (UK)**
Associate Professor, Division of Diabetes,
Endocrinology & Metabolism, Department of
Internal Medicine, Texas A&M Health Sciences
Center and College of Medicine; Director,
Cardiometabolic, Lipid Clinic and Medical
Weight Management Services, Scott and
White, Temple, Texas

JOEL D. SCHILLING, MD, PhD
Assistant Professor, Departments of Medicine,
Pathology and Immunology, Diabetic
Cardiovascular Disease Center, Division of
Cardiology, Washington University School
of Medicine, St Louis, Missouri

JAMES R. SOWERS, MD
Professor, Departments of Internal Medicine,
Medical Pharmacology and Physiology;
Director, Diabetes and Cardiovascular
Research Center, University of Missouri School
of Medicine; Harry S. Truman Memorial
Veterans' Hospital, Columbia, Missouri

VELLORE A.R. SRINIVASAN, MSc, PhD
Professor, Department of Biochemistry,
Mahatma Gandhi Medical College & Research
Institute, Sri Balaji Vidyapeeth University,
Puducherry, India

ALLAN D. STRUTHERS, MD, FRCP, FESC
Division of Cardiovascular and Diabetes
Medicine, Medical Research Institute,

Ninewells Hospital and Medical School,
University of Dundee, Dundee, United Kingdom

**PETER P. TOTH, MD, PhD, FAAFP, FNLA,
FCCP, FAHA, FACC**
Professor of Clinical Family and Community
Medicine, University of Illinois College of
Medicine, Peoria, Illinois; Director of
Preventive Cardiology, CGH Medical
Center, Sterling, Illinois

AARON K.F. WONG, MD, MRCP
Division of Cardiovascular and Diabetes
Medicine, Medical Research Institute,
Ninewells Hospital and Medical School,
University of Dundee, Dundee,
United Kingdom

Contents

Both glucose and fatty acids may have good/adaptive or toxic/maladaptive actions on the pancreatic beta cell, depending on their concentrations. Hyperglycemia, via metabolic intermediates, may result in multiple cellular effects that are toxic to the pancreatic beta cell and indeed other tissues. While free fatty acids may affect cellular processes beyond lipid metabolism by interacting with transcription factors, triglyceride rich lipoproteins are endothelial cell-toxic and facilitate atherogenesis. The paradigm of "glucolipotoxicity" espouses that increased glucose and fatty acid levels act synergistically in causing toxicity to pancreatic islets and other organs, a process that eventually leads to the multiple defects seen in the metabolic syndrome and diabetes mellitus.

Glucose lowering should be approached by managing overall cardiovascular risk. Glycemic goals should be individualized based on duration of diabetes, preexisting cardiovascular disease, age, and life expectancy. Intensive glycemic control has consistently been shown to produce a substantial benefit for preventing long-term microvascular complications in both type 1 and type 2 diabetes mellitus. Although cardiovascular disease is the major cause of death in patients with diabetes, microvascular complications cause substantial morbidity and disability. Thus, it is apparent that additional strategies on multimodal treatment options are necessary to promote effective management and prevention of diabetic complications.

The mechanisms for hyperglycemia-mediated harm in the hospitalized cardiac patient are poorly understood. Potential obstacles in the inpatient management of hyperglycemia in cardiac patients include rapidly changing clinical status, frequent procedures and interruptions in carbohydrate exposure, and short hospital length of stay. A patient's preadmission regimen is rarely suitable for inpatient glycemic control. Instead, an approach to a flexible, physiologic insulin regimen is described, which is intended to minimize glycemic excursions. When diabetes or hyperglycemia is addressed early and consistently, the hospital stay can serve as a potential window of opportunity for reinforcing self-care behaviors that reduce long-term complications.

a hallmark of atherosclerosis, hypertension, and coronary heart disease, which are major complications of metabolic disorders, including diabetes and obesity. Several therapeutic interventions, including changes in lifestyle as well as pharmacologic treatments, are useful for improving endothelial dysfunction in the face of lipotoxicity. This review discusses the current understanding of molecular and physiologic mechanisms underlying lipotoxicity-mediated endothelial dysfunction as well as relevant therapeutic approaches to ameliorate dyslipidemia and consequent endothelial dysfunction that have the potential to improve cardiovascular and metabolic outcomes.

Annayya R. Aroor, Chirag H. Mandavia, and James R. Sowers

This article addresses the issue of insulin resistance and associated reductions in cardiac insulin metabolic signaling, which is emerging as a major factor in the development of heart failure, and assumes more importance because of an epidemic increase in obesity and the cardiorenal metabolic syndrome in our aging population. The effects of cardiac insulin resistance are exacerbated by metabolic, endocrine, and cytokine alterations associated with systemic insulin resistance. Understanding the molecular mechanisms linking insulin resistance and heart failure may help to design new and more effective mechanism-based drugs to improve myocardial and systemic insulin resistance.

Joel D. Schilling and Douglas L. Mann

The study of diabetic cardiomyopathy is an area of significant interest given the strong association between diabetes and the risk of heart failure. Many unanswered questions remain regarding the clinical definition and pathogenesis of this metabolic cardiomyopathy. This article reviews the current understanding of diabetic cardiomyopathy with a particular emphasis on the unresolved issues that have limited translation of scientific discovery to patient bedside.

Tae-Sik Park and Ira J. Goldberg

In the setting of obesity and type 2 diabetes mellitus, the ectopic disposition of lipids may be a cause of heart failure. Clinical studies have clearly shown a correlation between the accumulation of triglycerides and heart dysfunction. In this process, it is likely that there are also changes in the contents of sphingolipids. Sphingolipids are important structural and signaling molecules. One specific sphingolipid, ceramide, may cause cardiac dysfunction, whereas another, sphingosine 1-phosphate, is cardioprotective. In this review, the authors focus on the role of sphingolipids in the development and prevention of cardiac failure.

Bernard P.C. Kok and David N. Brindley

Management of diabetes and insulin resistance in the setting of cardiovascular disease has become an important issue in an increasingly obese society. Besides the development of hypertension and buildup of atherosclerotic plaques, the derangement of fatty acid and lipid metabolism in the heart plays an important role in promoting cardiac dysfunction and oxidative stress. This review discusses the mechanisms by which metabolic inflexibility in the use of fatty acids as the preferred cardiac substrate in diabetes produces detrimental effects on mechanical efficiency, mitochondrial function, and recovery from ischemia. Lipid accumulation and the consequences of toxic lipid metabolites are also discussed.

Cardiac and hepatic fat are associated with insulin resistance and impaired suppression of lipolysis, ultimately leading to lipotoxicity. In the heart the lipotoxic effect translates into an impairment of energetic and mechanical efficiency, whereas in the liver a fibrogenic response is favored by the abundance of inflammatory cells. These features precede, and likely contribute to, left ventricular overload and cardiac hypertrophy through mechanisms similar to the ones observed in the progression of liver damage in nonalcoholic fatty liver disease (NAFLD). Collectively these findings suggest the presence of complex and intertwined interrelationships between NAFLD, myocardial steatosis, and coronary artery disease.

Insulin resistance (IR) is the accepted primary cause of the metabolic syndrome. Visceral obesity is inversely correlated with insulin sensitivity. Hyperinsulinemia (a surrogate for IR) is highly prevalent in patients with coronary artery disease (CAD). Abnormalities in lipid metabolism give rise to steatosis in multiple organs. Evidence is rapidly accumulating to show that epicardial steatosis and expansion of coronary fat pad volume are highly deleterious and associated with increased risk for CAD. This article explores such associations from biochemical and structural standpoints, focusing on changes in epicardial adiposity.

HEART FAILURE CLINICS

**DOWNLOAD
Free App!**

Review Articles
THE CLINICS

NOW AVAILABLE FOR YOUR iPhone and iPad

Editorial

β-Blockers in Heart Failure: Breaking Tradition to Avoid Diabetes?

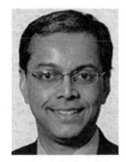 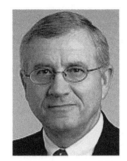

Ragavendra R. Baliga, MD, MBA   James B. Young, MD

Consulting Editors

A tradition without intelligence is not worth having.

— *T.S. Eliot*

β-Blockers are now a mainstay in the management of systolic heart failure.[1,2] The benefits of β-blockers include reversal of cardiac remodeling,[3] a decrease in rennin-angiotensin-aldosterone system activity,[4] improved myocardial perfusion in ischemic heart disease[5,6] (decreasing heart rate and blood pressure and prolongation of diastole with subsequent increase in coronary filling), anti-arrhythmic properties[5,6] (prevention of sudden death), and anti-atherogenic[6] properties (improved endothelial function with plaque stabilization). However, the long-term use of traditional β-blockers, such as atenolol and metoprolol, has been reported to have potentially detrimental metabolic side effects including weight increase,[7,8] adverse effects on lipid profiles[9] (may increase triglyceride levels and may lower high-density lipoprotein cholesterol levels), and an impact on insulin sensitivity[8,9] (attenuation of release of pancreatic insulin).

The Atherosclerosis Risk in Communities Study (ARIC) investigators were the first to report that long-term utilization of traditional β-blockers is associated with a 28% higher risk of subsequent diabetes [hazard ratio (HR), 1.28; 95% confidence interval (CI), 1.04-1.57],[10] whereas subjects who were taking angiotensin-converting-enzyme inhibitors and calcium-channel antagonists were not at greater risk than those not taking any medication. This effort was a prospective study of 12,550 adults 45 to 64 years old who did not have diabetes; the incidence of new cases of diabetes was assessed after 3 and 6 years by the measurement of fasting serum glucose concentrations.

The Anglo-Scandinavian Cardiac Outcomes Trial-Blood Pressure Lowering Arm (ASCOT-BPLA),[11] a multicenter randomized controlled trial of 19,257 patients with hypertension aged 40 to 79 years, also reported an increased onset of new diabetes when the traditional β-blocker atenolol was combined with diuretics compared to a combination of angiotensin-converting-enzyme inhibitor and calcium channel antagonist (HR = 0.70 [95% CI, 0.63–0.78] $P < 0.0001$) (**Fig. 1**).

Two meta-analyses also reported that utilization of traditional β-blockers was associated with increased risk of diabetes. Bangalore and coworkers studied 12 trials (n = 94,492) and found that older β-blockers increased the relative risk of new onset diabetes by 21% when compared to calcium channel antagonists ($P = 0.003$) and by 23% when compared to angiotensin-converting-enzyme inhibitors or angiotensin receptor blockers ($P = 0.007$).[12] This meta-analysis also reported that β-blockers were associated with a decrease in relative risk of new onset diabetes by 26% when

Heart Failure Clin 8 (2012) xiii–xvi
http://dx.doi.org/10.1016/j.hfc.2012.07.002

heartfailure.theclinics.com

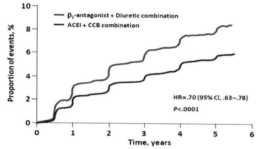

Fig. 1. ASCOT-BPLA and risk of new onset diabetes with β-blockers. HR, hazard ratio; CI, confidence interval. [*Adapted from* Dahlof B, Sever PS, Poulter NR, et al. Prevention of cardiovascular events with an antihypertensive regimen of amlodipine adding perindopril as required versus atenolol adding bendroflumethiazide as required, in the Anglo-Scandinavian Cardiac Outcomes Trial-Blood Pressure Lowering Arm (ASCOT-BPLA): a multicentre randomised controlled trial. Lancet 2005;366(9489):895–906 with permission.]

compared to thiazides (*P* = 0.002). The second meta-analysis, by Elliott and Meyers, of 22 trials of antihypertensive medications (n = 143,153), including 9 trials that utilized older β-blockers, reported that the association of antihypertensive drugs with incident diabetes is lowest for angiotensin receptor blockers and angiotensin-converting-enzyme inhibitors followed by calcium channel antagonists and placebo, β-blockers, and diuretics in rank order (**Fig. 2**).[13] The older and more traditional β-blocker, atenolol, was the primary β-blocker comparator for most of the trials included in the meta-analyses. Also noted was that when compared with atenolol, nonatenolol β-blockers reduced the risk of new myocardial infarction by 13%.[14] Vasodilating β-blockers such as

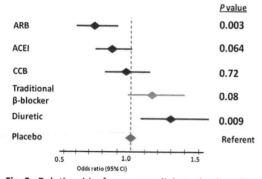

Fig. 2. Relative risk of new onset diabetes by drug class. [*Data from* Elliott WJ, Meyer PM. Incident diabetes in clinical trials of antihypertensive drugs: a network meta-analysis. Lancet 2007;369(9557):201–7.]

carvedilol and nebivolol only represented a small percentage of the data in the meta-analyses (1 trial).

Is there a clinically significant difference in β-adrenergic blocking drugs based on their different pharmacologic actions? The vasodilating β-blockers such as carvedilol[15] and nebivolol[16-18] have been shown efficacious in the management of heart failure due to left ventricular systolic dysfunction. The GEMINI study[19] (The Glycemic Effects in Diabetes Mellitus: Carvedilol-Metoprolol Comparison in Hypertensives) compared the effects of carvedilol (vasodilating β-blocker) and metoprolol tartrate (older and more traditional β-blocker) on glycemic and metabolic control in participants with diabetes mellitus and hypertension receiving renin-angiotensin system (RAS) blockade. This study was a randomized, double-blind, parallel-group trial that evaluated 1235 participants aged 36 to 85 years with hypertension (>130/80 mm Hg) and type 2 diabetes mellitus (glycosylated hemoglobin [HbA1c], 6.5%-8.5%) and receiving RAS blockers. The study subjects were randomized to receive a 6.25- to 25-mg dose of carvedilol (n = 498) or a 50- to 200-mg dose of metoprolol tartrate (n = 737), each twice daily. Open-label hydrochlorothiazide and a dihydropyridine calcium channel antagonist were added, when required, to achieve target blood pressures.

The study cohort was followed up for 35 weeks. The mean (SD) HbA1c increased with metoprolol (0.15% [0.04%]; *P* < 0.001) but not carvedilol (0.02% [0.04%]; *P* = 0.65). Insulin sensitivity improved with carvedilol (−9.1%; *P* = 0.004) but not metoprolol (−2.0%; *P* = 0.48); the between-group difference was −7.2% (95% CI, −13.8% to −0.2%; *P* = 0.004). Blood pressure was similar between groups. Progression to microalbuminuria was less frequent with carvedilol than with metoprolol (6.4% vs 10.3%; odds ratio, 0.60; 95% CI, 0.36-0.97; *P* = 0.04). This study suggests that traditional β-blockers make insulin sensitivity worse, whereas vasodilating β-blockers may have a beneficial effect. Small studies have shown that carvedilol improves insulin sensitivity compared to metoprolol[20] and atenolol.[21] It has been suggested that the α1-blocking properties of vasodilating β-blockers decrease total peripheral resistance (**Fig. 3**) when compared with traditional β-blockers, improve skeletal muscle blood flow, and increase insulin sensitivity.[22] It could be argued that vasodilating β-blockers should, indeed, be the β-blockers of choice for the long-term management of heart failure to avoid the 28% higher risk of subsequent diabetes reported after long-term utilization of these agents in the ARIC study.

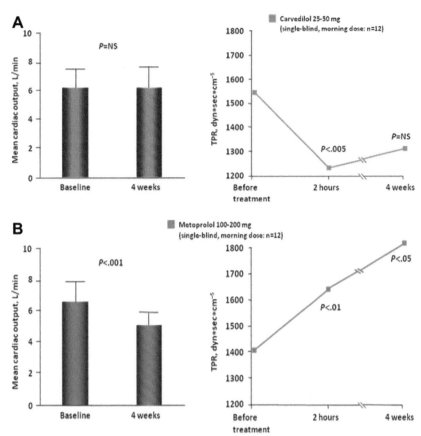

Fig. 3. (A) Effect of Carvedilol (vasodilating β-blocker) on cardiac output and total peripheral resistance. (B) Effect of Metoprolol (traditional β-blocker) on cardiac output and total peripheral resistance. [*From* Weber K, Bohmeke T, van der Does R, et al. Comparison of the hemodynamic effects of metoprolol and carvedilol in hypertensive patients. Cardiovasc Drugs Ther 1996;10(2):113–7; with kind permission from Springer Science+Business Media B.V.]

To discuss similar issues regarding glucolipotoxicity in heart failure, Vasudevan A. Raghavan, MD and Peter P. Toth, MD, PhD have assembled a world class team of experts. These articles shed light on the interface between glucose and lipid metabolism on cardiac function and heart failure. In our opinion, these articles support a break in some traditional practices in the management of heart failure, including the controversial recommendation of turning away from the older and more traditional β-blockers as first-line therapy and using vasodilating β-blockers instead. Perhaps it is time to break tradition to avoid the risk of diabetes associated with long-term utilization of some β-blockers.

Ragavendra R. Baliga, MD, MBA
Division of Cardiovascular Medicine
The Ohio State University Medical Center
Columbus, OH, USA

James B. Young, MD
Lerner College of Medicine and Endocrinology
& Metabolism Institute
Cleveland Clinic
Cleveland, OH, USA

E-mail addresses:
Ragavendra.baliga@osumc.edu (R.R. Baliga)
youngj@ccf.org (J.B. Young)

REFERENCES

1. Hunt SA, Abraham WT, Chin MH, et al. 2009 Focused update incorporated into the ACC/AHA 2005 Guidelines for the Diagnosis and Management of Heart Failure in Adults. A report of the American College of Cardiology Foundation/American Heart Association Task Force on Practice Guidelines developed in collaboration with the International Society for Heart and Lung Transplantation. J Am Coll Cardiol 2009;53(15):e1–90.

2. Hunt SA, Abraham WT, Chin MH, et al. ACC/AHA 2005 Guideline update for the diagnosis and management of chronic heart failure in the adult: a report of the American College of Cardiology/American Heart Association Task Force on Practice Guidelines (Writing Committee to Update the 2001 Guidelines for the Evaluation and Management of Heart Failure): developed in collaboration with the American College of Chest Physicians and the International Society for Heart and Lung Transplantation: endorsed by the Heart Rhythm Society. Circulation 2005;112(12):e154–235.

3. Hall SA, Cigarroa CG, Marcoux L, et al. Time course of improvement in left ventricular function, mass and geometry in patients with congestive heart failure treated with beta-adrenergic blockade. J Am Coll Cardiol 1995;25(5):1154–61.

4. Blumenfeld JD, Sealey JE, Mann SJ, et al. Beta-adrenergic receptor blockade as a therapeutic approach for suppressing the renin-angiotensin-aldosterone system in normotensive and hypertensive subjects. Am J Hypertens 1999;12(5):451–9.

5. Tse WY, Kendall M. Is there a role for beta-blockers in hypertensive diabetic patients? Diabet Med 1994;11(2):137–44.

6. Fonarow GC. Managing the patient with diabetes mellitus and heart failure: issues and considerations. Am J Med 2004;116(Suppl 5A):76S–88S.

7. Messerli FH, Bell DS, Fonseca V, et al. Body weight changes with beta-blocker use: results from GEMINI. Am J Med 2007;120(7):610–5.

8. Bangalore S, Messerli FH, Kostis JB, et al. Cardiovascular protection using beta-blockers: a critical review of the evidence. J Am Coll Cardiol 2007;50(7):563–72.

9. Bakris GL, Hart P, Ritz E. Beta blockers in the management of chronic kidney disease. Kidney Int 2006;70(11):1905–13.

10. Gress TW, Nieto FJ, Shahar E, et al. Hypertension and antihypertensive therapy as risk factors for type 2 diabetes mellitus. Atherosclerosis Risk in Communities Study. N Engl J Med 2000;342(13):905–12.

11. Dahlof B, Sever PS, Poulter NR, et al. Prevention of cardiovascular events with an antihypertensive regimen of amlodipine adding perindopril as required versus atenolol adding bendroflumethiazide as required, in the Anglo-Scandinavian Cardiac Outcomes Trial-Blood Pressure Lowering Arm (ASCOT-BPLA): a multicentre randomised controlled trial. Lancet 2005;366(9489):895–906.

12. Bangalore S, Parkar S, Grossman E, et al. A meta-analysis of 94,492 patients with hypertension treated with beta blockers to determine the risk of new-onset diabetes mellitus. Am J Cardiol 2007;100(8):1254–62.

13. Elliott WJ, Meyer PM. Incident diabetes in clinical trials of antihypertensive drugs: a network meta-analysis. Lancet 2007;369(9557):201–7.

14. Aursnes I, Osnes JB, Tvete IF, et al. Does atenolol differ from other beta-adrenergic blockers? BMC Clin Pharmacol 2007;7:4.

15. Young JB. Carvedilol for heart failure: renewed interest in beta blockers. Cleve Clin J Med 1997;64(8):415–22.

16. van Veldhuisen DJ, Cohen-Solal A, Bohm M, et al. Beta-blockade with nebivolol in elderly heart failure patients with impaired and preserved left ventricular ejection fraction: Data from SENIORS (Study of Effects of Nebivolol Intervention on Outcomes and Rehospitalization in Seniors With Heart Failure). J Am Coll Cardiol 2009;53(23):2150–8.

17. Tavazzi L. Nebivolol for heart failure in the elderly. Expert Rev Cardiovasc Ther 2007;5(3):423–33.

18. Edes I, Gasior Z, Wita K. Effects of nebivolol on left ventricular function in elderly patients with chronic heart failure: results of the ENECA study. Eur J Heart Fail 2005;7(4):631–9.

19. Bakris GL, Fonseca V, Katholi RE, et al. Metabolic effects of carvedilol vs metoprolol in patients with type 2 diabetes mellitus and hypertension: a randomized controlled trial. JAMA 2004;292(18):2227–36.

20. Jacob S, Rett K, Wicklmayr M, et al. Differential effect of chronic treatment with two beta-blocking agents on insulin sensitivity: the carvedilol-metoprolol study. J Hypertens 1996;14(4):489–94.

21. Giugliano D, Acampora R, Marfella R, et al. Metabolic and cardiovascular effects of carvedilol and atenolol in non-insulin-dependent diabetes mellitus and hypertension. A randomized, controlled trial. Ann Intern Med 1997;126(12):955–9.

22. Weber K, Bohmeke T, van der Does R, et al. Comparison of the hemodynamic effects of metoprolol and carvedilol in hypertensive patients. Cardiovasc Drugs Ther 1996;10(2):113–7.

Preface
Glucolipotoxicity and the Heart

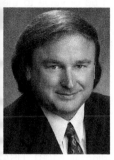
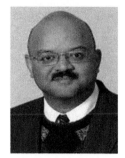

Peter P. Toth, MD, PhD   Vasudevan A. Raghavan, MBBS,
MD, MRCP (UK)

Guest Editors

Insulin resistance (IR) and type 2 diabetes mellitus are widely prevalent throughout the world and have reached epidemic proportions in both genders and in people of all racial and ethnic groups. IR has a metabolically complex and as yet incompletely understood etiology. Major driving forces for the rise of IR include obesity, sedentary lifestyle, excess caloric intake, and cigarette smoking, all of which have risen globally in prevalence. IR and diabetes mellitus (DM) increase the risk for all forms of atherosclerotic disease, heart failure, stroke, and microangiopathy, including proliferative retinopathy, nephropathy, and peripheral neuropathy. With over 340 million diabetic patients in the world, it is anticipated that this will result in a catastrophic rise in adult-onset blindness, end-stage renal disease, and need for dialysis, lower extremity amputation, as well as cardiovascular morbidity and premature mortality. Approximately 78% of diabetic patients will die of complications stemming from cardiovascular disease (CVD). The human, social, and economic costs of these clinical sequelae require urgent recognition and intervention.

It has recently been estimated that up to two-thirds of patients who present with myocardial infarction have either impaired glucose tolerance or DM. IR is frequently encountered in cardiology practice and it is important for cardiologists to have an in-depth understanding of how IR adversely impacts cardiac structure, function, and metabolism.

The term "glucolipotoxicity" is an apt descriptor for the overarching metabolic changes induced by IR. In this setting, systemic tissues do not internalize glucose appropriately in response to insulin and patients become progressively more hyperglycemic. Hyperglycemia and IR accelerate atherogenesis, induce endothelial dysfunction, promote inflammation and a pro-oxidative state, and are associated with multiple toxic, adverse changes in intracellular glucose metabolism. Despite the fact that aggressive glucose control in diabetic patients has not been shown to impact CVD risk favorably, trends toward event reduction have been shown in multiple trials. When patients from the Diabetes Control and Complications Trial and the United Kingdom Prospective Diabetes Study were followed up long term after the trials had been completed, both trials demonstrated statistically significant reductions in risk for CVD events. Thus, controlling serum glucose is important in preventing both microvascular and macrovascular complications of DM, although the beneficial effects on the former are more striking.

IR and DM are associated with significant changes in lipids and lipoprotein fractions resulting in the so-called atherogenic lipid triad: increased triglycerides and VLDL remnant particles, reduced HDL-C, and increased small, dense LDL-C. This most certainly augments risk for coronary artery disease. However, other profound changes in lipid handling and metabolism occur in parallel with the development of atherogenic dyslipidemia. Systemic tissue steatosis increases in organs such as the heart (myocardium and epicardium), liver, skeletal muscle, and pancreas. Increased intracellular lipid storage and toxicity result from exposure of tissues to high levels of fatty acids, diacylglycerol, and ceramide. In myocardium, the increased

Heart Failure Clin 8 (2012) xvii–xviii
http://dx.doi.org/10.1016/j.hfc.2012.07.001

heartfailure.theclinics.com

accumulation and storage of these lipids result in mitochondrial dysfunction, endoplasmic reticulum stress, and impaired intracellular energy and calcium ion metabolism. In the insulin-resistant state, myocardial function is compromised and the risk of nonischemic cardiomyopathy increases. Rates of atherogenesis in the epicardial vessels increase secondary to the accumulation of metabolically active epicardial fat that showers the surrounding vessels with lipid and inflammatory mediators. In the context of lipotoxicity, it is important to consider the adverse effects of lipids not just in terms of risk for atherosclerotic disease, but also for their capacity to induce myocardial functional impairment, myocyte apoptosis, cardiac fibrosis, and heart failure. Thus, the impact of dyslipidemia and the generation of excess cytotoxic lipid in the insulin-resistant state have much more far-reaching implications for cardiovascular function than previously assumed.

The goal of this issue of the *Heart Failure Clinics* is to raise awareness of the profound metabolic alterations induced by the glucolipotoxicity associated with IR and DM and the many ways in which these changes adversely affect the environment in which the vasculature and cardiac myocyte function. This issue also sheds light on the many potentially new therapeutic approaches available for preventing and/or managing the cardiovascular complications of glucolipotoxicity. We sincerely thank our contributors for devoting their time and effort in writing the various articles. We sincerely hope that the contents of this issue will be of value to the many cardiologists who care passionately about ever more refined approaches of reducing cardiovascular morbidity and mortality in their communities.

Peter P. Toth, MD, PhD
University of Illinois College of Medicine
Peoria, Illinois
CGH Medical Center
Sterling, IL 61081, USA

Vasudevan A. Raghavan, MBBS, MD, MRCP (UK)
Division of Diabetes, Endocrinology, and Metabolism
Texas A&M Health Sciences Center/
College of Medicine
Cardiometabolic and Medical Weight Management
Services
Scott and White
Temple, TX 76508, USA

E-mail addresses:
Peter.toth@cghmc.com (P.P. Toth)
raghavan@medicine.tamhsc.edu (V.A. Raghavan)

Biochemical Basis and Clinical Consequences of Glucolipotoxicity: A Primer

Vellore A.R. Srinivasan, MSc, PhD[a],
Vasudevan A. Raghavan, MBBS, MD, MRCP (UK)[b,c],
Sampath Parthasarathy, MSc, PhD[d,*]

KEYWORDS

- Glucolipotoxicity • Pancreatic β-cell dysfunction • Insulin resistance

KEY POINTS

- High glucose may have direct cellular toxicity by inducing specific cellular effects, including shift in energy source, and causing the accumulation of metabolic intermediates.
- Free fatty acids (lipids) may affect cellular processes beyond lipid metabolism by interacting with transcription factors. High triglyceride-carrying lipoproteins are toxic to endothelial cells.
- Glucose may increase oxygen free radical production, which may affect cellular macromolecules, thereby altering cellular behavior.
- Glucose-induced oxidative stress may promote lipid oxidation and thus could be a key factor in promoting atherosclerosis and renal diseases.

INTRODUCTION

The 2 main forms of diabetes mellitus (DM) are type 1 DM (T1DM) and type 2 DM (T2DM); T2DM is the more prevalent (90%–95%) form.[1] T2DM is characterized by β-cell failure in the setting of obesity-related insulin resistance (IR). Progressive β-cell dysfunction eventually supervenes regardless of the treatment modality used. There is mounting evidence that chronically increased circulating levels of glucose and fatty acids contribute to relentless β-cell function decline through processes commonly referred to as glucolipotoxicity.

T1DM is characterized by severe β-cell dysfunction and an absence of glucose-stimulated insulin secretion (GSIS).[2] After initial insulin treatment, many patients have a honeymoon phase of reduced insulin requirement. This phase tends to be variable in length, and sometimes insulin secretion is restored to the point that exogenous insulin treatment is rendered unnecessary, indicating that the diabetic milieu may be toxic to the β cell. Consistent with this view, transplantation of islets into streptozotocin-induced diabetic mice causes loss of GSIS by the islets in the absence of an immune reaction.[3] This finding suggests that circulating factors normalized by insulin treatment, perhaps increased free fatty acid (FFA) and glucose levels contribute, in addition to autoimmune attack to the development of T1DM.[3]

Although insulin deficiency is the primary defect in T1DM, several studies[4–7] suggest that IR is

a Department of Biochemistry, Mahatma Gandhi Medical College & Research Institute Sri Balaji Vidyapeeth University, Puduchery 607402, India; b Division of Endocrinology, Department of Internal Medicine, Texas A&M Health Sciences Center and College of Medicine, Temple, TX 76508, USA; c Cardiometabolic, Lipid Clinic and Medical Weight Management Services, Scott and White, Center for Diagnostic Medicine, 1605 S 31st Street, Temple, TX 76508, USA; d Burnett School of Biomedical Sciences, University of Central Florida, BBS 101G, 12722 Research Parkway, Orlando, FL 32826, USA
* Corresponding author.
E-mail address: spartha@ucf.edu

a salient feature and in part may contribute to the high incidence of cardiovascular disease (CVD) in this group.[8,9] IR to some extent is genetically inherited[10] and in nondiabetic patients and patients with T2DM is strongly related to abdominal fat independent of total adiposity.[11–13] Also, in T1DM, exogenous insulin administration in levels sufficient to achieve adequate portal levels and maintain euglycemia is almost always associated with (systemic) hyperinsulinemia. Hyperinsulinemia, by increasing the activity of 11β-hydroxysteroid dehydrogenase, may contribute to abdominal fat deposition in T1DM.[14] Insulin effects on omental adipocytes (and given the hypercortisolemic milieu) result in enhanced differentiation of adipose stromal cells to adipocytes, further promoting abdominal obesity.[15] Thus it seems that insulin secretory abnormalities and IR occur in both T1DM and T2DM, although as alluded to earlier, the time of occurrence of either pathophysiologic abnormality, relative to the natural history of disease progression, is different in the 2 types of DM.

Although hyperglycemia is the cardinal biochemical manifestation seen in DM, atherogenic dyslipidemia (combination of high serum triglycerides [TGs], low high-density lipoprotein cholesterol [HDL-C], increased low-density lipoprotein (LDL) particle numbers with small dense LDL cholesterol [sdLDL-c] predominance) is also a frequent occurrence in this condition and seems to be correlated with the degree of IR.[16] The various facets of glucolipotoxicity and its role in cardiac disease are discussed in detail in the articles by Drs Brindley and Sowers elsewhere in this issue. We intend to limit our discussion to the basic biochemical aspects of glucolipotoxicity and its overarching effects, contributing to organ dysfunction.

Experimental evidence suggests that glucolipotoxicity contributes to the steady decline of glucose homeostasis as seen in T2DM, and possibly in T1DM, contributing to both deterioration in β-cell function and peripheral IR. Thus, one may talk of glucotoxicity and lipotoxicity as separate but linked processes or as a combinatorial cellular event (glucolipotoxicity) with deleterious effects on both insulin secretion and insulin action.

GLUCOTOXICITY

Chronic hyperglycemia impairs glucose-induced pancreatic insulin secretion and insulin gene expression[16] through mechanisms that affect glucose desensitization, β-cell exhaustion and glucotoxicity. Glucose desensitization refers to the rapid and reversible refractoriness of the β-cell

exocytotic machinery that occurs after a short exposure to hyperglycemia[16] and is an adaptive mechanism that occurs even when insulin secretion is inhibited, thus differentiating it from β-cell exhaustion.[16] β-Cell exhaustion refers to depletion of the pool of intracellular insulin available for quick release, after prolonged exposure to a secretagogue.[17,18] In contrast, glucotoxicity describes the progressively irreversible effects of chronic hyperglycemia on β-cell function. The β-cell defects are reversible up to a point in time and become irreversible thereafter, suggesting a continuum between β-cell exhaustion and glucotoxicity, with the latter occurring because of prolonged hyperglycemia[19,20] Chronic hyperglycemia may also decrease β-cell mass by inducing islet cell apoptosis.[21,22]

HYPERGLYCEMIA BEGETS HYPERGLYCEMIA

Rats rendered diabetic by streptozotocin treatment or by partial pancreatectomy serve as models of fasting and postprandial hyperglycemia, with residual pancreatic islet (islet) β-cell function, but impaired glucose-induced insulin secretion.[23,24] That hyperglycemia per se may be toxic to the pancreatic islet is apparent from the fact that the insulin secretory defect was greater than could be expected from the surviving β-cell mass. Short-term (less than 48 hours) severe hyperglycemia in normal rats impaired acute glucose-induced insulin release.[25] In partially pancreatectomized diabetic rats, lowering blood glucose by phlorizin-induced renal glycosuria (without having any direct effect on the pancreas or peripheral insulin-responsive tissues), improved both glucose-induced insulin release and the effectiveness of insulin to lower glucose levels (insulin action or insulin sensitivity). This finding suggests that glucose itself may sustain the diabetogenic state.[26,27]

Glucotoxicity is more difficult to study in humans. Kosaka and colleagues[28] showed that lowering plasma glucose levels to the same extent in patients with adult-onset DM, through changes in diet, sulfonylurea, or insulin therapy resulted in similar degrees of improvement in insulin responsiveness to oral glucose, thereby suggesting that the poor insulin response in overt DM results from both relative insensitivity of β cells to glucose and the hyperglycemia inherent in poorly controlled DM. Glucotoxicity also induces IR, which is partially reversible with improved glycemic control. Yki-Jarvinen and colleagues[29] measured glucose uptake after 24 hours of hyperglycemia (281 ± 16 mg/dL; using intravenous glucose) and normoglycemia (99 ± 6 mg/dL; using normal saline) in 10 patients with T1DM (age 33 ± 3 years) treated with continuous subcutaneous insulin infusion. Insulin sensitivity (using the euglycemic clamp model) was significantly lower after the period of hyperglycemia than after normoglycemia. Because these patients lacked endogenous insulin production, this result was believed to represent impaired insulin sensitivity caused by previous exposure to hyperglycemia.

An element of glucotoxicity could also be inferred from the association of progressive hyperglycemia with worsening T2DM. If fasting insulin and glucose concentrations are plotted in patients with varying glucose intolerance and T2DM, an inverted U-shaped curve results (the so-called Starling curve of the pancreas), suggesting that initial compensation for hyperglycemia occurs through insulin hypersecretion, but eventually failure of islet β cells ensues, resulting in progressive worsening of DM.[30]

HYPERGLYCEMIA AND TISSUE TOXICITY: MOLECULAR MECHANISMS

Genetic susceptibility factors have been shown to underlie diabetic complications involving the kidneys, retina, and heart, although specific susceptibility (allelic) variants have not been described. Also important are comorbidities such as hypertension and hyperlipidemia, which tend to accelerate complications. Most tissues can protect themselves from hyperglycemia by reducing transcellular glucose transport, but many target tissues of diabetic complications, particularly vascular endothelial cells, lack this ability. Kaiser and colleagues[31] exposed smooth muscle cells and endothelial cells to varying concentrations of glucose. Smooth muscle cells exposed to high glucose were able to downregulate the rate of intracellular glucose transport, but endothelial cells preincubated with high glucose could not. High intracellular glucose concentration leads to reactive oxygen species (ROS) generation and oxidative stress. Further tissue toxicity, including a proatherogenic effect, could be caused by multiple mechanisms such as activation of protein kinase C (PKC) isoforms, increased flux through the hexosamine pathway, increased advanced glycation end products (AGE) formation, or increased polyol pathway flux.[32]

In laboratory studies, the defect in insulin gene expression after prolonged exposure to supraphysiologic glucose levels seems to be linked to the less than optimal activity of at least 2 key β-cell transcription factors, namely pancreatic-duodenum homeobox 1[33,34] and the activator of the rat insulin promoter element 3b1.[35,36] A loss of differentiation

of β cells exposed to increased glucose results in defective β-cell function.[37] This situation could be linked to the altered expression of the proto-oncogene C-myc.[37] Alternatively, an enhanced expression of the insulin gene transcriptional repressor CCAAT/enhancer-binding protein β has also been implicated in glucotoxicity of the β cell. ROS-mediated oxidative stress has also been implicated in glucolipotoxicity.[38–41] By using the insulin-secreting HIT-T15 cells, generation of ROS was observed in the presence of a reducing sugar[39] or sustained (chronic) exposure to increased glucose levels,[40] culminating in the decreased transcription of the insulin gene, a process readily reversed by the antioxidants aminoguanidine and N-acetyl-cysteine (NAC). Treatment of Zucker diabetic fatty (ZDF) rats with either aminoguanidine or NAC also seems to restore insulin mRNA level, insulin content, and insulin secretion, thereby normalizing blood glucose levels.[40] In vitro experiments on isolated islets reveal the accumulation of AGE, impaired β-cell function, and apoptosis-related reactions prevented by aminoguanidine and NAC.[38,42]

LIPOTOXICITY

T2DM is associated with a cluster of interrelated plasma lipid and lipoprotein abnormalities, including reduced HDL-C, increased TG levels, and a predominance of sdLDL-c particles.[43] IR has striking effects on lipoprotein size and subclass particle concentrations for very low-density lipoprotein (VLDL), LDL, and high-density lipoprotein,[44] and evidence suggests that each of these features is associated with increased risk of CVD. Altered metabolism of TG-rich lipoproteins is an integral part of the atherogenic dyslipidemia seen in DM. Increased hepatic secretion of VLDL and decreased clearance of VLDL and intestinally derived chylomicrons result in prolonged plasma retention of these particles and accumulation of highly atherogenic partially lipolyzed cholesterol-enriched intermediate-density lipoprotein remnants. Increased hepatic production or diminished plasma clearance of large VLDL results in increased production of precursors of sdLDL particles.[45–47] In addition to toxicity mediated by FFAs and their products, there is evidence to suggest that hypertriglyceridemia per se could result in direct cellular toxicity under some circumstances.[48] Chan and Pollard[49] showed that VLDL fractions from rats in the late stage of pregnancy are toxic to tumorigenic and nontransformed cells. Gianturco and colleagues[50] showed decreased viability of bovine aortic endothelial cells exposed to VLDL from hypertriglyceridemic humans, and Arbogast and colleagues[51] found that porcine aortic endothelial cells died when exposed to VLDL from diabetic rat serum. Although such concepts have not been extended to pancreatic β cells, it is possible that most organs and tissues of the body that are exposed to VLDL might experience similar toxic effects.

Several studies have established the association between LDL particle size or density and coronary artery disease.[44] sdLDL particles seem to arise from the progressive intravascular processing of specific larger VLDL precursors through a series of steps, including lipolysis. Hepatic LDL receptors have a reduced affinity for sdLDL, thereby facilitating prolonged plasma retention. Also, sdLDL are more vulnerable to oxidative modification in the subendothelial space, thereby facilitating atherogenesis.[52,53]

FFAs

Early humans typically went through cycles of relative food abundance and famine and the adipocyte perhaps evolved to enable them to store excess energy substrates in order to combat starvation, especially because the lean tissues lacked the ability to store triacylglycerols.[54] In contrast, modern humans, especially living in the western hemisphere, have easy and affordable access to high caloric food substrates and lead a sedentary lifestyle, resulting in a mismatch between energy intake and energy expenditure. The result is a burgeoning incidence of overweight (defined as body mass index [BMI, calculated as weight in kilograms divided by the square of height in meters] >25 kg/m^2 and <30 kg/m^2) and obesity (defined as BMI >30 kg/m^2), both of which are characterized by a pathologic increase in subcutaneous or visceral adiposity.

Hydrolysis of stored fat (common in insulin-resistant states) releases large amounts of FFA (nonesterified fatty acids) into the circulation. Although FFA subserves important physiologic functions, chronically increased plasma levels such as seen in obesity and T2DM are deleterious, largely because of the toxic effects of FFA in lean tissues. Even modest caloric excess may result in ectopic lipid deposition in the liver, heart, muscle, and endocrine pancreas, resulting in nonalcoholic fatty liver disease, lipotoxic heart disease (discussed elsewhere in this issue), myocellular IR, and DM. The excess presence of triacylglycerols beyond the oxidative needs of lean tissue (termed steatosis), leads to an FFA spillover effect, resulting in tissue lipotoxicity largely mediated by toxic end products of nonoxidative FFA metabolism.[55]

The deleterious consequences of lipid overload depend on the magnitude and duration of the imbalance between FFA influx and oxidation in any given tissue. For example, in diet-induced obesity, nonadipose tissues are protected by high leptin levels during the initial phase of FFA excess, but later, leptin resistance of undetermined cause sets in and seems to be responsible for gradual accrual of lipids in lean tissue, resulting in continuing lipotoxicity.[56] The prolonged exposure of β cells to FFAs enhances the release of basal insulin and impedes glucose-induced insulin secretion. Evidence obtained from recent studies (in vitro and ZDF rat islets) relate enhanced levels of FFAs with increased apoptosis of the β-cell mass.[57–59] The presence of high levels of glucose enables the FFAs to repress insulin gene expression,[60,61] possibly through the negative regulation of the transcription factor pancreatic-duodenum homeobox 1.

Thus, the abnormalities associated with defective β-cell function seem to occur when both glucose and circulating fatty acids are high.[62] This situation may be regarded as crucial in the manifestation of the pleiotropic defects in prediabetes and DM. Several enzymes in key metabolic pathways may be involved in the genesis of tissue toxicity in the context of excess glucose and fat exposure. The inhibition of release of insulin induced by sustained exposure to FFAs leads to the inhibition of glucose metabolism attributable to low pyruvate dehydrogenase (PDH) activity[63] and an increased activity of carnitine palmitoyltransferase I (CPT1).[64] The inhibitory actions on insulin release of the C_{16} saturated fatty acid palmitate are caused by the accumulation of long-chain fatty acyl coenzyme A (CoA) thioesters and subsequent enhancement in the activities of hexokinase and phosphofructokinase (PFK).[65,66] In contrast, the activity of glucokinase is decreased.[60] In addition, the accumulation of long-chain fatty acyl coenzyme thioesters has biochemical consequences, such as the activation of the adenosine triphosphate (ATP)-sensitive K$^+$ channel,[67] inhibition of glucose transporter 2,[60] and increased oxidation of FFAs.

FFAs have been implicated in the putative uncoupling of the mitochondrial respiratory chain in the mitochondria, with some of the projected actions being decreased generation of ATP and mitochondrial swelling.[68,69] There has been interest in mitochondrial uncoupling in the β cell as well. Using cultured rat pancreatic islets, Carlsson and colleagues[70] found that in the presence of palmitate, partial mitochondrial uncoupling could be induced and inhibition of insulin release was in tune with enhanced respiration, decreased

ATP content, and increased mitochondrial volume. This phenomenon of uncoupling was not observed with short-term exposure of the cells to FFA. β-Cell function was initially stimulated on exposure to FFAs, leading to the increased generation of ATP.[71,72]

Historically, the role of FFAs on inhibition of glucose-induced insulin secretion and biosynthesis as mediated through a glucose fatty acid cycle was advanced by Sir Phillip Randle almost half a century ago.[56] This principle evolved after a series of experiments that were designed to test the hypothesis that cardiac and skeletal muscle possessed mechanisms that allowed these tissues to shift readily back and forth between carbohydrate and fat as oxidative energy sources, depending primarily on the availability of FFAs. In particular, these experiments focused on the mechanisms involved in the switch from carbohydrate to fat oxidation. This model predicted that increased fat oxidation in muscle would inhibit both PDH and PFK by accumulation of acetyl CoA and citrate, respectively, thereby hindering the glycolytic pathway and resulting in enhanced glucose 6-phosphate concentration. This situation in turn would inhibit hexokinase, thereby reducing glucose uptake and oxidation.

Zhou and colleagues[73] tested effects of long-term exposure of pancreatic islets to FFAs in vitro on pancreatic β-cell function. Islets isolated from male Sprague-Dawley rats were exposed to palmitate (0.125 or 0.25 mM), oleate (0.125 mM), or octanoate (2.0 mM) during culture. Insulin responses were subsequently tested in the absence of FFA. After a 48-hour exposure to FFA, insulin secretion during basal glucose (3.3 mM) was increased several-fold. However, during stimulation with 27 mM glucose, secretion was inhibited by 30% to 50% and proinsulin biosynthesis by 30% to 40%. Total protein synthesis was similarly affected. Conversely, previous palmitate did not impair α-ketoisocaproic acid (5 mM)-induced insulin release. Induction and reversibility of the inhibitory effect on glucose-induced insulin secretion required between 6 and 24 hours. Addition of the CPT1 inhibitor etomoxir (1 μM) partially reversed (by >50%) FFA-associated decrease in secretory as well as proinsulin biosynthetic responses to 27 mM glucose. These investigators concluded that long-term exposure to FFAs inhibited glucose-induced insulin secretion and biosynthesis probably via the glucose fatty acid cycle.

This was an important study because several aspects suggested that the inhibitory effect of long-term FFAs was not caused by nonspecific damage of β-cell function: (1) the effect was reversible on removal of FFAs on a time scale comparable with that for induction; (2) responses to another nutrient secretagogue (α-ketoisocaproic acid) were not inhibited; and (3) an effect of FFAs on glucose-induced insulin release was rapidly reversible by a CPT1 inhibitor. Thus, the investigators showed that fatty acids time-dependently inhibited glucose-induced insulin secretion and biosynthesis and the specificity of this effect and its linkage to fatty acid oxidation indicated perhaps that a glucose-fatty acid cycle was operative in the pancreatic β cell as well.

ROS

The role of ROS on the inhibition of insulin secretion and IR was alluded to in the previous sections. Medical evidence exists both to support and to refute the notion that oxidative stress is a key player in this context.[74–78] Also, evidence supports the notion that FFAs may induce β-cell apoptosis by a mechanism distinct from the one that is mediated by cytokines.[79] Although apoptosis is probably the main form of β-cell death in both T1DM and T2DM, cytokines contribute to β-cell destruction in the former through nuclear factor κB (NF-κB) activation. Although previous studies suggested that in T2DM, high glucose and FFA levels are β-cell toxic also via NF-κB activation, there is some evidence that this is not the case. Kharroubi and colleagues[79] sought to clarify the mechanisms involved in FFA-induced and cytokine-induced β-cell apoptosis and determine if tumor necrosis factor α (TNF-α), an adipocyte-derived cytokine, potentiated FFA toxicity through enhanced NF-κB activation. Apoptosis was induced in insulinoma (INS)-1E cells, rat islets, and fluorescence-activated cell sorting-purified β cells by oleate, palmitate, or several cytokines. Palmitate and interleukin 1 β induced a similar percentage of apoptosis in INS-1E cells, whereas oleate was less toxic. TNF-α did not potentiate FFA toxicity in primary β cells. Findings also suggested that FFAs triggered an endoplasmic reticulum (ER) stress response. They concluded that apoptosis is the main mode of FFA-induced and cytokine-induced β-cell death but the mechanisms involved were different. Whereas cytokines induced NF-κB activation and ER stress (secondary to nitric oxide formation), FFAs activated an ER stress response via an NF-κB–independent and nitric oxide–independent mechanism.

Steroid Regulatory Element Binding Protein

In the context of the association of lipotoxicity with IR and β-cell failure, the role of the steroid regulatory element binding protein (SREBP-1C) bears mention. O'Rahilly and colleagues[80] detected 2 novel missense mutations in the SREBP-1C gene

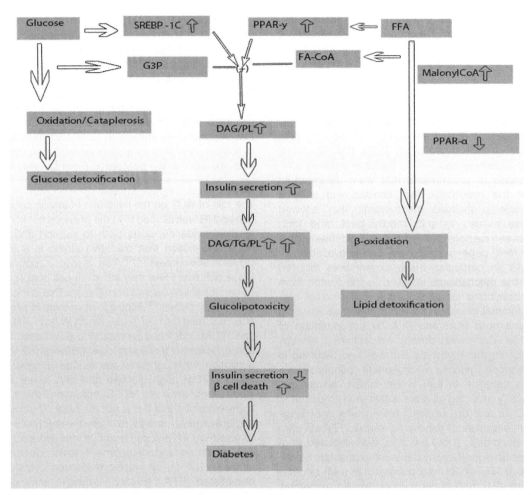

Fig. 1. Molecular events implicated in β-cell glucolipotoxicity. G3P, glycerol 3-phosphate; FA-CoA, fatty acyl CoA; PL, phospholipid; TAG, triacylglycerol or triglyceride.

(P87L and P416A), which was associated with an increased risk for T2DM, IR, and increased cholesterol levels. Kakuma and Unger[81] measured SREBP-1 mRNA in liver and islets of obese, leptin-unresponsive fa/fa ZDF rats. Hepatic SREBP-1 mRNA was 2.4 times higher than in lean +/+ controls, primarily because of increased SREBP-1c expression. Messenger RNA of lipogenic enzymes ranged from 2.4-fold to 4.6-fold higher than in lean controls, and TG content was 5.4 times higher. In pancreatic islets of fa/fa rats, SREBP-1c was 3.4 times higher than in lean +/+ ZDF rats. The increase of SREBP-1 in liver and islets of untreated fa/fa rats was blocked by peroxisome proliferator-activated receptor γ (PPAR-γ) agonist and thiazolidinedione (TZD) agent, troglitazone, and the diabetic phenotype was prevented. Upregulation of SREBP-1 also occurred in the livers of Sprague-Dawley rats with diet-induced obesity. Hyperleptinemia, induced in lean +/+ rats by adenovirus gene transfer, decreased

hepatic SREBP-1c by 74% and the lipogenic enzymes from 35% to 59%. These investigators concluded that overnutrition increases and adenovirus-induced hyperleptinemia decrease SREBP-1c expression in liver and islets. SREBP-1 overexpression, prevented by troglitazone, may play a role in the ectopic lipogenesis and lipotoxicity complicating obesity in ZDF rats. The direct antidiabetic action of leptin is manifest in the depletion of TGs in β cells of pancreas, liver, and skeletal muscle, which runs hand in hand with the intracellular oxidation of FFAs. This finding has been confirmed by the fact that leptin did not have any effect on obese rats with leptin receptor mutations.[82] Likewise, TZD drugs, which are PPAR agonists, perhaps improve IR in part through their effects on SREBP-1C.[83–85]

Thus, the overarching mechanisms by which lipotoxicity operates could be summarized as follows: (1) increased FFA oxidation and a resulting decline in glucose oxidation, suggesting a shift in

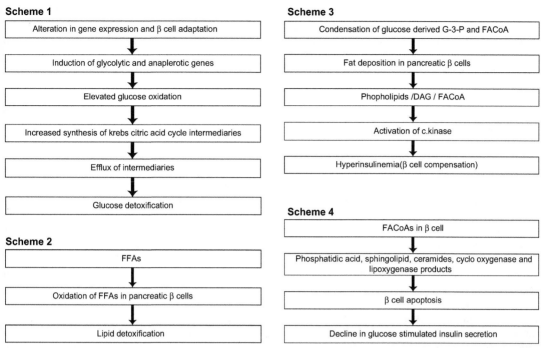

Fig. 2. (*Scheme 1*) Model for glucotoxicity (at slightly increased concentrations of glucose). β cell, pancreatic β cell. (*Scheme 2*) Model for lipotoxicity (low glucose levels and increased malonyl CoA). β cell, pancreatic β cell. (*Scheme 3*) Model depicting increasing IR (at increased levels of FFAs and TG-rich lipoproteins). β cell, pancreatic β cell; G3P, glycerol 3 phosphate; FACoA, fatty acyl CoA; c. kinase, protein kinase c. (*Scheme 4*) Model depicting molecular events at levels attributable to the progressive accumulation of fatty acyl CoAs in the β cell. β cell, pancreatic β cell.

energy source for cellular respiration (this oxidation is not connected directly to the generation of ROS or lipid peroxidation); and (2) generation of a cytosolic signal via esterification of FFA. Between these 2, the latter seems to be more plausible because the intermediary metabolites produced in the esterification pathway cause harmful effects of chronically increased FFA levels, because prolonged exposure to FFAs is associated with minimal changes in glucose metabolism. Segall and Prentki[86,87] have reviewed the basis for this hypothesis elsewhere. According to this hypothesis, the simultaneous presence of increased glucose and FFA levels leads to the accumulation of cytosolic citrate, the precursor of malonyl CoA (via acetyl CoA). This in turn inhibits CPT1, a key enzyme that facilitates transport of FFA into the mitochondria. Sustained inhibition of CPT1 results in the accumulation of long-chain fatty acyl CoAs (LC-CoAs), which are the mediators of several deleterious effects.[88] This model proposes that the glucose concentration plays a crucial role in the biochemical effects of FFAs. However, the exact molecular mechanisms by which LC-CoA accumulation induces β-cell dysfunction remains less clear. Some of the putative candidates

include diacylglycerols (DAGs) and phospholipids derived from LC-CoA and their deleterious effects on cell constituents such as the ATP-sensitive K^+ channel, PKC, uncoupling protein Z, exocytotic machinery, and even modulation of insulin gene expression.

SUMMARY

Figs. 1 and **2** depict key molecular events in glucotoxity, lipotoxicity, and glucolipotoxicity, both with respect to pancreatic β cells and other cell types. Glucose intolerance linked with hyperinsulinemia and IR are regarded as cardinal biochemical abnormalities in prediabetes and early T2DM.[89–91] Although hyperinsulinemia may be a direct consequence of IR,[89] it is unclear whether IR precedes hyperinsulinemia uniformly. However, based on current medical evidence, IR in the target tissues per se is not likely to result in DM without β-cell failure.[92] Yet another point that remains to be linked is the association between apoptosis and altered mitochondrial function on the one hand and altered insulin gene expression, particularly in the β cells, on the other. Although energy metabolism and mitochondrial functions are generally applicable to all cell types, insulin synthesis and secretion are unique to the β cells. Thus, more research is needed to tease out the relationships between generalized cellular effects of glucolipotoxicity and specific gene alterations in the genesis of DM. The emerging perspective is that glucose dramatically influences the metabolism of lipids in the β cells of islets of Langerhans. Thus arose the concept of glucolipotoxicity, several aspects of which have been described in earlier sections. Prentki and colleagues[93] have proposed a model of β-cell glucolipotoxicity, which brings to the interface several metabolic players such as malonyl CoA, PPAR-α and PPAR-γ, and SREBP-1C, as well as altered lipid partitioning. β Cells possess inherent mechanisms to adapt to overnutrition and the concentrations of glucose, fatty acids, and other fuels to maintain glucose homeostasis. However, this situation is counterbalanced by potentially harmful actions of the same nutrients. Both glucose and fatty acids may cause good/adaptive or toxic/maladaptive actions on the β cell, depending on their concentrations and the time during which they are increased. Chronic hyperglycemia influences β-cell lipid metabolism via substrate availability, changes in the activity and expression of enzymes of glucose and lipid metabolism, and modifications in the expression level of key transcription factors. In Prentki and colleagues' model, β-cell glucotoxicity may in part be indirectly caused by lipotoxicity, and these abnormalities become apparent when both glucose and circulating fatty acid levels are high. The model espouses the concept that increased glucose and fatty acid levels act synergistically in causing toxicity in islets and other organs, a process that may be instrumental in the multiple defects associated with the metabolic syndrome, T1DM, and T2DM. The various aspects of this glucolipotoxicity model are displayed in **Figs. 1** and **2** and implicate alterations in β-cell malonyl CoA concentrations, PPAR-α and PPAR-γ, and sterol regulatory element binding protein 1c expression and lipid partitioning.

ACKNOWLEDGMENTS

The authors wish to acknowledge the help of Ms Krithika Vasudevan (Westwood High School, Austin, TX) in the preparation of **Figs. 1** and **2**.

REFERENCES

1. Qaseem A, Humphrey LL, Sweet DE, et al. Oral pharmacologic treatment of type 2 diabetes mellitus: a clinical practice guideline from the American College of Physicians. Ann Intern Med 2012; 156(3):218–31.
2. Rabinovitch A. Immunoregulatory and cytokine imbalances in the pathogenesis of IDDM. Therapeutic intervention by immunostimulation? Diabetes 1994;43(5):613–21.
3. Ogawa Y, Noma Y, Davalli AM, et al. Loss of glucose-induced insulin secretion and GLUT2 expression in transplanted beta-cells. Diabetes 1995;44(1):75–9.
4. DeFronzo RA, Hendler R, Simonson D. Insulin resistance is a prominent feature of insulin-dependent diabetes. Diabetes 1982;31(9):795–801.
5. DeFronzo RA, Simonson D, Ferrannini E. Hepatic and peripheral insulin resistance: a common feature of type 2 (non-insulin-dependent) and type 1 (insulin-dependent) diabetes mellitus. Diabetologia 1982;23(4):313–9.
6. Pernet A, Trimble ER, Kuntschen F, et al. Insulin resistance in type 1 (insulin-dependent) diabetes: dependence on plasma insulin concentration. Diabetologia 1984;26(4):255–60.
7. Yki-Jarvinen H, Koivisto VA. Natural course of insulin resistance in type I diabetes. N Engl J Med 1986; 315(4):224–30.
8. Erbey JR, Kuller LH, Becker DJ, et al. The association between a family history of type 2 diabetes and coronary artery disease in a type 1 diabetes population. Diabetes Care 1998;21(4):610–4.
9. Martin FI, Hopper JL. The relationship of acute insulin sensitivity to the progression of vascular disease in long-term type 1 (insulin-dependent) diabetes mellitus. Diabetologia 1987;30(3):149–53.
10. Samaras K, Nguyen TV, Jenkins AB, et al. Clustering of insulin resistance, total and central abdominal fat: same genes or same environment? Twin Res 1999; 2(3):218–25.
11. Carey DG, Jenkins AB, Campbell LV, et al. Abdominal fat and insulin resistance in normal and overweight women: direct measurements reveal a strong relationship in subjects at both low and high risk of NIDDM. Diabetes 1996;45(5):633–8.
12. Chisholm DJ, Campbell LV, Kraegen EW. Pathogenesis of the insulin resistance syndrome (syndrome X). Clin Exp Pharmacol Physiol 1997;24(9–10):782–4.
13. Montague CT, O'Rahilly S. The perils of portliness: causes and consequences of visceral adiposity. Diabetes 2000;49(6):883–8.
14. Kabadi UM, Vora A, Kabadi M. Hyperinsulinemia and central adiposity: influence of chronic insulin therapy in type 1 diabetes. Diabetes Care 2000; 23(7):1024–5.
15. Bujalska IJ, Kumar S, Stewart PM. Does central obesity reflect "Cushing's disease of the omentum"? Lancet 1997;349(9060):1210–3.
16. Poitout V, Robertson RP. Minireview: secondary beta-cell failure in type 2 diabetes–a convergence

of glucotoxicity and lipotoxicity. Endocrinology 2002; 143(2):339–42.

17. Sako Y, Grill VE. Coupling of beta-cell desensitization by hyperglycemia to excessive stimulation and circulating insulin in glucose-infused rats. Diabetes 1990;39(12):1580–3.

18. Leahy JL, Bumbalo LM, Chen C. Diazoxide causes recovery of beta-cell glucose responsiveness in 90% pancreatectomized diabetic rats. Diabetes 1994;43(2):173–9.

19. Moran A, Zhang HJ, Olson LK, et al. Differentiation of glucose toxicity from beta cell exhaustion during the evolution of defective insulin gene expression in the pancreatic islet cell line, HIT-T15. J Clin Invest 1997;99(3):534–9.

20. Gleason CE, Gonzalez M, Harmon JS, et al. Determinants of glucose toxicity and its reversibility in the pancreatic islet beta-cell line, HIT-T15. Am J Physiol Endocrinol Metab 2000;279(5):E997–1002.

21. Pick A, Clark J, Kubstrup C, et al. Role of apoptosis in failure of beta-cell mass compensation for insulin resistance and beta-cell defects in the male Zucker diabetic fatty rat. Diabetes 1998;47(3):358–64.

22. Donath MY, Gross DJ, Cerasi E, et al. Hyperglycemia-induced beta-cell apoptosis in pancreatic islets of Psammomys obesus during development of diabetes. Diabetes 1999;48(4):738–44.

23. Bonner-Weir S, Trent DF, Honey RN, et al. Responses of neonatal rat islets to streptozotocin: limited B-cell regeneration and hyperglycemia. Diabetes 1981;30(1):64–9.

24. Bonner-Weir S, Trent DF, Weir GC. Partial pancreatectomy in the rat and subsequent defect in glucose-induced insulin release. J Clin Invest 1983;71(6):1544–53.

25. Leahy JL, Weir GC. Evolution of abnormal insulin secretory responses during 48-h in vivo hyperglycemia. Diabetes 1988;37(2):217–22.

26. Rossetti L, Shulman GI, Zawalich W, et al. Effect of chronic hyperglycemia on in vivo insulin secretion in partially pancreatectomized rats. J Clin Invest 1987;80(4):1037–44.

27. Rossetti L, Smith D, Shulman GI, et al. Correction of hyperglycemia with phlorizin normalizes tissue sensitivity to insulin in diabetic rats. J Clin Invest 1987;79(5):1510–5.

28. Kosaka K, Kuzuya T, Akanuma Y, et al. Increase in insulin response after treatment of overt maturity-onset diabetes is independent of the mode of treatment. Diabetologia 1980;18(1):23–8.

29. Yki-Jarvinen H, Helve E, Koivisto VA. Hyperglycemia decreases glucose uptake in type I diabetes. Diabetes 1987;36(8):892–6.

30. Most RS, Sinnock P. The epidemiology of lower extremity amputations in diabetic individuals. Diabetes Care 1983;6(1):87–91.

31. Kaiser N, Sasson S, Feener EP, et al. Differential regulation of glucose transport and transporters by glucose in vascular endothelial and smooth muscle cells. Diabetes 1993;42(1):80–9.

32. Du X, Matsumura T, Edelstein D, et al. Inhibition of GAPDH activity by poly(ADP-ribose) polymerase activates three major pathways of hyperglycemic damage in endothelial cells. J Clin Invest 2003; 112(7):1049–57.

33. Olson LK, Redmon JB, Towle HC, et al. Chronic exposure of HIT cells to high glucose concentrations paradoxically decreases insulin gene transcription and alters binding of insulin gene regulatory protein. J Clin Invest 1993;92(1):514–9.

34. Olson LK, Sharma A, Peshavaria M, et al. Reduction of insulin gene transcription in HIT-T15 beta cells chronically exposed to a supraphysiologic glucose concentration is associated with loss of STF-1 transcription factor expression. Proc Natl Acad Sci U S A 1995; 92(20):9127–31.

35. Sharma A, Olson LK, Robertson RP, et al. The reduction of insulin gene transcription in HIT-T15 beta cells chronically exposed to high glucose concentration is associated with the loss of RIPE3b1 and STF-1 transcription factor expression. Mol Endocrinol 1995;9(9):1127–34.

36. Poitout V, Olson LK, Robertson RP. Chronic exposure of betaTC-6 cells to supraphysiologic concentrations of glucose decreases binding of the RIPE3b1 insulin gene transcription activator. J Clin Invest 1996;97(4):1041–6.

37. Jonas JC, Sharma A, Hasenkamp W, et al. Chronic hyperglycemia triggers loss of pancreatic beta cell differentiation in an animal model of diabetes. J Biol Chem 1999;274(20):14112–21.

38. Tajiri Y, Moller C, Grill V. Long-term effects of aminoguanidine on insulin release and biosynthesis: evidence that the formation of advanced glycosylation end products inhibits B cell function. Endocrinology 1997;138(1):273–80.

39. Matsuoka T, Kajimoto Y, Watada H, et al. Glycation-dependent, reactive oxygen species-mediated suppression of the insulin gene promoter activity in HIT cells. J Clin Invest 1997;99(1):144–50.

40. Tanaka Y, Gleason CE, Tran PO, et al. Prevention of glucose toxicity in HIT-T15 cells and Zucker diabetic fatty rats by antioxidants. Proc Natl Acad Sci U S A 1999;96(19):10857–62.

41. Ihara Y, Toyokuni S, Uchida K, et al. Hyperglycemia causes oxidative stress in pancreatic beta-cells of GK rats, a model of type 2 diabetes. Diabetes 1999;48(4):927–32.

42. Kaneto H, Fujii J, Myint T, et al. Reducing sugars trigger oxidative modification and apoptosis in pancreatic beta-cells by provoking oxidative stress through the glycation reaction. Biochem J 1996; 320(Pt 3):855–63.

43. Haffner SM. Management of dyslipidemia in adults with diabetes. Diabetes Care 2003;26(Suppl 1):S83–6.

44. Garvey WT, Kwon S, Zheng D, et al. Effects of insulin resistance and type 2 diabetes on lipoprotein subclass particle size and concentration determined by nuclear magnetic resonance. Diabetes 2003; 52(2):453–62.

45. Austin MA, King MC, Vranizan KM, et al. Atherogenic lipoprotein phenotype. A proposed genetic marker for coronary heart disease risk. Circulation 1990;82(2):495–506.

46. Austin MA, Breslow JL, Hennekens CH, et al. Low-density lipoprotein subclass patterns and risk of myocardial infarction. JAMA 1988;260(13):1917–21.

47. Campos H, Genest JJ Jr, Blijlevens E, et al. Low density lipoprotein particle size and coronary artery disease. Arterioscler Thromb 1992;12(2):187–95.

48. Hessler JR, Morel DW, Lewis LJ, et al. Lipoprotein oxidation and lipoprotein-induced cytotoxicity. Arteriosclerosis 1983;3(3):215–22.

49. Chan SY, Pollard M. In vitro effects of lipoprotein-associated cytotoxic factor on rat prostate adenocarcinoma cells. Cancer Res 1978;38(9):2956–61.

50. Gianturco SH, Eskin SG, Navarro LT, et al. Abnormal effects of hypertriacylglycerolemic very low-density lipoproteins on 3-hydroxy-3-methylglutaryl-CoA reductase activity and viability of cultured bovine aortic endothelial cells. Biochim Biophys Acta 1980;618(1):143–52.

51. Arbogast BW, Lee GM, Raymond TL. In vitro injury of porcine aortic endothelial cells by very-low-density lipoproteins from diabetic rat serum. Diabetes 1982;31(7):593–9.

52. Vasudevan AR, Garber AJ. Diabetic dyslipidemia and the heart. Heart Failure Clinics 2006;2(1):37–52.

53. Berneis KK, Krauss RM. Metabolic origins and clinical significance of LDL heterogeneity. J Lipid Res 2002;43(9):1363–79.

54. Neel JV. Diabetes mellitus: a "thrifty" genotype rendered detrimental by "progress"? 1962. Bull World Health Organ 1999;77(8):694–703 [discussion: 692–3].

55. Lee Y, Hirose H, Ohneda M, et al. Beta-cell lipotoxicity in the pathogenesis of non-insulin-dependent diabetes mellitus of obese rats: impairment in adipocyte-beta-cell relationships. Proc Natl Acad Sci U S A 1994;91(23):10878–82.

56. Unger RH, Zhou YT. Lipotoxicity of beta-cells in obesity and in other causes of fatty acid spillover. Diabetes 2001;50(Suppl 1):S118–21.

57. Maedler K, Spinas GA, Dyntar D, et al. Distinct effects of saturated and monounsaturated fatty acids on beta-cell turnover and function. Diabetes 2001;50(1):69–76.

58. Cnop M, Hannaert JC, Hoorens A, et al. Inverse relationship between cytotoxicity of free fatty acids in pancreatic islet cells and cellular triglyceride accumulation. Diabetes 2001;50(8):1771–7.

59. Shimabukuro M, Higa M, Zhou YT, et al. Lipoapoptosis in beta-cells of obese prediabetic fa/fa rats. Role of serine palmitoyltransferase overexpression. J Biol Chem 1998;273(49):32487–90.

60. Gremlich S, Bonny C, Waeber G, et al. Fatty acids decrease IDX-1 expression in rat pancreatic islets and reduce GLUT2, glucokinase, insulin, and somatostatin levels. J Biol Chem 1997;272(48): 30261–9.

61. Jacqueminet S, Briaud I, Rouault C, et al. Inhibition of insulin gene expression by long-term exposure of pancreatic beta cells to palmitate is dependent on the presence of a stimulatory glucose concentration. Metabolism 2000;49(4):532–6.

62. Bergman RN, Ader M. Free fatty acids and pathogenesis of type 2 diabetes mellitus. Trends Endocrinol Metab 2000;11(9):351–6.

63. Zhou YP, Grill VE. Palmitate-induced beta-cell insensitivity to glucose is coupled to decreased pyruvate dehydrogenase activity and enhanced kinase activity in rat pancreatic islets. Diabetes 1995; 44(4):394–9.

64. Assimacopoulos-Jeannet F, Thumelin S, Roche E, et al. Fatty acids rapidly induce the carnitine palmitoyltransferase I gene in the pancreatic beta-cell line INS-1. J Biol Chem 1997;272(3):1659–64.

65. Hosokawa H, Corkey BE, Leahy JL. Beta-cell hypersensitivity to glucose following 24-h exposure of rat islets to fatty acids. Diabetologia 1997;40(4):392–7.

66. Liu YQ, Tornheim K, Leahy JL. Fatty acid-induced beta cell hypersensitivity to glucose. Increased phosphofructokinase activity and lowered glucose-6-phosphate content. J Clin Invest 1998;101(9): 1870–5.

67. Larsson O, Deeney JT, Branstrom R, et al. Activation of the ATP-sensitive K+ channel by long chain acyl-CoA. A role in modulation of pancreatic beta-cell glucose sensitivity. J Biol Chem 1996;271(18): 10623–6.

68. Wojtczak L, Schonfeld P. Effect of fatty acids on energy coupling processes in mitochondria. Biochim Biophys Acta 1993;1183(1):41–57.

69. Schonfeld P. Does the function of adenine nucleotide translocase in fatty acid uncoupling depend on the type of mitochondria? FEBS Lett 1990; 264(2):246–8.

70. Carlsson C, Borg LA, Welsh N. Sodium palmitate induces partial mitochondrial uncoupling and reactive oxygen species in rat pancreatic islets in vitro. Endocrinology 1999;140(8):3422–8.

71. Malaisse WJ, Malaisse-Lagae F, Sener A, et al. Participation of endogenous fatty acids in the secretory activity of the pancreatic B-cell. Biochem J 1985;227(3):995–1002.

72. Sako Y, Grill VE. A 48-hour lipid infusion in the rat time-dependently inhibits glucose-induced insulin secretion and B cell oxidation through a process

likely coupled to fatty acid oxidation. Endocrinology 1990;127(4):1580–9.

73. Zhou YP, Grill VE. Long-term exposure of rat pancreatic islets to fatty acids inhibits glucose-induced insulin secretion and biosynthesis through a glucose fatty acid cycle. J Clin Invest 1994;93(2):870–6.

74. Fridlyand LE, Philipson LH. Does the glucose-dependent insulin secretion mechanism itself cause oxidative stress in pancreatic beta-cells? Diabetes 2004;53(8):1942–8.

75. Ceriello A, Motz E. Is oxidative stress the pathogenic mechanism underlying insulin resistance, diabetes, and cardiovascular disease? The common soil hypothesis revisited. Arterioscler Thromb Vasc Biol 2004;24(5):816–23.

76. Evans JL, Goldfine ID, Maddux BA, et al. Are oxidative stress-activated signaling pathways mediators of insulin resistance and beta-cell dysfunction? Diabetes 2003;52(1):1–8.

77. Evans JL, Goldfine ID, Maddux BA, et al. Oxidative stress and stress-activated signaling pathways: a unifying hypothesis of type 2 diabetes. Endocr Rev 2002;23(5):599–622.

78. Moore PC, Ugas MA, Hagman DK, et al. Evidence against the involvement of oxidative stress in fatty acid inhibition of insulin secretion. Diabetes 2004; 53(10):2610–6.

79. Kharroubi I, Ladriere L, Cardozo AK, et al. Free fatty acids and cytokines induce pancreatic beta-cell apoptosis by different mechanisms: role of nuclear factor-kappaB and endoplasmic reticulum stress. Endocrinology 2004;145(11):5087–96.

80. Laudes M, Barroso I, Luan J, et al. Genetic variants in human sterol regulatory element binding protein-1c in syndromes of severe insulin resistance and type 2 diabetes. Diabetes 2004;53(3):842–6.

81. Kakuma T, Lee Y, Higa M, et al. Leptin, troglitazone, and the expression of sterol regulatory element binding proteins in liver and pancreatic islets. Proc Natl Acad Sci U S A 2000;97(15):8536–41.

82. Shimabukuro M, Koyama K, Chen G, et al. Direct antidiabetic effect of leptin through triglyceride depletion of tissues. Proc Natl Acad Sci U S A 1997;94(9):4637–41.

83. Inoue Y, Tanigawa K, Nakamura S, et al. Lack of effect of CS-045, a new antidiabetic agent, on insulin secretion in the remnant pancreas after 90% pancreatectomy in rats. Diabetes Res Clin Pract 1995;27(1):19–26.

84. Masuda K, Okamoto Y, Tsuura Y, et al. Effects of Troglitazone (CS-045) on insulin secretion in isolated rat pancreatic islets and HIT cells: an insulinotropic mechanism distinct from glibenclamide. Diabetologia 1995;38(1):24–30.

85. Wang H, Maechler P, Antinozzi PA, et al. The transcription factor SREBP-1c is instrumental in the development of beta-cell dysfunction. J Biol Chem 2003;278(19):16622–9.

86. Segall L, Lameloise N, Assimacopoulos-Jeannet F, et al. Lipid rather than glucose metabolism is implicated in altered insulin secretion caused by oleate in INS-1 cells. Am J Physiol 1999;277(3 Pt 1):E521–8.

87. Prentki M, Corkey BE. Are the beta-cell signaling molecules malonyl-CoA and cystolic long-chain acyl-CoA implicated in multiple tissue defects of obesity and NIDDM? Diabetes 1996;45(3):273–83.

88. Prentki M, Roduit R, Corkey BE, et al. Glucotoxicity, lipotoxicity and ß-cell function in diabetes: a role for altered lipid partitioning. Can J Diabetes Care 2001; 25:36–46.

89. Kahn CR. Banting lecture. Insulin action, diabetogenes, and the cause of type II diabetes. Diabetes 1994;43(8):1066–84.

90. Poitout V, Robertson RP. An integrated view of beta-cell dysfunction in type-II diabetes. Annu Rev Med 1996;47:69–83.

91. Porte D Jr. Banting lecture 1990. Beta-cells in type II diabetes mellitus. Diabetes 1991;40(2):166–80.

92. Polonsky KS, Sturis J, Bell GI. Seminars in Medicine of the Beth Israel Hospital, Boston. Non-insulin-dependent diabetes mellitus–genetically programmed failure of the beta cell to compensate for insulin resistance. N Engl J Med 1996;334(12): 777–83.

93. Prentki M, Joly E, El-Assaad W, et al. Malonyl-CoA signaling, lipid partitioning, and glucolipotoxicity: role in beta-cell adaptation and failure in the etiology of diabetes. Diabetes 2002;51(Suppl 3):S405–13.

Glucose Control and Cardiovascular Outcomes in Individuals with Diabetes Mellitus
Lessons Learned from the Megatrials

Nicholas A. Avitabile, MD*, Ajaz Banka, MD,
Vivian A. Fonseca, MD

KEYWORDS

- Diabetes mellitus • Glycemic control • Cardiovascular disease

KEY POINTS

- Rates of cardiovascular disease (CVD) mortality are 2 to 4 times higher in patients with diabetes than in those without diabetes.
- Epidemiologic studies have shown that aggressive glycemic control can reduce the risks of CVD in certain individuals, but it seems to be detrimental in other subgroups.
- The decreased incidence and progression of microvascular complications seen in both ADVANCE (Action in Diabetes and Vascular Disease Pretrax and Diamicron Modified Release Controlled Evaluation) and ACCORD (Action to Control Cardiovascular Risk in Diabetes) may have longer-term beneficial effects on CVD.
- Results from several meta-analyses, which have included results from the ACCORD, ADVANCE, and VADT (Veterans Affairs Diabetes Trial) studies, showed a benefit of improved glycemic control on nonfatal myocardial infarction, and no overall effect of intensive glucose control on cardiovascular or all-cause mortality.

Diabetes mellitus (DM) is associated with an increased risk of cardiovascular disease (CVD) including fatal and nonfatal myocardial infarction (MI), heart failure, and cerebrovascular disease (stroke). Regardless of the type of DM, there is substantial evidence supporting an increase in CVD risk with increasing hyperglycemia. CVD death rates that are 2 to 4 times higher in those with DM compared with those who are not diabetic, and about 68% of deaths in diabetic patients aged 65 years and older are attributable to CVD.[1] Several large outcomes trials studies have studied the effect of glucose control on CVD outcomes, both in those with type 1 diabetes mellitus (T1DM)[2] and type 2 diabetes mellitus (T2DM).[3] These include the Action to Control Cardiovascular Risk in Diabetes (ACCORD), Action in Diabetes and Vascular Disease: Preterax and Diamicron Modified Release Controlled Evaluation (ADVANCE), and Veterans Affairs Diabetes Trial (VADT) trials.[4–6] Although the latter trials have shown lack of benefit, or possibly even harm, with respect to intensive glycemic control on CVD outcomes, the low event rates in these 3 trials that enrolled high-risk patients must be borne in mind. Furthermore, several meta-analyses have provided combinatorial data,[7,8]

Section of Endocrinology, Department of Medicine, Tulane University Health Sciences Center, 1430 Tulane Avenue, SL-53, New Orleans, LA 70112, USA
* Corresponding author.
E-mail address: dr.avitable@gmail.com

Heart Failure Clin 8 (2012) 513–522
http://dx.doi.org/10.1016/j.hfc.2012.06.009
1551-7136/12/$ – see front matter © 2012 Elsevier Inc. All rights reserved.

although factors such as heterogeneity in the included studies render interpretation difficult. This article reviews both the common and unique features of each of the megatrials and highlights key aspects that may help clinicians set glycemic goals for patients and favorably influence both microvascular and macrovascular outcomes.

CARDIOVASCULAR DISEASE RISK IN DM: LESSONS LEARNED FROM THE PAST
European Prospective Investigation into Cancer in Norfolk

Despite rapid advances in the treatment of DM, CVD outcomes in these patients remain suboptimal and hyperglycemia remains an appropriate risk factor to target and treat for CVD prevention.[9] The European Prospective Investigation into Cancer in Norfolk (EPIC-NORFOLK) study looked at the association between glycosylated hemoglobin (Hb) A1c and incident mortality. An increase in HbA1c of 1% was associated with a hazard ratio for all-cause mortality of 1.24 (95% confidence interval [CI], 1.14–1.34; $P<.001$) in men and 1.28 (95% CI, 1.06–1.32; $P<.001$) in women. However, studies focusing on intensive glycemic control to reduce HbA1c levels have had incongruent results.[10]

United Kingdom Prospective Diabetes Study

Perhaps the most extensive epidemiologic analysis of glycemia and CVD risk is supported by data from the United Kingdom Prospective Diabetes Study (UKPDS). In this study, Stratton and colleagues[11] showed a significant reduction in MI and all-cause mortality in overweight newly diagnosed patients with T2DM who were randomized to intensified glycemic control with metformin. Secondary analysis showed that the microvascular risk reduction and trend toward reduction in MI in the intensive control group was offset by a nonsignificant increase in stroke risk and no statistically significant effect on macrovascular complications.[3] Long-term follow-up of 3277 patients showed that, although differences in HbA1c between the groups were lost within the first year after the trial ended, the intensive glycemic group had significant reductions in observed MI and all-cause mortality in all treatment groups (either sulfonylurea or insulin or metformin), as well as a sustained benefit in previously shown microvascular risk reduction.[12,13]

Diabetes Control and Complications Trial

The Diabetes Control and Complications Trial (DCCT) was a landmark study designed to assess the impact of intensive glycemic control on microvascular risk in T1DM. Although this trial was not intended to evaluate the impact of glycemic control on CVD risk, the overall rate of CVD was low in this young, healthy population with shorter duration of disease. The youth of the patients made the detection of treatment-related differences in rates of macrovascular events less likely. However, when major cardiovascular and peripheral vascular events were combined, intensive therapy reduced the risk of macrovascular disease by 41% (to 0.5 events per 100 patient-years, vs 0.8 event; 95% CI, −10% to 68%), although the result did not reach statistical significance.[2]

The findings from both UKPDS and DCCT provided support for the premise that intensive glycemic control may reduce CVD risk in patients with DM. In both trials, posttrial follow-up was conducted to assess the effect of the initial period of intervention on future risk of complications. The Epidemiology of Diabetes Interventions and Complications (EDIC) study, the 17-year follow-up of the DCCT cohort, showed that intensive treatment reduced the risk of any CVD event by 42% and the risk of nonfatal MI, stroke, or death from CVD by 57%.[12]

LESSONS LEARNED FROM RECENT MEGATRIALS

After the DCCT and UKPDS trials, several unanswered questions remained as to the benefits of intensive glycemic control on CVD outcomes. To resolve some of this uncertainty, the past decade has seen 3 randomized controlled trials. The ACCORD, ADVANCE, and the VADT have appreciably expanded understanding in this regard. Moreover, many new questions were raised regarding the risks and benefits of intensive glucose control on CVD outcomes. The key patient characteristics and study design of these trials, along with those of the UKPDS, are outlined in **Table 1**.

ACCORD

The ACCORD study randomized 10,251 patients (aged 55–79 years) with a history of a CVD event (aged 40–79 years) or at significant risk for CVD events to either intensive therapy (target HbA1c <6.0%) or standard therapy. Other CVD risk factors such as lipids and blood pressure were treated aggressively in both groups. Patients had a history of DM for at least 10 years before enrollment. Median baseline HbA1c values were approximately 8.3%. After a mean follow-up of 3.5 years, those in the intensive arm achieved a significantly greater reduction in median HbA1c (6.4% compared with 7.5%) compared with those

Table 1
Selected features of trials of intensive glucose control and cardiovascular outcomes

	UKPDS[3]	ACCORD[4]	ADVANCE[5]	VADT[6]
Number of subjects	3867	10,251	11,140	1791
Mean age (y)	53	62	66	60
Duration of T2DM (y)	Newly diagnosed	10	8	11.5
History of CVD (%)	Not reported (95% CI)	35	32	40
Mean baseline HbA1c (%)	7.0	8.1	7.5	9.4
BMI (kg/m^2)	28	32	28	31
Study design	Randomized, open label	Randomized, 2 × 2 factorial design	Factorial randomized trial	Randomized, open label
Primary end point	Aggregate of any diabetes-related clinical end point, diabetes-related death, and all-cause mortality	Composite of nonfatal MI, nonfatal stroke, or death from cardiovascular causes	Macrovascular events (composites of nonfatal stroke, nonfatal MI or CV death) and microvascular events	Major cardiovascular event
Intensive treatment protocol	Sulfonylurea, insulin, or metformin. Target FPG <90 mg/dL	Treatment with metformin, sulfonylurea, glinide, TZD, acarbose, insulin, or a combination of these. Target HbA1c concentration <6%	30–120 mg oral gliclazide modified release, with or without metformin, TZD, glinide, acarbose, or insulin. Target HbA1c ≤6.5%	Maximum dose of metformin, with either rosiglitazone (BMI >27) or glimepiride and rosiglitazone (BMI <27)
Standard treatment protocol	Standard diet. Drugs were added if there were hyperglycemic symptoms or FPG >270 mg/dL	Standard treatment. Target HbA1c level 7.0%–7.9%	Standard treatment as per local guideline	Half dose of intensive treatments
Duration of follow-up (y)	10	3.5	5	5.6
Achieved HbA1c for intensive vs standard (%)	7.0 vs 7.9	6.4 vs 7.5	6.3 vs 7.0	6.9 vs 8.5
RR CV events (95% CI)	0.84 (0.71–1.00); not significant	0.90 (0.78–1.04); not significant	0.94 (0.84–1.06); not Significant	0.88 (0.74–1.05); not Significant
HR mortality (95% CI)	0.94 (0.80–1.10); not significant	1.22 (1.01–1.46); P = .02	0.93 (0.83–1.06); not significant	1.07 (0.81–1.42); not significant

Abbreviations: ACCORD, Action to Control Cardiovascular Risk in Diabetes; ADVANCE, Action in Diabetes and Vascular Disease Pretrax and Diamicron Modified Release Controlled Evaluation; BMI, body mass index; CV, cardiovascular; FPG, fasting plasma glucose; HR, hazard ratio (95% CI); RR, relative risk; TZD, thiazolidinediones.

in the standard treatment arm. Although the trial was not designed to test the components of the strategies used to intensify glucose control, the intensive arm required multiple combinations of oral agents and were more likely to be treated with insulin.[4] In February 2008, the intensive glycemia intervention was terminated ahead of the planned 5.5 years of average follow-up because of increased all-cause mortality. Participants in the intensive-therapy group subsequently were transitioned to standard glycemic therapy, and the target HbA1c target changed from less than 6% to a target between 7% and 7.9%. The blood pressure and lipid arms of the study continued and patients were followed up at least every 4 months until June 2009.

During the 3.5 years of average follow-up, 1.42% of patients in the intensive arm died each year compared with 1.14% a year in the standard intervention arm (hazard ratio [HR] 1.22, 95% CI 1.01–1.46; P = .04). In addition, there was a higher CVD mortality (HR 1.35, 95% CI 1.04–1.76; P = .02). The underlying cause of the increased mortality in the intensive arm was unclear at the time that the intervention was stopped. Despite these increased mortalities in the first 3.5 years of the ACCORD trial, rates of nonfatal MI were significantly lower in the intensively treated group (HR 0.76; 95% CI 62–0.920; P = .004). Although there was no significant difference in the rate of either nonfatal stroke or congestive heart failure between the 2 groups, there was a nonsignificant trend toward a reduction in the primary outcome of the trial (a composite of nonfatal MI, nonfatal stroke, or death from cardiovascular causes) with intensive glucose control (HR 0.90; 95% CI 0.78–1.04; P = .16).[4]

Several hypotheses have been proposed to explain the higher mortality observed early in ACCORD. A key question pertains to general applicability to the broader population or to specific subgroups of patients with T2DM. Prespecified subgroup analyses in ACCORD suggested a significant benefit of intensive glycemic control on CVD events in those participants with lower HbA1c at entry or absence of CVD event by history, but there was no suggestion of a differential effect on mortality. However, these observations are based on only a few subgroup analyses at the time of the primary publication. To further explore the theory that the higher mortality in the intensive glycemic control group may have been modified by other characteristics of patients, a post hoc analysis was conducted in which subjects were stratified by specific baseline characteristics.[14] The goal of this study was to determine whether particular subgroups at higher or lower risk strata could be identified. Baseline characteristics studied were in 4 categories: (1) demographic and anthropometric characteristics, (2) medical history characteristics, (3) medication use, and (4) laboratory variables. None of the baseline demographic and anthropometric characteristics had a statistically significant interaction with glycemia group assignment on mortality. The highest body mass index (BMI) category (>35 kg/m^2) showed the highest HR for intensive versus standard glycemia (HR 1.70, 95% CI 1.20–2.41) compared with BMI of 30 to 34 kg/m^2 (HR 1.05, 95% CI 0.76–1.44) and BMI less than 30 kg/m^2 (HR 1.01, 95% CI 0.81–1.48; P for interaction = .078).The 2 highest quartiles for waist circumference also showed the highest HR for intensive versus standard glycemia (P for interaction <.10). There were no significant interactions for age, sex, race, living alone, clinical network, education level, or randomization year found. Among the baseline medical history subgroups, participants with a self-reported history of neuropathy had a greater risk of mortality in the intensive glycemia arm compared with the standard glycemia arm (P for interaction = .0008). However, the presence of peripheral neuropathy at baseline, as documented on the clinical examination, was not associated with increased mortality in the intensive arm compared with the standard arm. In the intensively treated arm, there were no associations between excess mortality and CVD disease, duration of diabetes, history of retinal surgery, smoking, depression, systolic blood pressure, electrocardiogram variables, or prior amputation. The analysis of medications reported at baseline found that use of aspirin was associated with excess mortality in the intensive group (HR 1.45, 95% CI 1.13–1.85) compared with nonusers (HR 0.96, 95% CI 0.72–1.27; P for interaction = .03). A similar but not statistically significant differential effect occurred for use of antidepressant medications at baseline (HR 1.87, 95% CI 1.10–3.20, for users compared with HR 1.15, 95% CI 0.94–1.40 for nonusers; P for interaction = .08). Use of a diabetic medication, either as monotherapy or in combination, did not predict higher mortality in the intensive group. Furthermore, no antilipidemic agent or antihypertensive medication had an interaction with group assignment in predicting mortality. This analysis concluded that the intensive treatment had a greater effect on mortality in subgroups defined by 3 baseline clinical variables: HbA1c greater than or equal to 8.5% (interaction P = .044), aspirin use (interaction P = .03), and self-reported history of neuropathy (interaction P = .0008).

Another post hoc analysis studied the relationship between 4 HbA1c-associated measures and all-cause mortality.[15] These were: (1) mean HbA1c levels over the follow-up period, (2) final HbA1c, (3) decrease in HbA1c in the first year, and (4) decrease in HbA1c in the first 4 months. HbA1c values declined rapidly from the 8.1% (median) baseline in both treatment groups during the first year of treatment. With standard treatment, a plateau value close to 7.5% was achieved and, in the intensive treatment group, a plateau at 6.4% was attained between 12 and 24 months. All-cause mortalities were equivalent with the 2 strategies in the first 2 years, but, in the third year, the rate with the intensive strategy was double that of the standard strategy. After adjustment for other covariates, a higher average HbA1c level was a stronger predictor of mortality than either the final HbA1c or the decreases in HbA1c in the first year. Higher average HbA1c level was associated with a higher risk for death: each percentage-point increase in mean HbA1c was associated with an approximate 20% increase in all-cause mortality. The risk for death with the intensive strategy increased almost linearly from HbA1c levels of 6.0% to 9.0%. Despite the limitations inherent in a post hoc analysis, the finding that mortality increased linearly with increasing HbA1c is reassuring as well as consistent with other studies.[11,16] Average HbA1c level was a better predictor of mortality than decline in HbA1c, because this negates the premise that rapid lowering of HbA1c may have been the reason for the excess mortality noted in the intensive arm. Also, this analysis indicates that a poor response (as opposed to a good response) to intensive therapy is perhaps linked to a higher risk for death, a hypothesis that would lend itself to further evaluation.

ACCORD: Is Hypoglycemia the Culprit?

The ACCORD clinical trial offers an opportunity to investigate the relationship between hypoglycemia and mortality. Special attention was given to monitoring and minimizing severe hypoglycemia in the ACCORD study because of a priori concern regarding the consequences of hypoglycemia in the older population. One or more hypoglycemic episodes requiring assistance was associated with an increased risk of death, although the effect size was lower in the intensively treated group, with an HR of 1.4 compared with 2.3 in the standard treatment group. The risk of death in intensively treated patients who had severe hypoglycemia requiring medical assistance had (counterintuitively) a lower HR of 0.55 for mortality compared with the standard treatment group. These seemingly paradoxic findings suggest that, with intensive monitoring, the adverse effects of intensive treatment might be mitigated, resulting in clinical benefits.[17] The mechanism(s) underlying the increased

mortality among patients with severe hypoglycemia are yet to be defined. However, a possible explanation is that myocardial ischemia or fatal arrhythmia during recognized or unrecognized episodes of hypoglycemia may be responsible, particularly in the setting of cardiac autonomic neuropathy.[18] In a detailed study using simultaneous continuous glucose monitoring and electrocardiogram monitoring among 19 insulin-treated patients with T2DM and coronary artery disease, 10 episodes of angina and 4 episodes of cardiac ischemia were observed in 26 recorded episodes of symptomatic hypoglycemia.[19] In addition, 2 occasions of ischemia were seen in 28 episodes of asymptomatic hypoglycemia. Change in QT interval and QT dispersion have been seen during controlled episodes of hypoglycemia in other studies.[20]

Taken together, patients with T2DM who experience symptomatic, severe hypoglycemia are at increased risk of death, regardless of the intensity of glucose control. The reasons for the higher mortality in the intensive-therapy group during the pretransition period are still unclear. Because the rates of hypoglycemia were similar in the posttransition period, the increased risk of death among participants in the intensive glycemia control arm cannot be attributed to the increased rate of severe hypoglycemia in participants in the intensive arm.

ADVANCE TRIAL

The ADVANCE trial randomized 11,140 patients with established T2DM to either intensive glucose control (achieving a mean HbA1c of 6.5%) or standard control (achieving an HbA1c of 7.2%). In contrast with ACCORD, the ADVANCE cohort had different characteristics. They were older (required to be at least 55 years) with either known vascular disease or at least 1 other vascular risk factor. The patients in ADVANCE were diabetic for about 8 years before randomization, had lower baseline HbA1c levels, and required little use of insulin. After a median follow-up of 5 years, significantly lower HbA1c values were attained in the intensive treatment group (6.5%) versus the standard treatment group (7.3%). The rate of HbA1c reduction in ADVANCE was substantially slower than that observed in ACCORD (decrease of 0.5% at 6 months vs 0.6% at 12 months). Severe hypoglycemia was more common in the intensive control arm, although the rate of hypoglycemia was lower compared with ACCORD (2.7% vs 1.5%, HR 1.86%, 95% CI 1.42–2.40, P<.001).[5]

The incidence of combined major macrovascular and microvascular events was significantly reduced in the intensive glucose control arm (HR 0.90, 95% CI 0.82–0.98, P = .01). This result was primarily caused by a 21% relative reduction in development of nephropathy. The component of new or worsening nephropathy that was most clearly reduced through intensive glucose control was the development of macroalbuminuria (2.9% vs 4.1% with standard control; HR 0.70, 95% CI 0.57–0.85, P<.001). By contrast, the CVD component of the primary end point (a composite of MI, stroke, and cardiovascular death), analyzed in isolation, was not significantly reduced by intensive glucose control (HR 0.94, 95% CI 0.84–1.06, P = .32), although, in absolute terms, CVD mortality was reduced by 12% in the intensive arm. There was no evidence that intensive glucose control increased cardiovascular or all-cause mortality.[21]

Participants in ADVANCE were drawn from 20 different countries. A study was conducted to determine whether the effects of intensive glycemic control on major outcomes in ADVANCE differed between participants from Asia, established market economies, and eastern Europe. Demographic and clinical characteristics were compared across regions using generalized linear and mixed models. Effects on outcomes of the gliclazide modified release–based intensive glucose control regimen, targeting an HbAlc less than or equal to 6.5%, were compared across regions using Cox proportional hazards models, and the effects of intensive glycemic control were not significantly different ($P \geq$.23) between regions for any outcome, including mortality, vascular end points, and severe hypoglycemic episodes. Likewise, differences in health care systems, clinical practice, and use of medications (including statins and blood pressure–lowering medication) did not have a significant bearing on the results.[22]

VADT

The VADT randomized 1791 military veterans (mean age 60.4 years) with suboptimal glycemic control (median HbA1c of 9.4% at enrollment) to either intensive or standard glucose-lowering treatment. Intensive therapy was designed to reduce HbA1c by 1.5% more than standard therapy alone. Other cardiovascular risk factors were treated uniformly in both groups. Forty percent of participants had a past history of CVD events. Enrollees had a history of DM for about 11.5 years at the time of randomization. The primary outcome of the study was occurrence of a major CVD event such as MI, stroke, death from cardiovascular causes, congestive heart failure, inoperable coronary artery disease, and ischemia leading to lower extremity amputation.

After a median of 5.6 years of treatment, HbA1c in the intensive-therapy group was 6.9% and 8.4% in the standard-therapy group. No differences in primary outcome and all-cause mortality were observed between the 2 groups (29.5% vs 33.5%, HR 0.88, 95% CI 0.74–1.05). Severe hypoglycemic episodes were significantly more frequent in the intensive-therapy group compared with the standard-therapy group (21.2% vs 9.9%, P<.001).[6] Intensive glucose control in patients with poorly controlled T2DM had no significant effect on the rates of major cardiovascular events and death. With intensive glucose-lowering therapy, the greatest attenuation of albuminuria was noted in participants with higher levels of baseline albuminuria, preexisting retinopathy, greater body weight, and lower diastolic blood pressure.[23]

In a subgroup analysis, 301 participants in VADT with T2DM were evaluated to determine whether the initial extent of vascular disease influenced responsiveness to glucose-lowering therapy. Baseline coronary atherosclerosis was assessed using coronary artery calcium (CAC) measured by computed tomography. Participants with lower CAC (<100 Agatston units) had better outcome with intensive glycemic control. No significant improvement in CVD outcome was noted between the 2 treatment groups when CAC scores were greater than 100. This subgroup analysis showed that intensive control is beneficial in patients with less extensive coronary atherosclerosis. This subgroup seemed to be representative of the VADT cohort, and 60% of this subset of VADT had CAC scores greater than 100 units, which may explain the overall negative results in VADT.[24] Post hoc subgroup analyses of the study revealed benefit from intensive glycemic control in patients with duration of diabetes less than 12 years. However, cardiovascular events were unchanged or even increased in patients with duration of diabetes more than 12 years at the time of study entry. Severe hypoglycemia was associated with increased cardiovascular events in both arms and increased CVD death in the subsequent 180 days following severe hypoglycemia (HR 3.72, P = .01).[25] Because the patient population in VADT had a long history of established DM, whether intensive treatment over a longer time period would have translated into meaningful cardiovascular benefits is unclear. In addition, because 97% of participants were men, these findings may have limited validity for the management of diabetes in women. One explanation for the lack of beneficial effects of intensive therapy in patients with longstanding uncontrolled diabetes is the accumulation of advanced glycation end products over prolonged periods that exert proatherogenic effects.[26]

These complications are irreversible, so and it may be unrealistic to expect that progression of advanced complications can be halted with intensive glycemic control. However, aggressive glycemic control in patients with newly diagnosed diabetes produces a legacy effect that may provide protection against cardiovascular events in future years.[27] This concept has also been referred to as metabolic memory, which implies that the early glycemic environment is remembered by cells of the vasculature and of target organs.[28]

Other Studies

The Prospective Pioglitazone Clinical Trial in Macrovascular Events (PROactive) study[29] was conducted to explore whether the addition of pioglitazone or placebo to a patient's normal glucose-lowering medications could reduce CVD events. Pioglitazone treatment was associated with a 0.6% lower HbA1c level compared with placebo treatment (7.0% vs 7.6%, respectively). The primary end point of the study, a composite of all-cause mortality, nonfatal MI, stroke, acute coronary syndrome, endovascular or surgical intervention for coronary or leg arterial disease, and amputation above the ankle, was nonsignificantly reduced by 10% with pioglitazone treatment (HR 0.90, 95% CI 0.8–1.02, P = .095).The study was, controversially, presented as having a positive outcome because the main secondary end point, a composite of all-cause mortality, nonfatal MI, and stroke was significantly reduced by 16% with pioglitazone treatment (HR 0.84, 95% CI 0.72–0.98, P = .027). Patients with New York Heart Association class II to IV heart failure at screening were excluded from the PROactive trial. However, all of the patients who were included had established macrovascular disease and were at high risk for heart failure, so any therapeutic advantage could possibly be lost by risk of associated heart failure mortality. To address this issue, Erdmann and colleagues[30] conducted an analysis from PROactive study data to assess the risk factors for serious heart failure and to evaluate the effects of treatment on morbidity and mortality after reports of serious heart failure. More patients taking pioglitazone (5.7%) than placebo (4.1%) had serious episodes of heart failure during the study (P = .007). However, mortality caused by heart failure was similar (25 of 2605 [0.96%] for pioglitazone vs 22 of 2633 [0.84%] for placebo, P = .639). Among patients with a serious heart failure event, subsequent all-cause mortality was proportionately lower with pioglitazone (40 of 149 [26.8%] vs 37 of 108 [34.3%] with placebo, P = .1338). Fewer patients with serious heart failure taking pioglitazone went on to have an event in the primary

end point (47.7% with pioglitazone vs 57.4% with placebo, P = .0593) or main secondary end point (34.9% with pioglitazone vs 47.2% with placebo, P = .025). Although the incidence of serious heart failure was increased with pioglitazone versus placebo in the total PROactive population of patients with T2DM and macrovascular disease, subsequent mortality or morbidity was not increased in patients with serious heart failure, which implies that thiazolidinediones such as pioglitazone may be contributing to signs of heart failure in patients at risk.[31]

META-ANALYSES OF INTENSIVE GLYCEMIC CONTROL TRIALS

As a result of the early termination of ACCORD and fewer events than anticipated in ADVANCE and VADT, there was concern that these studies were underpowered to truly appreciate the effects of intensive glucose control on CVD risk. Several meta-analyses have explored the relationship between glycemic control and CVD events in subjects with T2DM since 2009 (**Table 2**). The first analysis included 33,040 participants from UKPDS, ACCORD, ADVANCE, VADT, and PROactive.[8] Intensive glucose control decreased HbA1c levels by 0.9% compared with the standard-therapy group. There was an overall significant 17% reduction in nonfatal MI and a 15% reduction in coronary heart disease (CHD)–related events. Intensive control had no significant effect on stroke or all-cause mortality.

A second meta-analysis by Kelly and colleagues[7] that included 27,000 participants from UKPDS, ACCORD, ADVANCE, and VADT revealed that intensive glucose control decreased HbA1c levels by 0.8%. Moreover, intensive glucose control was associated with a significant 10% relative reduction in CVD events, primarily as result of an 11% reduction of CHD events. There was no effect on rates of stroke, cardiovascular mortality, congestive heart failure, or all-cause mortality. Nevertheless, when the combined results of the ACCORD, ADVANCE, and VADT studies were analyzed, there was only a 10% nonsignificant relative reduction in CHD events (odds ratio 0.9, 95% CI 0.83–1.01). The overall analysis indicated that the benefits of intensive glucose control were at the cost of an increased risk for severe hypoglycemia (odds ratio 2.3, 95% CI 1.46–2.81).

A third meta-analysis, by Mannucci and colleagues,[32] was conducted in a similar manner to the study mentioned earlier but also included results from the PROactive trial. Intensive glucose control was associated with a significant 11% relative reduction in cardiovascular events that was

Table 2
Summary of recent meta-analyses of intensive glucose control on cardiovascular outcomes

Meta-Analyses	Trials Included	Subjects	% of HbA1C Reduction with Intensive Glycemic Control	MI	Mortality	Hypoglycemia
Ray et al,[8] 2009	UKPDS PROactive ACCORD ADVANCE VADT	33,040	0.9	OR 0.85 (0.77–0.93)	OR 1.02 (0.87–1.19)	Not reported
Kelly et al,[7] 2009	UKPDS ACCORD ADVANCE VADT	27,802	0.8	OR 0.89 (0.81–0.96)	OR 0.98 (0.84–1.15)	OR 2.3 (1.46–2.81)
Mannucci et al,[32] 2009	UKPDS PROactive ACCORD ADVANCE VADT	32,632	0.9	OR 0.86 (0.78–0.93)	OR 0.98 (0.77–1.23)	OR 3.01 (1.47–4.60)
Turnbull et al,[33] 2009	UKPDS ACCORD ADVANCE VADT	27,049	0.9	HR 0.85 (0.76–0.94)	HR 1.04 (0.90–1.20)	HR 2.48 (1.91–3.21)

Abbreviations: NR, not reported; OR, odds ratio (95% CI); PROactive, Prospective Pioglitazone Clinical Trial in Macrovascular Events.[28]

attributed to a 14% reduction in MI rates. Again, there was no effect of intensive glucose control on rates of stroke, cardiovascular mortality, or all-cause mortality, and intensive glucose control significantly increased rates of severe hypoglycemic events compared with standard control (odds ratio 3.01, 95% CI 1.47–4.60).

Turnbull and colleagues[33] performed a meta-analysis that included a total of 27,049 participants with 2370 major vascular events. The overall difference in HbA1c levels between intensive and standard glycemic control was a 0.9%. Major cardiovascular events were decreased by 9% (HR 0.91, 95% CI 0.84–0.99) with intensive glycemic control, predominantly because of a significant 15% reduction in the rate of MI. Cardiovascular and total mortality were not significantly reduced with intensive glycemic control. Intensive glycemic control was associated with a 2-fold reduction in the risk of severe hypoglycemia.

SUMMARY

It is important to approach glucose lowering in the context of managing overall cardiovascular risk. The American Diabetes Association and American Heart Association issued a joint position statement providing additional guidance on glycemic targets for patients with DM. The HbA1c goal remains at less than 7% in most patients with DM. Nevertheless, glycemic goals should be individualized based on duration of diabetes, preexisting cardiovascular disease, age, and life expectancy. For example, more stringent goals are reasonable for a young patient with recent-onset DM and no underlying CVD. In contrast, less intensive goals should be recommended for an elderly patient with long-standing DM and established macrovascular disease. In addition, intensive glycemic control has consistently been shown to produce a substantial benefit for preventing long-term microvascular complications in both T1DM and T2DM. Although CVD disease is the major cause of death in patients with diabetes, microvascular complications cause substantial morbidity and disability. Thus, it is apparent that additional strategies on multimodal treatment options are necessary to promote effective management and prevention of diabetic complications.

REFERENCES

1. Centers for Disease Control and Prevention. National diabetes fact sheet: national estimates and general information on diabetes and prediabetes in the United States, 2011. Atlanta (GA): US

Department of Health and Human Services, Centers for Disease Control and Prevention; 2011.

2. The Diabetes Control and Complications Trial Research Group (DCCT). The effect of intensive treatment of diabetes on the development and progression of long-term complications in insulin-dependent diabetes mellitus. N Engl J Med 1993; 329(14):977–86.

3. UK Prospective Diabetes Study (UKPDS) Group. Intensive blood glucose control with sulphonylureas or insulin compared with conventional treatment and risk of complications in patients with type 2 diabetes (UKPDS 33). Lancet 1998;352:837–53.

4. The Action to Control Cardiovascular Risk in Diabetes Study Group. Effects of intensive glucose lowering in type 2 diabetes. N Engl J Med 2008; 358:2545–59.

5. The ADVANCE Collaborative Group. Intensive blood glucose control and vascular outcomes in patients with type 2 diabetes. N Engl J Med 2008;358: 2560–72.

6. Duckworth WC, Abraira C, Moritz T, et al. Glucose control and vascular complications in veterans with type 2 diabetes. N Engl J Med 2009;360:129–39.

7. Kelly TN, Bazzano LA, Fonseca VA, et al. Systematic review: glucose control and cardiovascular disease in type 2 diabetes. Ann Intern Med 2009; 151:394–403.

8. Ray KK, Seshasai SR, Wijesuriya S, et al. Effect of intensive control of glucose on cardiovascular outcomes and death in patients with diabetes mellitus: a meta-analysis of randomised controlled trials. Lancet 2009;373:1765–72.

9. Desouza C, Raghavan VA, Fonseca VA. The enigma of glucose and cardiovascular disease. Heart 2010; 96:649–51.

10. Myint PH, Sinha S, Wareham NJ, et al. Glycated hemoglobin and risk of stroke in people without known diabetes in the European Prospective Investigation into Cancer (EPIC)–Norfolk Prospective Population Study. Stroke 2007;38:271–5.

11. Stratton IM, Adler AI, Neil HA, et al. Association of glycaemia with macrovascular and microvascular complications of type 2 diabetes (UKPDS 35): Prospective observational study. BMJ 2000; 321(7258):405–12.

12. Nathan DM, Cleary PA, Backlund JY, et al, Diabetes Control and Complications Trial/Epidemiology of Diabetes Interventions and Complications (DCCT/EDIC) Study Research Group. Intensive diabetes treatment and cardiovascular disease in patients with type 1 diabetes. N Engl J Med 2005;353:2643–53.

13. Holman RR, Paul SK, Bethel MA, et al. 10-year follow-up of intensive glucose control in type 2 diabetes. N Engl J Med 2008;359:1577–89.

14. Calles-Escandón J, Lovato LC, Simons-Morton DG, et al. Effect of intensive compared with standard glycemia treatment strategies on mortality by baseline subgroup characteristics. Diabetes Care 2010; 33(4):721–7.

15. Riddle MC, Ambrosius WT, Brillon DJ, et al. Epidemiologic relationships between A1C and all-cause mortality during a median 3.4-year follow-up of glycemic treatment in the ACCORD trial. Diabetes Care 2010;33(5):983–90.

16. Gerstein HC, Pogue J, Mann JF, et al. The relationship between dysglycemia and cardiovascular and renal risk in diabetic and non-diabetic participants in the HOPE study: a prospective epidemiological analysis [abstract]. Diabetologia 2005;48:1749–55.

17. Bonds DE, Miller ME, Bergenstal RM, et al. The association between symptomatic, severe hypoglycaemia and mortality in type 2 diabetes: retrospective epidemiological analysis of The ACCORD study. BMJ 2010;340:b4909.

18. Adler GK, Bonyhay I, Failing H, et al. Antecedent hypoglycemia impairs autonomic cardiovascular function: implications for rigorous glycemic control. Diabetes 2009;58:360–6.

19. Desouza C, Salazar H, Cheong B, et al. Association of hypoglycemia and cardiac ischemia: a study based on continuous monitoring. Diabetes Care 2003;26:1485–9.

20. Landstedt-Hallin L, Englund A, Adamson U, et al. Increased QT dispersion during hypoglycaemia in patients with type 2 diabetes mellitus. J Intern Med 1999;246:299–307.

21. Fonseca VA. Ongoing clinical trials evaluating the cardiovascular safety and efficacy of therapeutic approaches to diabetes mellitus. Am J Cardiol 2011;108(Suppl 3):52B–8B.

22. Woodward M, Patel A, Zoungas S, et al. Does glycemic control offer similar benefits among patients with diabetes in different regions of the world? Diabetes Care 2011;34(12):2491–5.

23. Agarwal L, Azad N, Emamele N, et al. Observations on renal outcomes in VADT. Diabetes Care 2011; 34(9):2090–4.

24. Reaven P, Moritz T, Schwenke D, et al. Intensive glucose lowering therapy reduces cardiovascular disease events in Veterans Affairs trial participants with lower calcified coronary atherosclerosis. Diabetes 2009 Nov;58(11):2642–8.

25. Duckworth WC. VA diabetes trial (VADT) update. 69th scientific sessions. American Diabetes Association; Abstract 468-P. Presented June 9, 2009.

26. Goldin A, Beckman J, Schmidt A, et al. Advanced glycation end products: sparking the development of vascular injury. Circulation 2006;114(6):597–605.

27. Del Prato S. Megatrials in type 2 diabetes. From excitement to frustration? Diabetologia 2009;52:1219–26.

28. Ceriello A. Hypothesis: the "metabolic memory", the new challenge of diabetes. Diabetes Res Clin Pract 2009;86(Suppl 1):S2–6.

29. Dormandy JA, Charbonnel B, Eckland DJ, et al. Secondary prevention of macrovascular events in patients with type 2 diabetes in the PROactive Study (PROspective pioglitAzone Clinical Trial In macro-Vascular Events): a randomised controlled trial. Lancet 2005;366:1279–89.

30. Erdmann E, Charbonnel B, Wilcox RG, et al. Pioglita-zone use and heart failure in patients with type 2 diabetes and preexisting cardiovascular disease: data from the PROactive Study (PROactive 08). Diabetes Care 2007;30:2773–8.

31. Horwich TB, Fonarow GC. Glucose, obesity, meta-bolic syndrome, and diabetes: relevance to inci-dence of heart failure. J Am Coll Cardiol 2010; 55(4):283–93.

32. Mannucci E, Monami M, Lamanna C, et al. Prevention of cardiovascular disease through glycemic control in type 2 diabetes: a meta-analysis of randomized clin-ical trials. Nutr Metab Cardiovasc Dis 2009;19:604–12.

33. Turnbull FM, Abraira C, Anderson RJ, et al. Intensive glucose control and macrovascular outcomes in type 2 diabetes. Diabetologia 2009;52:2288–98.

Glycemic Variability and Glycemic Control in the Acutely Ill Cardiac Patient

Jared Moore, MD[a], Kathleen Dungan, MD[b],*

KEYWORDS

- Glucose • Glycemic control • Glycemic variability • Hospital • Cardiac

KEY POINTS

- Acute hyperglycemia is associated with worse outcomes in hospitalized cardiac patients.
- Hospitalized cardiac patients are at particular risk for developing hyperglycemia and hypoglycemia for a variety of reasons.
- Flexible physiologic insulin regimens are appropriate for most hospitalized patients.
- Hospitalization provides an opportunity for reinforcement of good diabetes-related self-care behaviors to prevent long-term complications.
- Well-designed studies addressing glycemic control in the hospitalized cardiac population are needed.

SCOPE OF THE PROBLEM

For the estimated 25.6 million Americans more than the age of 20 years who have diabetes, the risk of having a myocardial infarction or congestive heart failure is about twice as great as those without diabetes.[1,2] In addition, it is estimated that 20% to 30% of patients admitted to the hospital with acute coronary syndrome, and 20% to 40% of those admitted with congestive heart failure exacerbation, have diabetes.[3–5] Diabetes is believed to be an independent risk factor for heart failure.[6–8] However, the association between acute and chronic hyperglycemia and outcomes after acute cardiovascular events is less clear.

Published studies have used different diagnostic criteria for identification of diabetes and inpatient (or stress-induced) hyperglycemia.[9–11] Current estimates suggest that 37% of persons with diabetes are unaware of their diagnosis.[12] Within this context, studies have shown that 10% to 34% of patients with myocardial infarction who had hyperglycemia on admission (defined differently) with no known history of diabetes were subsequently diagnosed with diabetes within 1 week of discharge.[13–15] The remainder are assumed to have stress-induced hyperglycemia.

In addition, cardiovascular disease (and possibly inpatient outcomes) in patients with diabetes or prediabetes represents a complex interplay of disease processes that may not be adequately modeled by the current diagnostic criteria, which are based on the correlation of laboratory values with the onset and progression of microvascular disease processes over many years of exposure.[9,10,16,17] Cardiac risk increases before a patient becomes hyperglycemic by the traditional definition. Furthermore, as discussed later,

Disclosures: KD discloses receiving research support from Novo Nordisk, as well as consulting fees from Eli Lilly and Pfizer.
[a] Department of Internal Medicine, The Ohio State University, 2050 Kenny Road, Suite 2400, Columbus, OH 43221-3502, USA; [b] Division of Endocrinology, Diabetes and Metabolism, Department of Internal Medicine, The Ohio State University, 491 McCampbell Hall, 1581 Dodd Drive, Columbus, OH 43210, USA
* Corresponding author.
E-mail address: Kathleen.dungan@osumc.edu

Heart Failure Clin 8 (2012) 523–538
http://dx.doi.org/10.1016/j.hfc.2012.06.006
1551-7136/12/$ – see front matter © 2012 Elsevier Inc. All rights reserved.

short-term hyperglycemia or glycemic fluctuations may also have an important effect on outcomes in acutely ill patients, although this is less well established. This situation should be considered when evaluating studies that dichotomously categorize populations as either having or not having diabetes or hyperglycemia.

MECHANISMS FOR HYPERGLYCEMIA IN HOSPITALIZED PATIENTS

In the acutely ill cardiac patient, many reasons coexist for the development of hyperglycemia, whether or not a patient has known diabetes. Certain therapeutic interventions, such as vasopressor agents, glucocorticoids, and parenteral nutrition can worsen or precipitate hyperglycemia.[18] Patient-specific factors also probably contribute, including a patient's underlying insulin resistance and β-cell function. However, hyperglycemia may be exacerbated by the severity of illness itself, which is marked by a proportionate increase in counterregulatory hormones and cytokines that have an adverse effect on insulin sensitivity. For example, in patients without known diabetes who were admitted to the hospital with acute myocardial infarction, cortisol, epinephrine, and norepinephrine (not hemoglobin A1c [HbA1c] or infarct size) were reported to be the primary determinants of glucose levels.[19] In patients presenting with chest pain, plasma cortisol, catecholamines, glucose, and insulin were increased across the spectrum from noncardiac chest pain to unstable angina to myocardial infarction.[20] Cortisol was associated with glucose levels. Such neurohormonal abnormalities have been known for decades.[21,22]

Neurohormonal derangements lead to excessive hepatic glucose production and insulin resistance during critical illness.[23,24] Although hepatic glucose production seems to be the major player,[25,26] peripheral insulin-mediated glucose uptake and nonoxidative glucose disposal are also reduced, at least in sepsis, which parallels the hormonal response observed after myocardial infarction in some ways.[27,28] Acute illness is generally associated with a catabolic metabolism that is marked by hyperglycemia as well as lipolysis. Hyperglycemia, lipolysis, and hyperinsulinemia are known to interact in complex ways, contributing to exaggerated inflammatory and counterregulatory hormone responses.[29,30] Resolution of hyperglycemia is associated with normalization of the inflammatory response.[31]

In heart failure, metabolic abnormalities also reflect the severity of symptoms.[32,33] Low cardiac output leads to compensatory increases in hormones that are counterregulatory to insulin in patients with heart failure.[34,35] Moreover, inflammatory cytokines such as tumor necrosis factor α (TNF-α) are increased and have been shown to directly inhibit insulin signaling.[36,37] These changes mirror those observed in acute illness in general, but it is unclear whether harmful effects would be additive to abnormalities already present during heart failure. The question is whether hyperglycemia induced by such neurohormonal changes is harmful or whether it is simply a marker of severe illness.

MECHANISMS OF ACUTE HYPERGLYCEMIA-MEDIATED HARM
Diabetes

The presence of diabetes is believed to increase the risk of death for patients who are admitted with the diagnosis of myocardial infarction.[38–40] This risk is related both to the direct, short-term sequelae of the infarction itself as well as to the heart failure that may subsequently result from it. Microvascular perfusion abnormalities and impaired myocardial energy production are suspected to affect patients with diabetes more prominently than those without diabetes.[17] In part, these factors are suspected of predisposing patients with diabetes to larger infarct sizes, as measured by serologic biomarkers and magnetic resonance imaging, as well as rates of postinfarction heart failure that are 2 times greater than for those without diabetes.[8,39,41] In the case of heart failure, the correlates of chronic metabolic and neurohormonal derangements are already a feature, including activation of the sympathetic nervous system and renin-angiotensin system,[42,43] increased oxidative stress,[44–46] endothelial dysfunction,[47,48] inefficient myocardial substrate use, and catabolic metabolism.[34] Thus, it is less clear whether exacerbation worsens outcomes. The OPTIMIZE-HF (Organized Program to Initiate Lifesaving Treatment In Hospitalized Patients With Heart Failure) trial found no correlation between in-hospital, 30-day, and 60-day postdischarge mortality for patients who were admitted with both heart failure and diabetes, but this study did not examine the role of glycemic control.[5]

Hospital Hyperglycemia

The typical chronic complications of diabetes require several years to develop. Outside the hospital, cardiovascular benefits from glycemic control emerge only after long-term follow-up, and any mortality benefit from tight glycemic control seems be limited to patients with recently diagnosed diabetes.[49,50] However, it is unclear if these observations can be extended to acute hyperglycemia associated with acute illness. Limited evidence suggests preferential downregulation of glucose transporters under conditions of chronic hyperglycemia as opposed to intermittent hyperglycemia and acute illness, potentially allowing glucose to enter cells unchecked by normal downregulatory responses.[51,52] This situation provides a rationale for differential outcomes associated with stress hyperglycemia compared with chronic hyperglycemia. Stress hyperglycemia can also be considered to contribute to glycemic variability (**Fig. 1**). Outside the inpatient setting, intermittent glycemic excursions are associated with more profound endothelial toxicity than increases in tonic glucose level in vitro,[53–55] and glycemic variability is independently associated with higher levels of oxidative stress in patients with type 2 diabetes.[56] A study using a euinsulinemic, hyperglycemic clamp in patients with or without type 2 diabetes reported that oscillating glucose levels between 90 and 270 mg/dL resulted in increased endothelial dysfunction and oxidative stress that exceeded the effects of sustained hyperglycemia at 270 mg/dL in both groups.[57] This finding was confirmed in another study.[58]

Cardiovascular Harm

In the cardiac patient, other lines of evidence exist for a role of glycemic fluctuations in disease onset or modification. In patients admitted with chest pain, glycemic variability was an independent predictor of the severity of coronary artery disease on angiography and was superior to HbA1c.[59]

Glycemic variability was associated with coronary artery calcium scores in men but not women with type 1 diabetes.[60] In a mouse model of diabetes, induced glycemic variability impaired ischemia-induced angiogenesis, independently of mean glucose level, through alteration of the vascular endothelial growth factor pathway.[61] A prospective study of patients with type 2 diabetes and ischemic heart disease found that ischemic electrocardiographic changes were more common during rapid glucose changes (>100 mg/dL/h) than during normoglycemia or sustained hyperglycemia.[62] Glycemic variability was associated with sympathovagal balance, endothelial function, and left ventricular mass index in patients with type 2 diabetes.[63] Thus, it makes sense to consider short-term and long-term glycemic control separately in the hospitalized cardiac patient.

DIABETES, HYPERGLYCEMIA, AND OUTCOMES IN CARDIAC PATIENTS
Chronic Hyperglycemia

The lower limit at which chronic glycemic control (determined by HbA1c) becomes insignificant in acute cardiovascular disease is unknown.[10] For example, a recent observational study of patients hospitalized for myocardial infarction found that stepwise increases in HbA1c, even if they were less than 6.5%, were associated with higher 1-year and 3-year mortality.[64] On the other hand, a study of 827 patients with diabetes and average HbA1c levels near 8.0% who were admitted with a diagnosis of myocardial infarction found that HbA1c was not associated with in-hospital mortality.[65] Therefore, chronic hyperglycemia

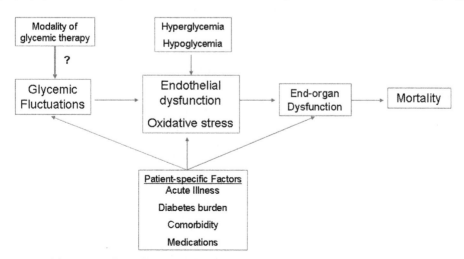

Fig. 1. Conceptual framework for a theoretic role of glycemic variability in the acutely ill patient. Glycemic variability may be influenced by patient-specific factors such as acute illness, duration of diabetes, presence of comorbidities, and other medications. Sustained hyperglycemia, hypoglycemia, and glycemic variability may lead to endothelial dysfunction and oxidative stress, which in turn contribute to end-organ dysfunction and death.

may be more reflective of long-term outcomes. In heart failure, HbA1c was a progressive risk factor for mortality and hospitalization for heart failure in patients with or without diabetes[66] but a U-shaped relationship may exist.[67] Heart failure readmission has been associated with increasing HbA1c.[68]

Acute Hyperglycemia

Increasing admission blood glucose levels have also been shown to have an inverse relationship with in-hospital and long-term postmyocardial infarction survival, independent of a diagnosis of diabetes.[64,65,69–71] More specifically, larger deviations of admission glucose level from a patient's preillness glycemic control, defined by HbA1c (suggesting the presence of stress hyperglycemia), are correlated with 30-day and 1-year mortality.[65,72–74] Thus, acute hyperglycemia seems to be a better predictor of mortality than chronic hyperglycemia for myocardial infarction. It is also sometimes difficult to know whether outcomes are observed with improved glycemic control per se or because of secondary effects of insulin itself. In 1 study of 141,680 patients admitted with an acute myocardial infarction,[65] three-quarters of the patients with diabetes and admission glucose levels greater than 240 mg/dL received insulin therapy, compared with only 22% of those without diabetes. Thirty-day and 1-year mortality were greater in the patients without diabetes. By comparison, 1 study found no correlation between admission glucose levels and 30-day and 1-year mortality in patients admitted with heart failure.[75]

Most retrospective studies rely heavily on admission glucose level for analysis, which provides only a snapshot of glycemic control. A recent study of approximately 17,000 patients admitted with myocardial infarction showed that increasing in-hospital mean glucose level was associated with increasing inpatient mortality.[76] The effect was observed in patients with and without diabetes, although a higher threshold for harm was identified in those with diabetes. Furthermore, mean hospital glucose level was a better predictor of mortality than admission glucose level. The importance of acute hyperglycemia, relative to chronic hyperglycemia, may be further supported by a study that showed that among intensive care unit (ICU) patients with diabetes who had poor chronic glycemic control (determined by HbA1c), rapid achievement of normoglycemia in the ICU was associated with higher mortality.[77] Thus, the unique role of stress hyperglycemia deserves further attention in prospective studies.

Glycemic Variability

One factor that is receiving increasing attention both in the inpatient and outpatient setting is glycemic variability. A large review of more than 7000 medical and surgical ICU patients found that the standard deviation of glucose level was a better predictor of mortality than mean glucose level.[78] This finding has been observed in other critical care settings,[79,80] but has not been well studied in myocardial infarction. In patients admitted with heart failure exacerbation, glycemic variability, but not mean hospital glucose level, was associated with inpatient mortality.[81] There are currently no prospective studies specifically examining outcomes through the pharmacologic manipulation of glycemic variability in the hospital. Moreover, such a study would be technically difficult to perform.

Clinical Trials Data

Over the past decade, awareness has increased about the need to find appropriate management strategies for treating hyperglycemia in hospitalized patients. Recent reports in the medical and surgical ICU have tempered any enthusiasm for strict glycemic control (target of 80–110 mg/dL), because of what has been considered an unacceptable risk of hypoglycemia and possible increase in mortality.[82–85] The ACCORD (Action to Control Cardiovascular Risk in Diabetes) trial added another layer of complexity when it was ended early because of higher all-cause and cardiovascular mortality in the intensive therapy group compared with the standard therapy group.[50] However, in both settings, tight glycemic control was compared with what many consider acceptable glycemic control, not poor control. Therefore, it does not follow that glycemic control should be abandoned in the hospital. For example, in a smaller multicenter randomized controlled trial of 211 surgical patients,[86] basal bolus insulin resulted in lower mean glucose level compared with sliding scale insulin (147 vs 172 mg/dL, $P <$ .01), and there was a reduction in the composite outcome of wound infection, pneumonia, bacteremia, and respiratory and acute renal failure (odds ratio [OR] 3.4, 95% confidence interval [CI] 1.5–7.7). In addition, a meta-analysis of clinical trials aiming for at least less than 180 mg/dL also showed benefits in multiple outcomes after cardiac surgery.[87]

Studies evaluating the management of hyperglycemia in patients with acute nonsurgical cardiovascular disease have been difficult to interpret. DIGAMI (Diabetes Mellitus Insulin-Glucose Infusion in Acute Myocardial Infarction) 1 and DIGAMI

2 trials attempted to determine if improved inpatient glucose control would decrease mortality after acute myocardial infarction. DIGAMI 1 evaluated the effectiveness of immediate intravenous (IV) insulin therapy followed by insulin-based long-term therapy for patients with diabetes who were admitted with an acute myocardial infarction. Whereas 1-year mortality was reduced, in-hospital and 3-month mortality were not significantly reduced in the group treated with IV insulin.[88] DIGAMI 2 was designed to determine whether the mortality benefit was caused by acute IV insulin or long-term subcutaneous insulin.[89] Low enrollment and a failure to reach statistically significant differences in plasma glucose and HbA1c levels amongst the 3 groups hampered the study and no difference in short-term and long-term mortality was observed.

GIPS 1 (Glucose-Insulin-Potassium Study-1), GIPS 2 (Glucose-Insulin-Potassium Study-2), and CREATE-ECLA (The Clinical Trial of Reviparin and Metabolic Modulation in Acute Myocardial Infarction Treatment and Evaluation-Estudios Clinicos Latino America) are examples of trials that attempted to determine whether insulin itself had a beneficial impact on mortality in patients suffering from acute myocardial infarction.[90–92] The impetus for conducting these trials was held in the theory that high-dose glucose-insulin-potassium (GIK) infusion after a myocardial infarction would increase glucose use by myocytes and decrease use of free fatty acids. This situation would result in a decreased production of free oxygen radicals, which may cause further injury to ischemic myocytes. These trials failed to show a consistent benefit, and results were confounded by hyperglycemia in the intervention arms, which exceeded that of control arms. However, post hoc analyses did show that hyperglycemia, defined by a glucose level more than 140 mg/dL at 6 or 24 hours, was associated with increased mortality in patients without known diabetes and

in patients who did not receive GIK.[93] This finding suggests that a different threshold of harm may exist for patients with or without diabetes, and possibly that GIK may still mitigate the harm. Postadmission hypoglycemia (<70 mg/dL) was not associated with mortality.

Given the limitations of data to guide clinicians in the management of hyperglycemia in acute cardiovascular disease, it is not surprising that from 1997 to 2006, there was no improvement in mortality related to glycemic control in patients hospitalized with acute myocardial infarction.[94]

MANAGEMENT
Targets

The current American Diabetes Association (ADA)/ American Association of Clinical Endocrinology hospital guidelines recommend a target glucose level of 140 to 180 mg/dL based on the control arm of the NICE-SUGAR ICU study in both ICU and non-ICU settings until further data are available (**Fig. 2**).[95] However, NICE-SUGAR did not address whether glycemic control targeting a more modest glucose range (110–140 mg/dL) is better. In particular, hypoglycemia is less common when a more modest target (100–150 mg/dL) is attempted (frequency of blood glucose of <60 mg/dL was 5% in both medical and cardiac care units).[96] As a result, an intermediate target glucose range between 110 and 140 mg/dL may be reasonable in certain populations (for example, after cardiac surgery) and institutions and patients in whom it can be performed safely. By comparison, the Endocrine Society recommends meal-specific targets, including a fasting glucose level less than 140 mg/dL and postprandial target of less than 180 mg/dL in noncritical care settings.[97] Regardless, a target glucose range attempting to achieve normoglycemia (80–110 mg/dL) is not recommended because of the unacceptable risk of hypoglycemia. Furthermore, this tight glucose

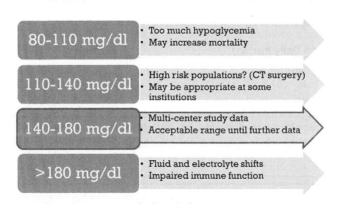

Fig. 2. Rationale for current glycemic targets in the hospital.

range is probably not technically feasible in most circumstances because of limitations of IV infusion algorithms and glucose monitoring.[98] Improvements in technology, such as more precise methods of glucose monitoring and computerized (or even closed loop) IV infusion algorithms, are needed to determine whether achievement of normoglycemia is beneficial.[99] Until more data are available, separate targets for acute and chronic hyperglycemia are not advocated.

General Approach

Current hospital and outpatient guidelines as well as large clinical studies focus mainly on the achievement of specific mean glucose targets and not necessarily on how those targets are achieved. The tendency for preoccupation with average glucose level neglects details in overall glucose control that may be linked to outcomes. One cannot just extrapolate successful approaches from the outpatient arena to the inpatient arena, because the dynamic nature of acute illness and the effects of other variables such as nutritional status and renal function necessitate constant vigilance and a flexible management plan. For these reasons, it is of interest to determine whether management of hyperglycemia is better viewed through the lens of minimizing glycemic variability rather than mean glucose level.

It is unknown whether measures that specifically minimize illness-induced glycemic excursions improve outcomes. In addition, some evidence suggests that glycemic variability is a function of patient-specific factors that are difficult to manipulate. Patients with glycemic lability may have long-standing diabetes with both β cell and counterregulatory hormone failure.[100] In hospitalized patients, glycemic variability has been associated with age, diabetes, and total insulin requirements.[101] However, measures that minimize fluctuations are more likely to achieve overall glycemic control without increasing the risk of hypoglycemia.[102,103] Studies in the outpatient setting suggest that physiologic insulin regimens reduce both mean glucose level and glycemic fluctuations.[104–106] Physiologic regimens, particularly when used in lieu of traditional sliding scale insulin, could also reduce glycemic variability in the hospital. Dozens of studies have investigated the efficacy of various IV insulin protocols.[107,108] However, efficacy is usually not defined in terms of glycemic variability. Computerized IV insulin protocols show reductions in hypoglycemia and hyperglycemia, indicating that they may also reduce glycemic variability.[109–111] More studies are needed to recommend for or against specific measures to reduce glycemic variability outside the traditional framework for tight glycemic control in the hospital. The remainder of this section focuses on strategies to provide physiologic glycemic control in hospitalized patients, with particular attention to the needs of the cardiac patient.

Insulin

The current ADA guidelines recommend insulin as the primary modality of therapy in most hospitalized patients with hyperglycemia.[96,98] In general, a physiologic regimen containing basal, prandial, and supplemental (correction) insulin components is advised to obtain glycemic control (**Table 1**).[96,98]

IV insulin

IV insulin is advised in patients with severe hyperglycemia and in patients who are critically ill, particularly those with hypotension or who are undergoing major surgery. Issues unique to the acutely ill cardiac patient, such as poor perfusion and edema, may render IV insulin a safer, more effective choice because of slower absorption of subcutaneous insulin and the potential for insulin stacking and delayed hypoglycemia (**Table 2**).[112]

Table 1
Approaches to physiologic insulin use in the hospital

	% of Total Daily Insulin[a]	Examples
Basal	<50% (if eating)	Long-acting insulin analogue Neutral protamine Hagedorn Continuous subcutaneous insulin (pump) IV insulin infusion
Prandial	≥50% divided evenly over meals (if eating)	Rapid-acting insulin analogue Regular insulin (tube feeds)
Correction	Varies	See prandial insulin IV insulin infusion

[a] Total estimate insulin per day from all sources. If patient is not eating, then basal insulin may account for most insulin requirements.

Table 2
Comparison of IV and SQ insulin in the hospital

	IV	SQ
Frequency of titration	Hourly	Daily
Time to target glucose	~12 h	~3 d
Adaptability to clinical status	+++	++
Absorption issues	No	Yes
Duration of hypoglycemia	<1 h	Hours
Labor	+++	++

IV insulin is often necessary for treatment of hyperglycemia associated with high-dose steroids and total parenteral nutrition. Multiple algorithms have been published,[108,109] but few randomized trials comparing algorithms are available.[113] In general, a validated protocol should be used, keeping in mind the ease of implementation and use as well as its efficacy and safety.[114]

Another issue of importance is the patient who is eating while receiving an insulin infusion. Even the most sophisticated insulin infusion algorithms are perturbed in patients who are eating,[115,116] likely representing the inability of standardized algorithms to adapt to the rapid glucose level changes induced by eating. In such patients, subcutaneous rapid-acting insulin may be provided to cover meals.[117] An alternative is to use an infusion algorithm that provides a programmable temporary step-up in infusion rate after a meal.[111,118]

Moving patients from IV to subcutaneous insulin should be deferred ideally until a patient is hemodynamically stable, off pressors, extubated, and eating.[119] Among patients undergoing postcardiac surgery, those with good glycemic control on stable or minimal insulin requirements meeting the aforementioned criteria are more successful with the transition. In surgical patients, an initial basal insulin dose of 50% to 65% of the daily IV insulin requirements (calculated from the average infusion rate during fasting or adequate subcutaneous prandial insulin coverage) is adequate for many patients 48 hours after surgery.[118,120] Inadequate prandial insulin coverage during an infusion may also lead to an overestimation of basal insulin necessary for transitioning a patient off an insulin infusion.[118] On the other hand, patients with more chronic hyperglycemia, marked insulin resistance, or shorter duration of infusion after the initial event may require a higher conversion factor or weight-based dosing.[121,122] The dosing regimen should be compared with the patient's home insulin requirements, HbA1c level, and weight (see later discussion).

Subcutaneous insulin
Initiation of insulin Subcutaneous insulin is the mainstay of treatment of hospitalized patients with diabetes. However, the initiation of insulin can be a challenging proposition for patients who are acutely ill, because a variety of factors, including altered eating habits and a rapidly changing clinical course, may significantly affect insulin requirements over time. It may be helpful to stratify the approach by preadmission glycemic control and therapy (**Fig. 3**).

Insulin-naive patients
- Poor baseline control: in patients with severe hyperglycemia (>300 mg/dL) refractory to intervention or who have other indications, IV insulin is an efficient means of calculating total insulin requirements, as

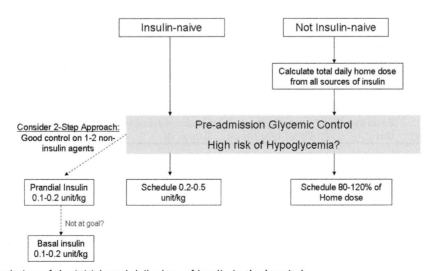

Fig. 3. Calculation of the initial total daily dose of insulin in the hospital.

noted earlier. In patients with moderate hyperglycemia or stable patients with more advanced hyperglycemia, a weight-based algorithm has been used for the initiation of subcutaneous insulin. The total daily dose is calculated as 0.4 to 0.5 units/kg and 50% is administered as basal insulin and 50% as prandial insulin, divided evenly over 3 meals. A lower dose (0.2–0.3 unit/kg) should be considered in patients at risk for hypoglycemia, such as elderly patients or those with renal or liver impairment.[98]

- Mild to moderate baseline control: there are few studies supporting approaches to insulin therapy in insulin-naive patients with more mild to moderate (<200 mg/dL) or intermittent hyperglycemia. These patients may be best treated with a step-wise approach. Outside the hospital, basal insulin is typically initiated before prandial insulin, but in the hospital, prandial insulin may be the preferred first-line therapy in patients who periodically must receive nothing by mouth for tests. If the fasting glucose level remains increased, a low dose of basal insulin can be implemented at 0.1 to 0.2 unit/kg.

Noninsulin-naive patients In noninsulin-naive patients, continuation of the home insulin regimen requires special consideration. First, it must be emphasized that patients with type 1 diabetes require basal insulin without exception at all times. Otherwise, one must inquire about the patient's level of adherence, the frequency of glucose self-monitoring, and patterns of hypoglycemia. In all cases, basal insulin is administered at no more than 50% of the total home daily dose (basal plus prandial) and the rest of the total daily requirements are spread out over meals.[87,123] In particular, nonphysiologic insulin regimens (particularly in cases in which basal insulin accounts for a large proportion of the total daily dose) need adjustment because patients must often receive nothing by mouth or otherwise may not be eating in the same way with hospital food. In such cases, basal insulin may require reduction in favor of more prandial insulin.

- Poor baseline control: the total daily dose may be increased 10% to 20% in patients who are adherent and uncontrolled.
- Good baseline control: the total daily dose may be continued without adjustment provided that hypoglycemia is not a significant problem and that a physiologic regimen is used.

Special considerations for prandial and correction insulin In general, a patient who is eating reasonably well should receive no more than 50% of the total daily insulin dose as basal insulin (**Table 3**).[87,123] Ideally, the prandial insulin dose is tailored to carbohydrate intake (flexible insulin dosing or carbohydrate counting starting at 1 unit per 10 or 15 g of carbohydrates). If fixed meal dosing is used, a consistent carbohydrate diet is necessary. Special precautions should accompany the order (cut dose in half if patient eats 50% of the tray or if glucose level is 70–90 mg/dL, hold dose if <50% of the tray is eaten, and so forth). Correction (supplemental) insulin should also be adjusted based on the patient's total daily insulin requirements. Coverage for enteral and parenteral feeding requires additional consideration, which is beyond the scope of this article.

Adjustment of therapy Daily adjustment of therapy should be directed at hypoglycemia first. Targeted reduction in insulin doses should be commensurate with the degree and frequency of hypoglycemia and

Table 3
Distribution of insulin dosing in hospitalized patients with normal oral intake[a] based on the total estimated daily dose

Total Daily Dose[b] (Units)	Basal Insulin Dose	Fixed Meal Dose[c] (Per Meal)	Insulin: Carbohydrate (Units: g)	Correction Factor (1 Unit per __ mg/dL More Than 150 mg/dL)
<20	≤10	2–3	1:20	100
20–40	10–20	4–5	1:15	50 (standard dose)
41–50	20–25	6–8	1:10 (standard dose)	50 (standard dose)
51–80	25–40	9–13	1:8	25
>80	40+	14+	1:5	25

[a] Assumes patient is eating a typical (carbohydrate-controlled) diet.
[b] Total estimated insulin per day from all sources.
[c] Accompany with appropriate hold parameters (eg, hold if patient eats less than half of tray or if glucose level <80 mg/dL).

risk of adverse consequences. In patients whose illness is marked by significant stress hyperglycemia (such as after cardiac surgery or large myocardial infarction), one must also allow for continued reduction in insulin requirements as the stress of the illness dissipates.[118,122] Continued preemptive dose reduction (10%–20% per day) may be required in patients who are tightly controlled (glucose level consistently <100 mg/dL) with severe illness.[98] Patients with chronic hyperglycemia or less acute illness may require less aggressive dose reduction.[123] Home insulin requirements may be a helpful guide. In patients with persistent hyperglycemia, randomized controlled trials have indicated that daily dose adjustment of 10% to 20% per day is reasonable in patients receiving basal bolus insulin analogues.[87,124]

Periprocedural care

The cardiac patient is particularly prone to changes in oral intake because of the need for frequent procedures. In general, it is not necessary to withhold basal insulin entirely. Although limited prospective data are available, 1 retrospective review reported that among patients who were told to take 50% of their home dose of basal insulin before surgery, hypoglycemia was uncommon (2% among patients with a preoperative glucose level <200 mg/dL; 0% among those with preoperative hyperglycemia).[124] However, postoperative hyperglycemia was persistent in most patients with preoperative hyperglycemia. By comparison, patients who are undergoing procedures such as cardiac stress testing or catheterization may have a smaller stress response, and a reduction of 50% may still be reasonable.

However, the necessity for dose reduction may be negligible and omissions may be minimized by prophylactically adjusting the home regimen to a more physiologic distribution at the time of admission, as discussed earlier. In patients with type 1 diabetes, minimal reductions (<20%), are necessary, and generally only in patients with tight glycemic control.[125]

Noninsulin Therapy

Oral agents

As stated earlier, for a variety of reasons guidelines advise discontinuation of oral agents in most hospitalized patients with diabetes (**Table 4**). Oral sulfonylureas may result in prolonged hypoglycemia in patients with even modest renal dysfunction, a common comorbidity in the cardiac patient, or nil-by-mouth status.[126,127] Metformin is associated with lactic acidosis in a variety of conditions, such as renal insufficiency (which is especially relevant in patients receiving IV contrast), decompensated heart failure, or hypoxia.[128–131] Although the risk is low, the estimated mortality is still high.[129,130,132] Thiazolidinediones are well known to be associated with congestive heart failure.[132,133] Furthermore, they have a slow onset of action and thus have limited use in the inpatient setting.

GLP-1 based therapy

Glucagonlike peptide 1 (GLP-1)-based therapies have garnered increasing interest for the treatment of diabetes or hyperglycemia in patients with diabetes. These agents do not generally cause hypoglycemia in the absence of other therapies that cause hypoglycemia.[134,135] There are GLP-1

Table 4
Comparison of insulin and noninsulin hypoglycemic agents in the hospital

	Noninsulin Agents	Insulin[a]
Frequency of titration	Days to weeks	Daily
Adaptability to changes in nutritional status	+	+++
Duration of hypoglycemia	None (M, T, G) Days (S)	Hours
Other cautions	Renal dysfunction (M, S) Liver disease (M, S, T) Lactic acidosis[b] (M) Nausea/vomiting/pancreatitis (G) Heart failure (T, M) Elderly (M, S)	Rare

DPP-4 inhibitors are generally safe but have limited efficacy and there are limited data for use in the hospital.
 Abbreviations: G, GLP-1 (exenatide, liraglutide, pramlintide); M, metformin; S, sulfonylureas; T, thiazolidinediones.
 [a] Using a physiologic regimen.
 [b] Metformin-associated lactic acidosis is increased in patients with renal dysfunction (and IV contrast administration), acidosis, respiratory failure, acute heart failure, and hemodynamic compromise.

receptors in the myocardium, and preclinical and early clinical studies raise the possibility that there may be beneficial cardiac effects, such as reduction of ischemic preconditioning and improved left ventricular function.[136] Furthermore, these therapies counteract the effects of inappropriate glucagon release, a pathologic feature of diabetes and stress hyperglycemia alike.[72] There are 2 main approaches to augmenting GLP-1 to treat hyperglycemia: (1) GLP-1 receptor agonists or mimetics and (2) inhibition of dipeptidyl peptidase IV (DPP-IV), the enzyme that degrades GLP-1.

- GLP-1 receptor agonists are generally more potent and have the advantage of promoting weight loss long-term.[137,138] These agents have been studied intravenously in small studies of hospitalized cardiac patients, but nausea is a major potential side effect and it is too early too tell if cardiac benefits are present.[139–143]
- DPP-IV inhibitors are generally well tolerated but have more limited efficacy.[136] However, in some patients with mild hyperglycemia, they may be considered. Meta-analyses from randomized controlled trials suggest cardiovascular benefits from these agents versus active comparators, although most studies were short-term.[144,145]

The long-term safety of these agents is unknown and the safety and efficacy of GLP-1–based therapies have not been extensively tested in hospitalized patients. Further study therefore is warranted.

Other approaches

Many other noninsulin therapies are under investigation for the treatment of diabetes in the outpatient setting.[146] There has been little interest in developing targeted therapies for inpatient use, possibly because of the complexity of the patients and the lack of randomized controlled trials that establish an appropriate glucose target. Noninsulin agents that lower glucose level without causing hypoglycemia are candidates for inpatient therapy. Agents that target major components of stress-induced hyperglycemia, such as hepatic glucose output or insulin resistance in general, are needed. These agents must be safe, effective, and ideally compatible with other IV medications. Until such therapies become available, insulin remains the mainstay of therapy.

Discharge

Sustained glycemic control after discharge may be facilitated with proper planning that begins at the time of hospital admission. Patients should be

Table 5
Home-going strategy based on HbA1c[a]

HbA1c (%)	Suggested Regimen
>9	Basal + oral or basal + bolus insulin
7–9	1-step to 2-step increase in therapy: oral → 2 oral → oral + basal insulin → basal bolus
<7	Resume home regimen

[a] Strategy assumes that patient is resuming a normal diet and that there are no contraindications.

screened for medication adherence and discharge needs with appropriate social work input early. Diabetes education should be considered early in the hospital course when needed, because education is best received when there is time for continued follow-up and reinforcement.[147,148] Likewise, diabetes physician consultation should be considered early in the course when necessary, because the attainment of glycemic control typically requires several days to achieve.[87,124] The HbA1c may be used to guide hospital discharge regimens such that those who are well controlled before admission may resume their preadmission therapy, provided there are no contraindications and oral intake has resumed to normal (**Table 5**). In other patients, 1-step or 2-step intensification of therapy is necessary based on the severity of hyperglycemia, comorbidities, and contraindications.[149] Written communication of changes in the diabetes regimen is crucial for patients at the time of discharge, and outpatient follow-up should be ensured.

SUMMARY

More studies are needed to recommend for or against specific measures to reduce glycemic excursions outside the traditional framework for tight glycemic control. However, measures to stabilize glucose through physiologic insulin regimens may have the potential to preserve or enhance the benefits of glycemic control and reduce the risks of hypoglycemia in the hospital. Such efforts also serve to build a united front with outpatient providers in reinforcing the importance of glycemic control for reducing the long-term risk of microvascular complications.

REFERENCES

1. Yusuf S, Hawken S, Ounpuu S, et al. Effect of potentially modifiable risk factors associated with

myocardial infarction in 52 countries (the INTER-HEART study): case-control study. Lancet 2004; 364(9438):937–52.

2. Nichols GA, Hillier TA, Erbey JR. Congestive heart failure in type 2 diabetes: prevalence, incidence, and risk factors. Diabetes Care 2001;24(9):1614–9.

3. Canto JG, Kiefe CI, Rogers WJ, et al. Number of coronary heart disease risk factors and mortality in patients with first myocardial infarction. JAMA 2011;306(19):2120–7.

4. Kapoor JR, Fonarow GC, Zhao X, et al. Diabetes, quality of care, and in-hospital outcomes in patients hospitalized with heart failure. Am Heart J 2011;162(3):480–486.e3.

5. Greenberg BH, Abraham WT, Albert NM, et al. Influence of diabetes on characteristics and outcomes in patients hospitalized with heart failure: a report from the organized program to initiate lifesaving treatment in hospitalized patients with heart failure (OPTIMIZE-HF). Am Heart J 2007;154(2):277.e1–8.

6. Lewis EF, Velazquez EJ, Solomon SD, et al. Predictors of the first heart failure hospitalization in patients who are stable survivors of myocardial infarction complicated by pulmonary congestion and/or left ventricular dysfunction: a VALIANT study. Eur Heart J 2008;29(6):748–56.

7. Khot UN, Khot MB, Bajzer CT, et al. Prevalence of conventional risk factors in patients with coronary heart disease. JAMA 2003;290(7):898–904.

8. Roy B, Pawar PP, Desai RV, et al. A propensity-matched study of the association of diabetes mellitus with incident heart failure and mortality among community-dwelling older adults. Am J Cardiol 2011;108(12):1747–53.

9. American Diabetes Association. Standards of medical care in diabetes–2011. Diabetes Care 2011;34(Suppl 1):S11–61.

10. International Expert Committee. International expert committee report on the role of the A1C assay in the diagnosis of diabetes. Diabetes Care 2009;32(7):1327–34.

11. Clement S, Braithwaite SS, Magee MF, et al. Management of diabetes and hyperglycemia in hospitals. Diabetes Care 2004;27(2):553–91.

12. Centers for Disease Control and Prevention. National diabetes fact sheet: national estimates and general information on diabetes and prediabetes in the United States, 2011. Atlanta, GA: U.S. Department of Health and Human Services, Centers for Disease Control and Prevention; 2011.

13. Hashimoto K, Ikewaki K, Yagi H, et al. Glucose intolerance is common in Japanese patients with acute coronary syndrome who were not previously diagnosed with diabetes. Diabetes Care 2005; 28(5):1182–6.

14. Ishihara M, Inoue I, Kawagoe T, et al. Is admission hyperglycaemia in non-diabetic patients with acute myocardial infarction a surrogate for previously undiagnosed abnormal glucose tolerance? Eur Heart J 2006;27(20):2413–9.

15. Wallander M, Malmberg K, Norhammar A, et al. Oral glucose tolerance test: a reliable tool for early detection of glucose abnormalities in patients with acute myocardial infarction in clinical practice: a report on repeated oral glucose tolerance tests from the GAMI study. Diabetes Care 2008;31(1):36–8.

16. DECODE Study Group, European Diabetes Epidemiology Group. Is the current definition for diabetes relevant to mortality risk from all causes and cardiovascular and noncardiovascular diseases? Diabetes Care 2003;26(3):688–96.

17. von Bibra H, St John Sutton M. Impact of diabetes on postinfarction heart failure and left ventricular remodeling. Curr Heart Fail Rep 2011;8(4):242–51.

18. Rady MY, Johnson DJ, Patel BM, et al. Influence of individual characteristics on outcome of glycemic control in intensive care unit patients with or without diabetes mellitus. Mayo Clin Proc 2005;80:1558–67.

19. Oswald GA, Smith CC, Betteridge DJ, et al. Determinants and importance of stress hyperglycaemia in non-diabetic patients with myocardial infarction. Br Med J (Clin Res Ed) 1986;293(6552):917–22.

20. Stubbs PJ, Laycock J, Alaghband-Zadeh J, et al. Circulating stress hormone and insulin concentrations in acute coronary syndromes: identification of insulin resistance on admission. Clin Sci (Lond) 1999;96:589–95.

21. Kurt TL, Genton E, Chidsey C 3rd, et al. Carbohydrate metabolism and acute myocardial infarction: circulating glucose, insulin, cortisol and growth hormone responses and excretion of catecholamines. Chest 1973;64(1):21–5.

22. Vetter NJ, Strange RC, Adams W, et al. Initial metabolic and hormonal response to acute myocardial infarction. Lancet 1974;1(7852):284–8 No abstract available.

23. Barth E, Albuszies G, Baumgart K, et al. Glucose metabolism and catecholamines. Crit Care Med 2007;35:S508–18.

24. Andrewq RC, Walker BR. Glucocorticoids and insulin resistance: old hormones, new targets. Clin Sci 1999;96:513–23.

25. Jeevanandam M, Young DH, Schiller WR. Glucose turnover, oxidation, and indices of recycling in severely traumatized patients. J Trauma 1990;30: 582–9.

26. McGuinness OP, Fugiwara T, Murrell S, et al. Impact of chronic stress hormone infusion on hepatic carbohydrate metabolism in the conscious dog. Am J Physiol 1993;265:E314–22.

27. Fan J, Li YH, Wojnar MM, et al. Endotoxin-induced alterations in insulin-stimulated phosphorylation of insulin receptor, IRS-1, and MAP kinase in skeletal muscle. Shock 1996;6:164–70.

28. Green CJ, Campbell IT, O'Sullivan E, et al. Septic patients in multiple organ failure can oxidize infused glucose, but non-oxidative disposal (storage) is impaired. Clin Sci (Lond) 1995;89:601–9.

29. Stegenga ME, van der Crabben SN, Blümer RM, et al. Hyperglycemia enhances coagulation and reduces neutrophil degranulation, whereas hyperinsulinemia inhibits fibrinolysis during human endotoxemia. Blood 2008;112:82–9.

30. Soop M, Duxbury H, Agwunobi AO, et al. Euglycemic hyperinsulinemia augments the cytokine and endocrine responses to endotoxin in humans. Am J Physiol Endocrinol Metab 2002;282:E1276–85.

31. Stentz FB, Umpierrez GE, Cuervo R, et al. Proinflammatory cytokines, markers of cardiovascular risks, oxidative stress, and lipid peroxidation in patients with hyperglycemic crises. Diabetes 2004;53:2079–86.

32. Sabelis LW, Senden PJ, Zonderland ML, et al. Determinants of insulin sensitivity in chronic heart failure. Eur Heart J 2003;5:759–65.

33. Tenenbaum A, Motro M, Fisman EZ, et al. Functional class in patients with heart failure is associated with the development of diabetes. Am J Med 2003;114:271–5.

34. Norrelund H, Wiggers H, Halbirk M, et al. Abnormalities of whole body protein turnover, muscle metabolism and levels of metabolic hormones in patients with chronic congestive heart failure. J Intern Med 2006;260:11–21.

35. Anker SD, Chua TP, Ponikowski P, et al. Hormonal changes and catabolic/anabolic imbalance in chronic heart failure and their importance for cardiac cachexia. Circulation 1997;96(2):526–34.

36. Anker SD, Clark AL, Kemp M, et al. Tumor necrosis factor and steroid metabolism in chronic heart failure: possible relation to muscle wasting. J Am Coll Cardiol 1997;30(4):997–1001.

37. Feinstein R, Kanety H, Papa MZ, et al. Tumor necrosis factor-alpha suppresses insulin-induced tyrosine phosphorylation of insulin receptor and its substrates. J Biol Chem 1993;268(35):26055–8.

38. Stranders I, Diamant M, van Gelder RE, et al. Admission blood glucose level as risk indicator of death after myocardial infarction in patients with and without diabetes mellitus. Arch Intern Med 2004;164(9):982–8.

39. Mathew V, Gersh BJ, Williams BA, et al. Outcomes in patients with diabetes mellitus undergoing percutaneous coronary intervention in the current era: a report from the prevention of REStenosis with tranilast and its outcomes (PRESTO) trial. Circulation 2004;109(4):476–80.

40. Shah AM, Uno H, Kober L, et al. The interrelationship of diabetes and left ventricular systolic function on outcome after high-risk myocardial infarction. Eur J Heart Fail 2010;12(11):1229–37.

41. Mather AN, Crean A, Abidin N, et al. Relationship of dysglycemia to acute myocardial infarct size and cardiovascular outcome as determined by cardiovascular magnetic resonance. J Cardiovasc Magn Reson 2010;12:61.

42. Pliquett RU, Fasshauer M, Bluher M, et al. Neurohumoral stimulation in type-2-diabetes as an emerging disease concept. Cardiovasc Diabetol 2004;3:4.

43. Gaboury CL, Simonson DC, Seely EW, et al. Relation of pressor responsiveness to angiotensin II and insulin resistance in hypertension. J Clin Invest 1994;94:2295–300.

44. Lopez Farre A, Casado S. Heart failure, redox alterations, and endothelial dysfunction. Hypertension 2001;38(6):1400–5.

45. Polidori MC, Pratico D, Savino K, et al. Increased F2 isoprostane plasma levels in patients with congestive heart failure are correlated with antioxidant status and disease severity. J Card Fail 2004; 10(4):334–8.

46. Tsutsui T, Tsutamoto T, Wada A, et al. Plasma oxidized low-density lipoprotein as a prognostic predictor in patients with chronic congestive heart failure. J Am Coll Cardiol 2002;39(6):957–62.

47. Heitzer T, Baldus S, von Kodolitsch Y, et al. Systemic endothelial dysfunction as an early predictor of adverse outcome in heart failure. Arterioscler Thromb Vasc Biol 2005;25(6):1174–9.

48. Williams SB, Cusco JA, Roddy MA, et al. Impaired nitric oxide-mediated vasodilation in patients with non-insulin-dependent diabetes mellitus. J Am Coll Cardiol 1996;27(3):567–74.

49. Holman RR, Paul SK, Bethel MA, et al. 10-year follow-up of intensive glucose control in type 2 diabetes. N Engl J Med 2008;359(15):1577–89.

50. ACCORD Study Group, Gerstein HC, Miller ME, Genuth S, et al. Long-term effects of intensive glucose lowering on cardiovascular outcomes. N Engl J Med 2011;364:818–28.

51. Vanhorebeek I, Van den Berghe G. Diabetes of injury: novel insights. Endocrinol Metab Clin North Am 2006;35:859–72.

52. Cohen G, Riahi Y, Alpert E, et al. The roles of hyperglycaemia and oxidative stress in the rise and collapse of the natural protective mechanism against vascular endothelial cell dysfunction in diabetes. Arch Physiol Biochem 2007;113:259–67.

53. Quagliaro L, Piconi L, Assaloni R, et al. Intermittent high glucose enhances apoptosis related to oxidative stress in human umbilical vein endothelial cells: the role of protein kinase C and NAD(P)H-oxidase activation. Diabetes 2003;52(11):2795–804.

54. Inhat M, Green D, Ross K, et al. Reduced antioxidant response of retinal and endothelial cells in response to chronic oscillating glucose levels. Diabetes 2005;54(Suppl 1):2314A.

55. Risso A, Mrecuri F, Quagliaro L, et al. Intermittent high glucose enhances apoptosis in human umbilical vein endothelial cells in culture. Am J Physiol Endocrinol Metab 2001;281:924–30.

56. Monnier L, Mas E, Ginet C, et al. Activation of oxidative stress by acute glucose fluctuations compared with sustained chronic hyperglycemia in patients with type 2 diabetes. JAMA 2006;295(14):1681–7.

57. Ceriello A, Esposito K, Piconi L, et al. Oscillating glucose is more deleterious to endothelial function and oxidative stress than mean glucose in normal and type 2 diabetic patients. Diabetes 2008;57(5):1349–54.

58. Buscemi S, Re A, Batsis JA, et al. Glycaemic variability using continuous glucose monitoring and endothelial function in the metabolic syndrome and in type 2 diabetes. Diabet Med 2010;27:872–8.

59. Su G, Mi S, Tao H, et al. Association of glycemic variability and the presence and severity of coronary artery disease in patients with type 2 diabetes. Cardiovasc Diabetol 2011;10:19.

60. Snell-Bergeon JK, Roman R, Rodbard D, et al. Glycaemic variability is associated with coronary artery calcium in men with type 1 diabetes: the Coronary Artery Calcification in Type 1 Diabetes study. Diabet Med 2010;27:1436–42.

61. Biscetti F, Pitocco D, Straface G, et al. Glycaemic variability affects ischaemia-induced angiogenesis in diabetic mice. Clin Sci (Lond) 2011;121(12):555–64.

62. Desouza C, Salazar H, Cheong B, et al. Association of hypoglycemia and cardiac ischemia: a study based on continuous monitoring. Diabetes Care 2003;26(5):1485–9.

63. Di Flaviani A, Picconi F, Di Stefano P, et al. Impact of glycemic and blood pressure variability on surrogate measures of cardiovascular outcomes in type 2 diabetic patients. Diabetes Care 2011;34:1605–9.

64. Timmer JR, van der Horst IC, Ottervanger JP, et al. Prognostic value of admission glucose in non-diabetic patients with myocardial infarction. Am Heart J 2004;148(3):399–404.

65. Cao JJ, Hudson M, Jankowski M, et al. Relation of chronic and acute glycemic control on mortality in acute myocardial infarction with diabetes mellitus. Am J Cardiol 2005;96(2):183–6.

66. Gerstein HC, Swedberg K, Carlsson J, et al, CHARM Program Investigators. The hemoglobin A1c level as a progressive risk factor for cardiovascular death, hospitalization for heart failure, or death in patients with chronic heart failure: an analysis of the Candesartan in Heart failure: Assessment of Reduction in Mortality and Morbidity (CHARM) program. Arch Intern Med 2008;168(15):1699–704.

67. Aguilar D, Bozkurt B, Ramasubbu K, et al. Relationship of hemoglobin A1C and mortality in heart failure patients with diabetes. J Am Coll Cardiol 2009;54(5):422–8.

68. Dungan KM, Osei K, Nagaraja HN, et al. Relationship between glycemic control and readmission rates in patients hospitalized with congestive heart failure during implementation of hospital-wide initiatives. Endocr Pract 2010;16(6):945–51.

69. Capes SE, Hunt D, Malmberg K, et al. Stress hyperglycaemia and increased risk of death after myocardial infarction in patients with and without diabetes: a systematic overview. Lancet 2000;355(9206):773–8.

70. Shah B, Amoroso NS, Sedlis SP. Hyperglycemia in nondiabetic patients presenting with acute myocardial infarction. Am J Med Sci 2012;343(4):321–6.

71. Kosiborod M, Rathore SS, Inzucchi SE, et al. Admission glucose and mortality in elderly patients hospitalized with acute myocardial infarction: implications for patients with and without recognized diabetes. Circulation 2005;111(23):3078–86.

72. Dungan KM, Braithwaite SS, Preiser JC. Stress hyperglycaemia. Lancet 2009;373(9677):1798–807.

73. Petursson P, Herlitz J, Caidahl K, et al. Admission glycaemia and outcome after acute coronary syndrome. Int J Cardiol 2007;116(3):315–20.

74. Ishihara M, Kagawa E, Inoue I, et al. Impact of admission hyperglycemia and diabetes mellitus on short- and long-term mortality after acute myocardial infarction in the coronary intervention era. Am J Cardiol 2007;99(12):1674–9.

75. Kosiborod M, Inzucchi SE, Spertus JA, et al. Elevated admission glucose and mortality in elderly patients hospitalized with heart failure. Circulation 2009;119(14):1899–907.

76. Kosiborod M, Inzucchi SE, Krumholz HM, et al. Glucometrics in patients hospitalized with acute myocardial infarction: defining the optimal outcomes-based measure of risk. Circulation 2008;117:1018–27.

77. Egi M, Bellomo R, Stachowski E, et al. The interaction of chronic and acute glycemia with mortality in critically ill patients with diabetes. Crit Care Med 2011;39:105–11.

78. Egi M, Bellomo R, Stachowski E, et al. Variability of blood glucose concentration and short-term mortality in critically ill patients. Anesthesiology 2006;105(2):244–52.

79. Wintergerst KA, Buckingham B, Gandrud L, et al. Association of hypoglycemia, hyperglycemia, and glucose variability with morbidity and death in the pediatric intensive care unit. Pediatrics 2006;118(1):173–9.

80. Ali NA, O'Brien JM, Dungan K, et al. Glucose variability and mortality in patients with sepsis. Crit Care Med 2008;36(8):2316–21.

81. Dungan KM, Binkley P, Nagaraja HN, et al. The effect of glycaemic control and glycaemic variability on mortality in patients hospitalized with

congestive heart failure. Diabetes Metab Res Rev 2011;27(1):85–93.

82. NICE-SUGAR Study Investigators, Finfer S, Chittock DR, Su SY, et al. Intensive versus conventional glucose control in critically ill patients. N Engl J Med 2009;360(13):1283–97.

83. Brunkhorst FM, Engel C, Bloos F, et al. Intensive insulin therapy and pentastarch resuscitation in severe sepsis. N Engl J Med 2008;358(2):125–39.

84. Preiser JC, Devos P, Ruiz-Santana S, et al. A prospective randomised multi-centre controlled trial on tight glucose control by intensive insulin therapy in adult intensive care units: the Glucontrol study. Intensive Care Med 2009;35(10):1738–48.

85. Marik PE, Preiser JC. Toward understanding tight glycemic control in the ICU: a systematic review and metaanalysis. Chest 2010;137(3):544–51.

86. Umpierrez GE, Smiley D, Jacobs S, et al. Randomized study of basal-bolus insulin therapy in the inpatient management of patients with type 2 diabetes undergoing general surgery (RABBIT 2 surgery). Diabetes Care 2011;34(2):256–61.

87. Haga KK, McClymont KL, Clarke S, et al. The effect of tight glycaemic control, during and after cardiac surgery, on patient mortality and morbidity: a systematic review and meta-analysis. J Cardiothorac Surg 2011;6:3.

88. Malmberg K, Ryden L, Efendic S, et al. Randomized trial of insulin-glucose infusion followed by subcutaneous insulin treatment in diabetic patients with acute myocardial infarction (DIGAMI study): effects on mortality at 1 year. J Am Coll Cardiol 1995;26(1):57–65.

89. Malmberg K, Ryden L, Wedel H, et al. Intense metabolic control by means of insulin in patients with diabetes mellitus and acute myocardial infarction (DIGAMI 2): effects on mortality and morbidity. Eur Heart J 2005;26(7):650–61.

90. van der Horst IC, Zijlstra F, van 't Hof AW, et al. Glucose-insulin-potassium infusion inpatients treated with primary angioplasty for acute myocardial infarction: the glucose-insulin-potassium study: a randomized trial. J Am Coll Cardiol 2003;42(5):784–91.

91. Timmer JR, Svilaas T, Ottervanger JP, et al. Glucose-insulin-potassium infusion in patients with acute myocardial infarction without signs of heart failure: the glucose-insulin-potassium study (GIPS)-II. J Am Coll Cardiol 2006;47(8):1730–1.

92. Mehta SR, Yusuf S, Diaz R, et al. Effect of glucose-insulin-potassium infusion on mortality in patients with acute ST-segment elevation myocardial infarction: the CREATE-ECLA randomized controlled trial. JAMA 2005;293(4):437–46.

93. Goyal A, Mehta SR, Díaz R, et al. Differential clinical outcomes associated with hypoglycemia and hyperglycemia in acute myocardial infarction. Circulation 2009;120(24):2429–37.

94. Holper EM, Abbott JD, Mulukutla S, et al. Temporal changes in the outcomes of patients with diabetes mellitus undergoing percutaneous coronary intervention in the National Heart, Lung, and Blood Institute dynamic registry. Am Heart J 2011;161(2):397–403.e1.

95. Moghissi ES, Korytkowski MT, DiNardo M, et al, American Association of Clinical Endocrinologists; American Diabetes Association. American Association of Clinical Endocrinologists and American Diabetes Association consensus statement on inpatient glycemic control. Diabetes Care 2009;32(6):1119–31.

96. Barth M, Oyen L, Warfield K, et al. Comparison of a nurse initiated insulin infusion protocol for intensive insulin therapy between adult surgical trauma, medical and coronary care intensive care patients. BMC Emerg Med 2007;7:14.

97. Umpierrez GE, Hellman R, Korytkowski MT, et al. Management of hyperglycemia in hospitalized patients in non-critical care setting: an endocrine society clinical practice guideline. J Clin Endocrinol Metab 2012;97(1):16–38.

98. Dungan K, Chapman J, Braithwaite SS, et al. Glucose measurement: confounding issues in setting targets for inpatient management. Diabetes Care 2007;30:403–9.

99. Hirsch IB. Intravenous bolus insulin delivery: implications for closed-loop control and hospital care. Diabetes Technol Ther 2012;14(1):6–7.

100. Murata GH, Duckworth WC, Shah JH, et al. Sources of glucose variability in insulin-treated type 2 diabetes: the Diabetes Outcomes in Veterans Study (DOVES). Clin Endocrinol (Oxf) 2004;60:451–6.

101. Al-Dorzi HM, Tamim HM, Arabi YM. Glycaemic fluctuation predicts mortality in critically ill patients. Anaesth Intensive Care 2010;38(4):695–702.

102. Monnier L, Wojtusciszyn A, Colette C, et al. The contribution of glucose variability to asymptomatic hypoglycemia in persons with type 2 diabetes. Diabetes Technol Ther 2011;13(8):813–8.

103. Kauffmann RM, Hayes RM, Buske BD, et al. Increasing blood glucose variability heralds hypoglycemia in the critically ill. J Surg Res 2011;170(2):257–64.

104. Colombel A, Murat A, Krempf M, et al. Improvement of blood glucose control in type 1 diabetic patients treated with lispro and multiple NPH injections. Diabet Med 1999;16(4):319–24.

105. Lepore G, Dodesini AR, Nosari I, et al. Effect of continuous subcutaneous insulin infusion vs multiple daily insulin injection with glargine as basal insulin: an open parallel long-term study. Diabetes Nutr Metab 2004;17(2):84–9.

106. Saudek CD, Duckworth WC, Giobbie-Hurder A, et al. Implantable insulin pump vs multiple-dose

insulin for non-insulin-dependent diabetes mellitus: a randomized clinical trial. Department of Veterans Affairs Implantable Insulin Pump Study Group. JAMA 1996;276(16):1322–7.

107. Meijering S, Corstjens AM, Tulleken JE, et al. Towards a feasible algorithm for tight glycaemic control in critically ill patients: a systematic review of the literature. Crit Care 2006;10(1):R19.

108. Wilson M, Weinreb J, Hoo GW. Intensive insulin therapy in critical care: a review of 12 protocols. Diabetes Care 2007;30(4):1005–11.

109. Vogelzang M, Loef BG, Regtien JG, et al. Computer-assisted glucose control in critically ill patients. Intensive Care Med 2008;34(8):1421–7.

110. Plank J, Blaha J, Cordingley J, et al. Multicentric, randomized, controlled trial to evaluate blood glucose control by the model predictive control algorithm versus routine glucose management protocols in intensive care unit patients. Diabetes Care 2006;29:271–6.

111. Cavalcanti AB, Silva E, Pereira AJ, et al. A randomized controlled trial comparing a computer-assisted insulin infusion protocol with a strict and a conventional protocol for glucose control in critically ill patients. J Crit Care 2009;24(3):371–8.

112. Ariza-Andraca CR, Altamirano-Bustamante E, Frati-Munari AC, et al. Delayed insulin absorption due to subcutaneous edema. Arch Invest Med 1991; 22(2):229–33.

113. Blaha J, Kopecky P, Matias M, et al. Comparison of three protocols for tight glycemic control in cardiac surgery patients. Diabetes Care 2009;32(5):757–61.

114. Krikorian A, Ismail-Beigi F, Moghissi ES. Comparisons of different insulin infusion protocols: a review of recent literature. Curr Opin Clin Nutr Metab Care 2010;13(2):198–204.

115. Davidson PC, Steed RD, Bode BW. Glucommander: a computer-directed intravenous insulin system shown to be safe, simple, and effective in 120,618 h of operation. Diabetes Care 2005; 28:2418–23.

116. Smiley D, Rhee M, Peng L, et al. Safety and efficacy of continuous insulin infusion in noncritical care settings. J Hosp Med 2010;5:212–7.

117. Dungan K, Hall C, Schuster D, et al. Comparison of 3 algorithms for basal insulin in transitioning from intravenous to subcutaneous insulin in stable patients after cardiothoracic surgery. Endocr Pract 2011;17(5):753–8.

118. Juneja R, Roudebush C, Kumar N, et al. Utilization of a computerized intravenous insulin infusion program to control blood glucose in the intensive care unit. Diabetes Technol Ther 2007;9:232–40.

119. Furnary AP, Braithwaite SS. Effects of outcome on in-hospital transition from intravenous insulin infusion to subcutaneous therapy. Am J Cardiol 2006; 98(4):557–64.

120. Schmeltz LR, DeSantis AJ, Schmidt K, et al. Conversion of intravenous insulin infusions to subcutaneously administered insulin glargine in patients with hyperglycemia. Endocr Pract 2006; 12:641–50.

121. Dungan K, Hall C, Schuster D, et al. Differential response between diabetes and stress-induced hyperglycaemia to algorithmic use of detemir and flexible mealtime aspart among stable postcardiac surgery patients requiring intravenous insulin. Diabetes Obes Metab 2011;13(12):1130–5.

122. Shomali ME, Herr DL, Hill PC, et al. Conversion from intravenous insulin to subcutaneous insulin after cardiovascular surgery: transition to target study. Diabetes Technol Ther 2011;13(2):121–6.

123. Umpierrez GE, Hor T, Smiley D, et al. Comparison of inpatient insulin regimens with detemir plus aspart versus neutral protamine hagedorn plus regular in medical patients with type 2 diabetes. J Clin Endocrinol Metab 2009;94(2):564–9.

124. DiNardo M, Donihi AC, Forte P, et al. Standardized glycemic management and perioperative glycemic outcomes in patients with diabetes mellitus who undergo same-day surgery. Endocr Pract 2011; 17:404–11.

125. Mucha GT, Merkel S, Thomas W, et al. Fasting and insulin glargine in individuals with type 1 diabetes. Diabetes Care 2004;27:1209–10.

126. Holstein A, Plaschke A, Hammer C, et al. Characteristics and time course of severe glimepiride-versus glibenclamide-induced hypoglycaemia. Eur J Clin Pharmacol 2003;59(2):91–7.

127. Holstein A, Hammer C, Hahn M, et al. Severe sulfonylurea-induced hypoglycemia: a problem of uncritical prescription and deficiencies of diabetes care in geriatric patients. Expert Opin Drug Saf 2010;9(5):675–81.

128. Yeung CW, Chung HY, Fong BM, et al. Metformin-associated lactic acidosis in Chinese patients with type II diabetes. Pharmacology 2011;88(5–6):260–5.

129. van Berlo-van de Laar IR, Vermeij CG, Doorenbos CJ. Metformin associated lactic acidosis: incidence and clinical correlation with metformin serum concentration measurements. J Clin Pharm Ther 2011;36(3):376–82.

130. Biradar V, Moran JL, Peake SL, et al. Metformin-associated lactic acidosis (MALA): clinical profile and outcomes in patients admitted to the intensive care unit. Crit Care Resusc 2010;12(3):191–5.

131. Seidowsky A, Nseir S, Houdret N, et al. Metformin-associated lactic acidosis: a prognostic and therapeutic study. Crit Care Med 2009;37(7):2191–6.

132. Lago RM, Singh PP, Nesto RW. Congestive heart failure and cardiovascular death in patients with prediabetes and type 2 diabetes given thiazolidinediones: a meta-analysis of randomised clinical trials. Lancet 2007;370:1129–36.

133. Kaul S, Bolger AF, Herrington D, et al. Thiazolidinedione drugs and cardiovascular risks: a science advisory from the American Heart Association and American College of Cardiology Foundation. J Am Coll Cardiol 2010;55(17): 1885–94.

134. Garber AJ. Long-acting glucagon-like peptide 1 receptor agonists: a review of their efficacy and tolerability. Diabetes Care 2011;34:S279–84.

135. Baetta R, Corsini A. Pharmacology of dipeptidyl peptidase-4 inhibitors: similarities and differences. Drugs 2011;71:1441–67.

136. Davidson MH. Cardiovascular effects of glucagon-like peptide-1 agonists. Am J Cardiol 2011; 108(Suppl 3):33B–41B.

137. Vilsbøll T, Christensen M, Junker AE, et al. Effects of glucagon-like peptide-1 receptor agonists on weight loss: systematic review and meta-analyses of randomised controlled trials. BMJ 2012;344:d7771.

138. Shyangdan DS, Royle P, Clar C, et al. Glucagon-like peptide analogues for type 2 diabetes mellitus. Cochrane Database Syst Rev 2011;(10):CD006423.

139. Halbirk M, Nørrelund H, Møller N, et al. Cardiovascular and metabolic effects of 48-h glucagon-like peptide-1 infusion in compensated chronic patients with heart failure. Am J Physiol Heart Circ Physiol 2010;298(3):H1096–102.

140. Deane AM, Chapman MJ, Fraser RJ, et al. The effect of exogenous glucagon-like peptide-1 on the glycaemic response to small intestinal nutrient in the critically ill: a randomised double-blind placebo-controlled cross over study. Crit Care 2009;13(3):R67.

141. Sourij H, Schmölzer I, Kettler-Schmut E, et al. Efficacy of a continuous GLP-1 infusion compared with a structured insulin infusion protocol to reach normoglycemia in nonfasted type 2 diabetic patients: a clinical pilot trial. Diabetes Care 2009; 32(9):1669–71.

142. Read PA, Hoole SP, White PA, et al. A pilot study to assess whether glucagon-like peptide-1 protects the heart from ischemic dysfunction and attenuates stunning after coronary balloon occlusion in humans. Circ Cardiovasc Interv 2011;4(3):266–72.

143. Sokos GG, Bolukoglu H, German J, et al. Effect of glucagon-like peptide-1 (GLP-1) on glycemic control and left ventricular function in patients undergoing coronary artery bypass grafting. Am J Cardiol 2007;100(5):824–9.

144. Johansen OE, Neubacher D, von Eynatten M, et al. Cardiovascular safety with linagliptin in patients with type 2 diabetes mellitus: a pre-specified, prospective, and adjudicated meta-analysis of a phase 3 programme. Cardiovasc Diabetol 2012;11(1):3.

145. Frederich R, Alexander JH, Fiedorek FT, et al. A systematic assessment of cardiovascular outcomes in the saxagliptin drug development program for type 2 diabetes. Postgrad Med 2010; 122(3):16–27.

146. Tahrani AA, Bailey CJ, Del Prato S, et al. Management of type 2 diabetes: new and future developments in treatment. Lancet 2011;378(9786):182–97.

147. Cook CB, Seifert KM, Hull BP, et al. Inpatient to outpatient transfer of diabetes care: planning for an effective hospital discharge. Endocr Pract 2009;15:263–9.

148. Kimmel B, Sullivan MM, Rushakoff RJ. Survey on transition from inpatient to outpatient for patients on insulin: what really goes on at home? Endocr Pract 2010;16(5):785–91.

149. Rodbard HW, Jellinger PS, Davidson JA, et al. Statement by an American Association of Clinical Endocrinologists/American College of Endocrinology consensus panel on type 2 diabetes mellitus: an algorithm for glycemic control. Endocr Pract 2009;15(6):540–59.

Insulin Sensitization Therapy and the Heart
Focus on Metformin and Thiazolidinediones

Aaron K.F. Wong, MD, MRCP,
Allan D. Struthers, MD, FRCP, FESC
Anna Maria J. Choy, MD, FRCP, Chim C. Lang, MD, FRCP*

KEYWORDS

- Insulin resistance • Chronic heart failure • Thiazolidinedione • Metformin

KEY POINTS

- Chronic heart failure (CHF) is an insulin-resistant state and the degree of insulin resistance is associated with disease severity and poor clinical outcome.
- Insulin resistance may be pathophysiologically linked to the disease in CHF and may be a target for therapy.
- Although thiazolidinediones are potent insulin sensitizers, their use in CHF has been limited because they have the potential to exacerbate CHF.
- There is evidence from observational studies and from animal models of CHF suggesting that metformin use is safe and may be beneficial in CHF.
- Randomized controlled trials of metformin are needed in patients with CHF identified to have insulin resistance.

INTRODUCTION

Diabetes and chronic heart failure (CHF) often coexist such that each condition may affect the other in terms of causation and outcome. This bidirectional interrelationship between CHF and diabetes also extend to insulin resistance (IR). Longitudinal epidemiologic data such as the Uppsala study of 1187 middle-aged and elderly men showed that IR precedes and predicts the development of CHF, independently of established risk factors for CHF, including diabetes itself.[1] In contrast, CHF has been shown to predict the development of diabetes and abnormal glucose metabolism. In the Bezafibrate Infarction Prevention (BIP) study, the mean baseline glucose measurement

was shown to increase during 7.7 years of follow-up in 2616 nondiabetic patients, and diabetes developed in these patients in a stepwise manner, from 13% with New York Heart Association (NYHA) class I to 20% in patients with NYHA functional class III.[2] IR and abnormalities in glucose metabolism have been shown to be highly prevalent in nondiabetic patients with CHF. Swan and colleagues[3] reported reduced insulin sensitivity as assessed during a weight-adjusted intravenous glucose tolerance test in patients with both ischemic and nonischemic CHF (58% reduction in insulin sensitivity in patients with CHF compared with healthy control subjects). In the Randomized Evaluation of Strategies for Left Ventricular Dysfunction (RESOLVD) pilot study, 33% had IR

This work was funded by the British Heart Foundation (grant number PG/06/143/21,897).
Division of Cardiovascular and Diabetes Medicine, Medical Research Institute, Ninewells Hospital and Medical School, University of Dundee, Dundee DD1 9SY, United Kingdom
* Corresponding author. Division of Cardiovascular and Diabetes Medicine, Medical Research Institute, Mailbox 2, Ninewells Hospital and Medical School, University of Dundee, Dundee DD1 9SY, United Kingdom.
E-mail address: c.c.lang@dundee.ac.uk

Heart Failure Clin 8 (2012) 539–550
http://dx.doi.org/10.1016/j.hfc.2012.06.002

as assessed by the Fasting Insulin Resistance Index (FIRI).[4] Using FIRI, we reported a higher prevalence of IR of 61% in a cohort of nondiabetic patients with CHF that had a greater proportion of patients who were NYHA functional class III to IV (**Fig. 1**).[5] We found a significant correlation between IR and waist circumference ($r = 0.37$; $P<.01$) and serum leptin ($r = 0.39$; $P = .03$).

RELATIONSHIPS BETWEEN IR AND SEVERITY OF CHF

The degree of IR seems to be related to the severity of CHF. In the RESOLVD study and in our study (**Fig. 2**), IR was positively related to NYHA functional class.[4,5] IR is also related to established prognostic indicators such as plasma BNP[6] and peak oxygen consumption (V_{O_2}).[3–5] IR has been reported to be an independent predictor of poor clinical outcome in CHF. Doehner and colleagues[7] showed in multivariable-adjusted models that the presence and the severity of IR in patients with CHF was independently associated with poorer outcome, characterized by reduced peak V_{O_2} and NYHA classes. More recently, Berry and colleagues[8] showed that abnormal glucose tolerance was a strong predictor of in-hospital mortality in patients admitted with acute decompensated CHF. In their study of 454 consecutive patients admitted with acute heart failure, abnormal glucose tolerance predicted in-hospital mortality (hazard ratio [HR] 5.90; 95% confidence interval [CI] 1.03–34.0).

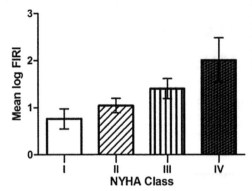

Fig. 2. Relationship between FIRI and NYHA. (*From* AlZadjali MA, Godfrey V, Khan F, et al. Insulin resistance is highly prevalent and is associated with reduced exercise tolerance in nondiabetic patients with heart failure. J Am Coll Cardiol 2009;53:750; with permission.)

PATHOPHYSIOLOGIC LINK OF IR TO CHF

The mechanisms underlying the development of IR in patients with CHF have not been defined. Several mechanisms have been proposed and these include sympathetic activation, endothelial dysfunction, loss of skeletal mass, and the influence of cytokines and adiponectins.[9,10]

Is there a pathophysiologic link between IR and the disease in CHF? The observation that IR is associated with disease severity and poor clinical outcome suggests this. The prognostic impact of IR is independent of other variables, including peak V_{O_2} and left ventricular ejection fraction, which may imply that IR may be pathogenic rather than simply a marker for worsened CHF.[4] It is likely that IR may play a mechanistic role in CHF because IR is associated with activation of neurohormones,[11,12] endothelial dysfunction, inflammation,[13] increased oxidative stress,[14] myocardial remodeling,[15,16] and altered myocardial metabolism[9,10]; processes that accelerate the progression of disease in CHF. A complete review of the molecular processes underlying this is beyond the scope of this article and has been reviewed in detail elsewhere.[9,10] However, this article briefly discusses the emerging evidence that IR may be central to altered myocardial metabolism in advanced CHF because this is relevant in the discussion on targeting myocardial IR and the altered myocardial metabolism in CHF. Under pathologic stress, the heart switches from free fatty acid (FFA) oxidation to more fuel-efficient glucose metabolism.[17] This provides the failing heart with 40% to 50% more adenosine triphosphate (ATP) per unit of O_2 consumed, which remains the case as long as the myocardium is responsive to insulin and the

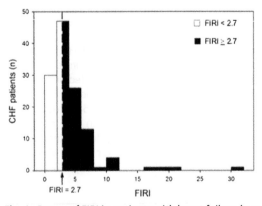

Fig. 1. Range of FIRI in patients with heart failure (n = 129). Patients were considered to be insulin resistant if they had an FIRI greater than or equal to 2.7. (*From* AlZadjali MA, Godfrey V, Khan F, et al. Insulin resistance is highly prevalent and is associated with reduced exercise tolerance in nondiabetic patients with heart failure. J Am Coll Cardiol 2009;53:750; with permission.)

glucose transport system is functional. When IR develops, glucose uptake is downregulated and FFA becomes the preferred oxidized substrate.[18] The consequent high supply of FFA can exceed the heart's oxidative capacity and could lead to accumulation of intramyocardial triglycerides and lipotoxicity that worsens CHF.[17,19–21] The high level of FFA also impairs the heart's ability to use glucose as a main source of ATP generation in several ways. First, it impairs insulin-mediated glucose uptake through inhibition of insulin receptor substrates (IRS) and protein kinase-B. Second, PPAR-α is activated and this leads to promotion of genes involved in FFA oxidation and pyruvate dehydrogenase kinase-4 (PDK-4), which inhibits pyruvate dehydrogenase (PDH) and influx of pyruvate into mitochondria. Third, high levels of acetyl-coenzyme A (CoA) from β-oxidation of FFA further activates PDK-4, leading to further inhibition of PDH and increased pyruvate influx. Fourth, augmented acetyl-CoA production also leads to the accumulation of citrate, which subsequently inhibits phosphofructose kinase-1 (PK1), the rate-limiting enzyme of glycolysis. Increased FFA level has been shown to correlate with decreased myocardial phosphocreatine/ATP (PCr/ATP) ratios, suggesting impaired ATP production.[22] A decreased PCr/ATP ratio has been shown to be a reliable, independent predictor of cardiovascular mortality.[23] In severe CHF, myocardial IR results in decreased membrane translocation of the glucose transport protein GLUT-4 (decreased glucose uptake) and decreased phosphorylation of Akt-1 (decreased glucose metabolism), resulting in decreased ATP production. It also prevents transition to the heart's adaptive response to stress (deriving ATP from glucose metabolism rather than FFA oxidation). The relationship between IR and abnormal myocardial metabolism has been shown clinically in studies using positron emission tomography scanning, which have shown that FFA uptake and myocardial β-oxidation were positively correlated to the presence of IR.[24] CHF in the setting of IR is probably the worst of all possibilities for myocardial energy metabolism.

IR AS A NEW THERAPEUTIC STRATEGY IN CHF

If IR is pathophysiologically linked to the disease in CHF, then IR might represent a new target for therapy in CHF. This article focuses on the insulin sensitizers metformin and thiazolidinediones (TZDs). However, standard lifestyle recommendations are important, most notably exercise, which has been shown to improve IR in patients with impaired glucose tolerance in the Diabetes Prevention Program (DPP) study.[25] Exercise training has

been shown to improve muscle glucose uptake and IR in patients with idiopathic dilated cardiomyopathy.[26] Studies of both diet and drug-induced weight loss have also been shown to improve functional status in patients with CHF.[27] However, there have been no studies of exercise therapy in patients with CHF identified to have IR.

DO CHF MEDICATIONS HAVE THE POTENTIAL TO IMPROVE IR?

Post hoc analysis of large randomized clinical trials in patients with CHF or at risk for coronary artery disease show that both angiotensin-converting enzyme (ACE) inhibitors and angiotensin receptor blockers (ARBs) may decrease the incidence of new-onset diabetes.[28] However, new-onset diabetes was not an end point of these trials. There are prospective trials of ACE inhibitors and ARBs in prediabetic individuals. In the Diabetes Reduction Assessment with Ramipril and Rosiglitazone Medication (DREAM) study, treatment with the ACE inhibitor ramipril did not significantly reduce the incidence of new-onset diabetes in patients with impaired fasting glucose (IFG) (18.1% vs 19.5%, $P = .15$).[29] However, in the NAVIGATOR (Nateglinide and Valsartan in Impaired Glucose Tolerance Outcomes Research) study, valsartan modestly reduced the incidence of diabetes (33.1% vs 36.8%, HR in the valsartan group 0.86, 95% CI 0.80–0.92, $P<.001$).[30] Some β-blockers, such as carvedilol, have been reported to have modest insulin-sensitizing properties.[31] In the COMET (Carvedilol or Metoprolol European Trial) study, carvedilol was also associated with reduced incidence of new-onset diabetes (HR 0.78, 95% CI 0.64–0.96, $P = .02$) in patients with CHF when compared with metoprolol.[32] The effect of the aldosterone antagonist on glucose metabolism seems to be complex. Endogenous aldosterone can suppress insulin secretion through a mineralocorticoid receptor (MR)–independent mechanism.[33] However, during treatment with aldosterone antagonists, plasma angiotensin II and aldosterone concentrations increase because of loss of feedback inhibition and induction of aldosterone-synthesizing enzymes. If aldosterone decreases insulin secretion through an MR-independent mechanism, then the increased aldosterone concentrations (which can suppress insulin secretion) during treatment with an aldosterone antagonist could potentially result in hyperglycemia in patients. In 1 randomized, placebo-controlled, crossover study of 50 patients with diabetes and resistant hypertension, spironolactone improved blood pressure but increased circulating angiotensin II concentrations and significantly worsened glycemic control.[34] Among patients with CHF, treatment with spironolactone resulted in increased hemoglobin A1C and cortisol concentrations and decreased adiponectin, whereas these findings were not seen in the eplerenone-treated group.[35] In a recent observational study of hypertensive patients, the incidence of diabetes was increased in spironolactone-treated patients compared with patients treated with the ARB losartan.[36] Additional prospective clinical studies are needed to elucidate the effect of aldosterone antagonism on glucose metabolism and insulin secretion.

It seems that CHF medications may have modest beneficial effects on glucose metabolism (such as with ACE inhibitors and ARBs and with carvedilol) and the effect of aldosterone antagonists on glucose metabolism is still not clear. However, there have been no specific studies of CHF therapies in patients with CHF with diabetes or those identified to have IR to further clarify these issues.

DIABETIC THERAPIES AND CHF: FOCUS ON TZDs AND METFORMIN

Metformin and TZDs are effective antidiabetic therapies that have a proven efficacy to reduce IR and are true insulin sensitizers.

TZDs

The TZDs rosiglitazone and pioglitazone bind to the peroxisome proliferator-activator receptor-γ (PPAR-γ) and modulate the transcription of the insulin-sensitive genes involved in the control of glucose and lipid metabolism in adipose tissue, muscle tissue, and in the liver.[37] They improve insulin sensitivity and decrease circulating FFAs. PPAR-γ is expressed in the liver and peripheral tissue and is weakly expressed in the myocardium.

POTENTIAL BENEFICIAL EFFECTS OF TZDs IN CHF

TZDs may have several effects that are of potential benefit to patients with CHF, including blood pressure lowering, reduction in angiotensin II, improvement in endothelial function, and slowing the progression of atherosclerosis.[38–40]

In Animal Models

In rodent models, TZDs had previously been shown to improve systolic function and myocardial contractility, improve diastology, and regress ventricular hypertrophy independently of loading conditions.[41–43] Pioglitazone has also been shown experimentally to attenuate angiotensin-induced

cardiac fibrosis by inhibiting myocardial macrophage infiltration,[44] and Shoghi and colleagues[45] reported that rosiglitazone enhances glucose use and diminishes FFA metabolism.

However, not all in vitro and animal studies have found beneficial effects with TZDs. Baranowski and colleagues[46] found increased lipid accumulation in the rat heart despite concomitant reduction of plasma FFA availability after administration of pioglitazone, suggesting that a mismatch between the rate of FFA uptake and oxidation was responsible for lipid accumulation. More recently, in a genetic model of spontaneously hypertensive insulin-resistant (spontaneously hypertensive heart failure [SHHF]) rats, pioglitazone exerted deleterious effects on the myocardium: augmented perivascular fibrosis and reduced capillary density, markedly potentiated myocardial lipid accumulation, inhibited endothelial nitric oxide synthase (eNOS) expression and increased the phospholamban/sarcoplasmic reticulum Ca^{2+}-adenosinetriphosphatase 2 ratio.[47]

Clinical Studies of TZDs and CHF

Several proof-of-concept studies have examined the effect of TZDs on surrogate markers and these showed that TZDs may beneficially lessen the accumulation of harmful saturated FFAs in the myocardium in patients with diabetes.[48,49] In a study of 78 diabetic individuals without structural heart disease and normal ejection fraction (60%), van der Meer and colleagues[49] showed that pioglitazone improved diastolic dysfunction and increased whole-body insulin sensitivity and myocardial glucose uptake as measured by magnetic resonance imaging, proton and phosphorus magnetic resonance spectroscopy, and 18F-2-fluoro-2-deoxy-D-glucose and 11C-palmitate positron emission tomography.

TZDs have been little studied in patients with CHF. Dargie and colleagues[50] investigated the effects of rosiglitazone on left ventricular ejection fraction in 224 patients with type 2 diabetes mellitus and NYHA functional class I to II CHF with ejection fraction less than or equal to 45%. Patients were randomized to a 52-week treatment with rosiglitazone (n = 110) or placebo (n = 114) in addition to background antidiabetic treatment. After 52 weeks of treatment, although glycemic control was significantly better in the rosiglitazone-treated group (mean difference in hemoglobin A1c −0.65%, $P<.0001$), there were significantly more adjudicated events of new or worsening edema ($P = .005$) and increased use of CHF medications ($P = .037$), but no significant difference between groups for other adjudicated end points.

The withdrawal rate of medications was similar between rosiglitazone and placebo. There was an echocardiographic substudy that did not show any change in left ventricular mass index, ejection fraction, and left ventricular end-diastolic volume between rosiglitazone and glyburide. In the rosiglitazone-treated group, there was a reduction in ambulatory diastolic blood pressure that was greater in rosiglitazone-treated patients than in those with glyburide, which might support a pleiotropic effect of rosiglitazone on the cardiovascular system.[51] In another study, Giles and colleagues[52] compared the effects of pioglitazone and glyburide for 6 months in a double-blind randomized multicenter study involving patients with symptomatic CHF (NYHA II/III) and showed that pioglitazone was associated with a higher incidence of hospitalization for CHF without a worsening of cardiac function on echocardiography. This CHF safety signal and other cardiovascular safety signals have emerged that have stopped any further exploratory studies of TZDs in CHF. An increased risk of ischemic cardiovascular events was found for rosiglitazone in meta-analyses of randomized controlled trials (RCTs).[53–55] In contrast, pioglitazone was reported to have a statistically significant lower risk in a composite endpoint of death, myocardial infarction (MI) and stroke from findings of another meta-analysis.[56] These reports were supported by a US Food and Drug Administration (FDA) meta-analysis of RCTs, which found that the risk of all-cause and cardiovascular mortality and MI tended to be lower with pioglitazone and higher with rosiglitazone (although most results did not reach statistical significance).[57] This same analysis also highlighted that the risk of CHF was increased with both TZDs. Another study also noted the increase in numbers of CHFs with both TZDs.[58] In this meta-analysis, 360 of 20,191 patients with diabetes who took part in these RCTs had CHF events (214 with TZDs and 146 with comparators). The results showed no heterogeneity of effects across studies (I^2 index = 22.8%; P for interaction = .26), which indicated a class effect for TZDs. However, the risk of cardiovascular death was not increased with either of the 2 TZDs (0.93, 0.67–1.29; P = .68).

However, there are limitations of these meta-analyses, most notably the low number of events and the pooling of data from clinical trials that have varying study designs and study populations. More recently, there have been observational studies of real-world prescribing. In a study of 227,571 US Medicare patients, Graham and colleagues[59] compared pioglitazone with rosiglitazone and showed that the latter is associated with a 25% increase in the risk of CHF and 14% increased mortality. Most patients were more than 70 years old, whereas 90% had hypertension and 37% had cardiovascular diseases before TZD treatment. By contrast, another recent study found equal event rates with the 2 TZDs in 36,628 people of mean age 54 years of whom less than 4% had had previous cardiovascular events.[60] However, a recent study commissioned by the UK Medicines and Healthcare products Regulatory Agency (MHRA) that used the UK General Practice Research Database (GPRD) showed that, among 206,940 patients, rosiglitazone users had an increased risk of death (relative risk [RR] 1.20; 95% CI 1.08–1.34) and of hospitalization for CHF (adjusted RR 1.73; 95% CI 1.19–2.51) compared with pioglitazone users.[61] This study supports the suspension of rosiglitazone by European regulatory authorities in September 2010.

HOW DO TZDs CAUSE EXACERBATION OF CHF?

The detailed mechanisms for how the TZDs potentiate CHF have yet to be defined. Echocardiographic studies have not shown a decrease in systolic function.[50,52] BNP levels have been shown to be increased following TZD therapy, which suggests an increase in left ventricular wall stress.[62] Fluid retention is a well-documented side effect of TZDs that may be explained by the effects of PPAR-γ agonists on the epithelial sodium channel of the distal collecting duct and also increased vascular permeability.[63–65] If latent diastolic dysfunction is present, which occurs in many patients with diabetes, it is plausible that the fluid retention may result in an increase in ventricular filling pressure that could induce symptoms requiring hospitalization with CHF. The cases of CHF reported in these clinical trials might have been caused by the unmasking of occult cardiac dysfunction in at-risk patients. In the DREAM trial, patients who developed CHF were older, had higher systolic blood pressure, and more often had a past medical history of hypertension.[66] A high prevalence of hypertension at baseline was also observed in other TZD trials that had shown an increased risk of CHF.[67,68]

Current US guidance from the American Heart Association/American Diabetes Association recommends caution in using TZDs in patients with class I to II CHF and complete avoidance in NYHA class III to IV.[63] When initiating TZDs in patients with mild CHF, they advise initiating therapy at the lowest doses and observing for side effects closely, with gradual dose escalation. European guidance through the European

Medicines Agency is more cautious because it advocates that TZDs be contraindicated in all diabetic patients with CHF or history of CHF, irrespective of NYHA functional class.[69]

METFORMIN

Another insulin-sensitizing drug that may have potential use in CHF is metformin. Metformin has been on the market for almost 50 years and is widely prescribed in diabetic populations. It was first described in the scientific literature in 1957 and was first marketed in France in 1979, but did not receive approval by the FDA for the treatment of type 2 diabetes until 1994 in the United States. Its precise mode of action is not known but it has a potent insulin-sensitizing effect.[70] It is the preferred antidiabetic medication for obese patients with type 2 diabetes mellitus because of its ability to stabilize weight and reduce cardiovascular events when used as monotherapy.[71]

The use of metformin in CHF has previously been discouraged because of concern about the risk of lactic acidosis. This concern stems from previous reports of severe lactic acidosis with phenformin, another biguanide that was removed from the market after 306 cases of lactic acidosis were reported in the 1970s. However, evidence of the risk of lactic acidosis with metformin is lacking.[72,73] The reported incidence of lactic acidosis related to metformin has been extremely low in large observational studies, and metformin levels do not correlate with lactate levels in individuals who develop lactic acidosis, which may support the notion that metformin may be an innocent bystander in sick patients, rather than the causal agent.[74,75] A recent systematic review of metformin use in type 2 diabetes with more than 70,000 patient years of follow-up showed no cases of fatal or nonfatal lactic acidosis, although specific effects in those with CHF were not assessed.[73]

Despite this cautionary labeling of its use in CHF, there has been off-label use of metformin in diabetic patients with CHF.[76] This may reflect the lack of certainty about the potential risk of lactic acidosis and also the general level of comfort among clinicians who frequently use metformin in treating diabetic individuals. This off-label use of metformin has allowed key observational studies to analyze the safety of metformin use in patients with CHF.

In 2005, a retrospective cohort analysis by Masoudi and colleagues[77] of a large group (n = 16,417) of Medicare beneficiaries with diabetes discharged after hospitalization with the principle discharge diagnosis of CHF showed not only the safe use but also a potential mortality benefit associated with its

use. Patients prescribed metformin experienced a 13% lower mortality over a year compared with those treated with sulfonylurea or insulin therapy after adjustment for a wide variety of baseline characteristics. There was no excess of admissions for lactic acidosis in patients treated with metformin. In that same year, Eurich and colleagues[78] reported their findings from the Saskatchewan Health database, which showed that patients with diabetes and incident CHF who took metformin experienced less mortality than those treated with sulfonylureas or insulin. These 2 large observational studies represent a major step that subsequently led to a change in the product labeling of metformin.[79]

We performed a similar observational study of a prescribing database in the population of Tayside, United Kingdom, with patients having diabetes and incident CHF who had received oral hypoglycemic agents. Fewer deaths occurred in metformin users, alone or in combination with sulfonylureas, compared with the sulfonylurea monotherapy cohort at 1 year (0.59, 95% CI 0.36–0.96) and over long-term follow-up (0.67, 95% CI 0.51–0.88) (**Fig. 3**).[78] The observation suggested that metformin is not only safe but could potentially be beneficial, a finding reported in other observational studies.[80–85] The initial observational reports of 2005 persuaded the FDA to remove the CHF contraindication from product labeling for metformin, although a black-box warning for the cautious use of metformin in this population still exists. One

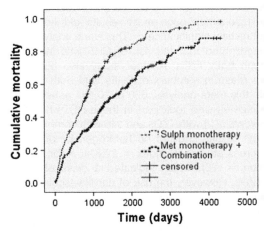

Fig. 3. Kaplan-Meier plot for 1-year follow-up comparing mortality in the sulfonylureas cohort (light dashed line) to mortality in the metformin-only and metformin plus sulfonylureas cohorts (heavy dashed line). Censored data (+) are displayed. (*From* Evans JM, Doney AS, AlZadjali MA, et al. Effect of Metformin on mortality in patients with heart failure and type 2 diabetes mellitus. Am J Cardiol 2010;106:1006–10, with permission.)

Table 1
Comparison between TZDs and metformin in heart failure

	TZDs	Metformin
Pleiotropic effects	Lowers blood pressure Inhibits renin-angiotensin system Improves endothelial function Slows progression of atherosclerosis	AMPK activation Improvement in left ventricular function and remodeling Attenuates oxidative stress–induced apoptosis Improves endothelial function Improves myocardial mechanical efficiency Antiinflammatory
Animal studies	Improves systolic and diastolic function Improves cardiac function Attenuates angiotensin-induced fibrosis Regresses left ventricle hypertrophy Enhances glucose and diminishes FFA metabolism in myocardium Increases lipid accumulation in myocardium Inhibits eNOS expression Augments perivascular fibrosis	Improves cardiac function Reduces myocyte apoptosis Enhances glucose and diminishes FFA metabolism in myocardium Improves left ventricle remodeling Improves myocardial mitochondrial biogenesis and improves cell survival

Clinical studies	Improvement of diastolic function, insulin sensitivity, and myocardial glucose uptake
	Reduced diastolic blood pressure and no change in left ventricular ejection fraction and volume
	Concerns regarding cardiovascular risks
	Exacerbates CHF
	    Increased vascular permeability
	    Reduced urinary sodium excretion
		Improves glycemic control
		Weight reduction
		Large observational studies show lower mortality in metformin users
		No excess of lactic acidosis in patients with CHF compared with other antidiabetic therapy

Undesirable effects	Weight gain Water retention Exacerbates CHF Osteoporosis	Lactic acidosis (in renal failure and unstable patients) Gastrointestinal upset Taste disturbance Decrease absorption of vitamin B_{12} (rare, <1 in 10,000) Skin rashes (rare)

major caution relates to its use in patients with renal failure or renal dysfunction (estimated glomerular filtration rate [GFR] <60 mL/min).[57] However, there have been studies that suggest that metformin is safe up to a GFR of 30 mL/min.[86] This renal caution may subject the observational studies described earlier to selection bias, which must be taken into account when interpreting these studies. Patients with renal disease who are at higher mortality risk would have been selected for sulfonylurea or insulin therapy rather than metformin. Because of selection bias and other limitations that are derived from the observational design, there is a need for a carefully conducted RCT of metformin in

CHF. However, this may not be feasible because a pilot clinical trial of metformin in patients with CHF with diabetes was attempted but abandoned in Canada because of the failure to recruit study patients with the widespread use of metformin.[87] However, we think that a study of metformin is still plausible in patients with CHF with IR or those identified to have dysglycemia, because metformin would not have been used in this population. The Metformin in Insulin-Resistant Left Ventricular Dysfunction (TAYSIDE) study is a proof-of-concept study that will investigate whether metformin increases exercise capacity in patients with CHF identified to have IR based on an FIRI greater than 2.7 (http://clinicaltrials.gov/ct2/show/NCT00473876).

HOW COULD METFORMIN BE BENEFICIAL IN CHF?

It may be difficult to determine whether there are any plausible mechanistic explanations for a benefit of metformin in CHF because the mechanism of action of metformin remains incompletely understood.[70] Metformin is endowed with pleiotropic effects that are predominantly mediated through activation of AMP-activated protein kinase (AMPK) (Table 1).[70] It could be argued that results from the UK. Prospective Diabetes Study, which show that metformin is the only hypoglycemic agent to reduce cardiovascular outcomes in primary prevention, suggest that the cardioprotective effects of metformin may be partly independent of glycemic control.[71]

Metformin has been reported to improve endothelial dysfunction,[88] and to have antiinflammatory properties[89] and reduce oxidative stress,[90] processes that contribute to the disease process in CHF. Metformin may also have effects on the myocardium, such as an impact on myocardial metabolism and left ventricular remodeling. With respect to the former, the heart with IR is exposed to high plasma FFA concentrations[9,10,91] and metformin has been shown to enhance basal and insulin-stimulated glucose uptake in IR cardiomyocytes.[92]

There have been several studies of metformin in animal models of CHF to explore the potential benefits of metformin in CHF. In these studies, metformin has been shown to activate eNOS via AMPK, which resulted in the improvement of left ventricular function and remodeling.[93] Metformin has also been shown to attenuate oxidative stress-induced cardiac myocyte apoptosis, resulting in improved survival.[94,95] In a recent study that compared metformin with rosiglitazone in a genetic model of SHHF rats, chronic treatment with metformin over 12 months had a profound beneficial effect on left ventricular remodeling and function, whereas rosiglitazone had deleterious effects.[46] Metformin reduced IR, FFA, myocardial lipid accumulation, and perivascular fibrosis.[47] These beneficial effects of metformin were ablated in AMPK-deficient mice, suggesting the key role of AMPK in the action of metformin. Metformin has been shown to increase phosphorylation of eNOS in an AMPK-dependent manner.[95,96] In CHF, peroxisome proliferator–activated receptor-γ coactivator 1α (PGC-1α) is induced in response to oxygen demand to increase myocardial ATP synthesis.[97] Gundewar and colleagues[95] showed that metformin treatment increased the expression of PGC-1α during heart failure in an AMPK-dependent manner, and improves mitochondrial oxygen consumption and ATP synthesis. These observations highlighted the key role of AMPK activation and its downstream pathways involving eNOS phosphorylation and PGC1-α expression for the cardioprotective effects of metformin. However, there is still a need for clinical studies. For example, although metformin has been shown to enhance basal and insulin-stimulated glucose uptake in IR cardiomyocytes,[92] in an imaging study of patients with diabetes, metformin did not improve myocardial glucose uptake.[98] Carefully conducted RCTs are needed in patients with CHF identified to have IR to help fully define a role for metformin in these patients.

SUMMARY

IR and CHF form an intricate pair that are in a vicious cycle in which they worsen each other at both tissue and cellular levels. Increased understanding of the relationships between IR and CHF provides the rationale for targeting IR in the development of new CHF therapy. However, there seems to be a conundrum in the choice of available insulin sensitizers because there are safety issues regarding TZDs and metformin. Although the concerns regarding TZDs seem to be justified, there is emerging evidence to suggest that metformin is not only safe in CHF but may be beneficial.

REFERENCES

1. Ingelsson E, Sundstrom J, Arnlov J, et al. Insulin resistance and risk of congestive heart failure. JAMA 2005;294:334–41.
2. Tenenbaum A, Motro M, Fisman EZ, et al. Functional class in patients with heart failure is associated with the development of diabetes. Am J Med 2003;114: 271–5.
3. Swan JW, Anker SD, Walton C, et al. Insulin resistance in chronic heart failure: relation to severity and etiology of heart failure. J Am Coll Cardiol 1997;30:527–32.
4. Suskin N, McKelvie RS, Burns RJ, et al. Glucose and insulin abnormalities relate to functional capacity in patients with congestive heart failure. Eur Heart J 2000;21:1368–75.
5. AlZadjali MA, Godfrey V, Khan F, et al. Insulin resistance is highly prevalent and is associated with reduced exercise tolerance in nondiabetic patients with heart failure. J Am Coll Cardiol 2009;53:747–53.
6. Tassone F, Gianotti L, Rolfo F, et al. B-type natriuretic peptide levels and insulin resistance in patients with severe ischemic myocardial dysfunction. J Endocrinol Invest 2009;32:805–9.

7. Doehner W, Rauchhaus M, Ponikowski P, et al. Impaired insulin sensitivity as an independent risk factor for mortality in patients with stable chronic heart failure. J Am Coll Cardiol 2005;46:1019–26.

8. Berry C, Brett M, Stevenson K, et al. Nature and prognostic importance of abnormal glucose tolerance and diabetes in acute heart failure. Heart 2008;94:296–304.

9. Witteles RM, Fowler MB. Insulin-resistant cardiomyopathy clinical evidence, mechanisms, and treatment options. J Am Coll Cardiol 2008;51:93–102.

10. Wong AK, AlZadjali MA, Choy AM, et al. Insulin resistance: a potential new target for therapy in patients with heart failure. Cardiovasc Ther 2008; 26:203–13.

11. Anderson EA, Hoffman RP, Balon TW, et al. Hyperinsulinemia produces both sympathetic neural activation and vasodilation in normal humans. J Clin Invest 1991;87:2246–52.

12. Gaboury CL, Simonson DC, Seely EW, et al. Relation of pressor responsiveness to angiotensin II and insulin resistance in hypertension. J Clin Invest 1994;94: 2295–300.

13. Wisniacki N, Taylor W, Lye M, et al. Insulin resistance and inflammatory activation in older patients with systolic and diastolic heart failure. Heart 2005;91:32–7.

14. Berdichevsky A, Guarente L, Bose A. Acute oxidative stress can reverse insulin resistance by inactivation of cytoplasmic JNK. J Biol Chem 2010;285: 21581–9.

15. Sartori M, Ceolotto G, Papparella I, et al. Effects of angiotensin II and insulin on ERK1/2 activation in fibroblasts from hypertensive patients. Am J Hypertens 2004;17:604–10.

16. Kosmala W, Jedrzejuk D, Derzhko R, et al. Left ventricular function impairment in patients with normal weight obesity: contribution of abdominal fat deposition, profibrotic state, reduced insulin sensitivity and proinflammatory activation. Circ Cardiovasc Imaging 2012;5(3):349–56.

17. Sokos GG, Nikolaidis LA, Mankad S, et al. Glucagon-like peptide-1 infusion improves left ventricular ejection fraction and functional status in patients with chronic heart failure. J Card Fail 2006;12:694–9.

18. Avogaro A, Nosadini R, Doria A, et al. Myocardial metabolism in insulin-deficient diabetic humans without coronary artery disease. Am J Physiol 1990; 258:E606–18.

19. Chiu HC, Kovacs A, Ford DA, et al. A novel mouse model of lipotoxic cardiomyopathy. J Clin Invest 2001;107:813–22.

20. Park TS, Yamashita H, Blaner WS, et al. Lipids in the heart: a source of fuel and a source of toxins. Curr Opin Lipidol 2007;18:277–82.

21. Vikramadithyan RK, Hirata K, Yagyu H, et al. Peroxisome proliferator-activated receptor agonists modulate heart function in transgenic mice with lipotoxic cardiomyopathy. J Pharmacol Exp Ther 2005;313:586–93.

22. Neubauer S, Horn M, Cramer M, et al. Myocardial phosphocreatine-to-ATP ratio is a predictor of mortality in patients with dilated cardiomyopathy. Circulation 1997;96:2190–6.

23. Neubauer S. The failing heart–an engine out of fuel. N Engl J Med 2007;356:1140–51.

24. Tuunanen H, Engblom E, Naum A, et al. Decreased myocardial free fatty acid uptake in patients with idiopathic dilated cardiomyopathy: evidence of relationship with insulin resistance and left ventricular dysfunction. J Card Fail 2006;12:644–52.

25. Knowler WC, Barrett-Connor E, Fowler SE, et al. Reduction in the incidence of type 2 diabetes with lifestyle intervention or metformin. N Engl J Med 2002;346:393–403.

26. Kemppainen J, Tsuchida H, Stolen K, et al. Insulin signalling and resistance in patients with chronic heart failure. J Physiol 2003;550:305–15.

27. Beck-da-Silva L, Higginson L, Fraser M, et al. Effect of orlistat in obese patients with heart failure: a pilot study. Congest Heart Fail 2005;11:118–23.

28. Scheen AJ. Prevention of type 2 diabetes mellitus through inhibition of the renin-angiotensin system. Drugs 2004;64:2537–65.

29. Potter BJ, LeLorier J. Effect of ramipril on the incidence of diabetes. N Engl J Med 2007;356:522–3 author reply: 523–4.

30. McMurray JJ, Holman RR, Haffner SM, et al. Effect of valsartan on the incidence of diabetes and cardiovascular events. N Engl J Med 2010;362:1477–90.

31. Bakris GL, Fonseca V, Katholi RE, et al. Metabolic effects of carvedilol vs metoprolol in patients with type 2 diabetes mellitus and hypertension: a randomized controlled trial. JAMA 2004;292:2227–36.

32. Torp-Pedersen C, Metra M, Charlesworth A, et al. Effects of metoprolol and carvedilol on pre-existing and new onset diabetes in patients with chronic heart failure: data from the Carvedilol or Metoprolol European Trial (COMET). Heart 2007;93:968–73.

33. Luther JM, Luo P, Kreger MT, et al. Aldosterone decreases glucose-stimulated insulin secretion in vivo in mice and in murine islets. Diabetologia 2011;54:2152–63.

34. Swaminathan K, Davies J, George J, et al. Spironolactone for poorly controlled hypertension in type 2 diabetes: conflicting effects on blood pressure, endothelial function, glycaemic control and hormonal profiles. Diabetologia 2008;51:762–8.

35. Yamaji M, Tsutamoto T, Kawahara C, et al. Effect of eplerenone versus spironolactone on cortisol and hemoglobin A(c) levels in patients with chronic heart failure. Am Heart J 2010;160:915–21.

36. Arase Y, Suzuki F, Suzuki Y, et al. Losartan reduces the onset of type 2 diabetes in hypertensive

Japanese patients with chronic hepatitis C. J Med Virol 2009;81:1584–90.

37. Kahn CR, Chen L, Cohen SE. Unraveling the mechanism of action of thiazolidinediones. J Clin Invest 2000;106:1305–7.

38. Vasudevan AR, Balasubramanyam A. Thiazolidinediones: a review of their mechanisms of insulin sensitization, therapeutic potential, clinical efficacy, and tolerability. Diabetes Technol Ther 2004;6:850–63.

39. Diep QN, El Mabrouk M, Cohn JS, et al. Structure, endothelial function, cell growth, and inflammation in blood vessels of angiotensin II-infused rats: role of peroxisome proliferator-activated receptor-gamma. Circulation 2002;105:2296–302.

40. Mazzone T, Meyer PM, Feinstein SB, et al. Effect of pioglitazone compared with glimepiride on carotid intima-media thickness in type 2 diabetes: a randomized trial. JAMA 2006;296:2572–81.

41. Furuse Y, Ogino K, Shimoyama M, et al. Ca(2+)-sensitizing effect is involved in the positive inotropic effect of troglitazone. Br J Pharmacol 2001;133: 1307–13.

42. Tsuji T, Mizushige K, Noma T, et al. Pioglitazone improves left ventricular diastolic function and decreases collagen accumulation in prediabetic stage of a type II diabetic rat. J Cardiovasc Pharmacol 2001;38:868–74.

43. Asakawa M, Takano H, Nagai T, et al. Peroxisome proliferator-activated receptor gamma plays a critical role in inhibition of cardiac hypertrophy in vitro and in vivo. Circulation 2002;105:1240–6.

44. Caglayan E, Stauber B, Collins AR, et al. Differential roles of cardiomyocyte and macrophage peroxisome proliferator-activated receptor gamma in cardiac fibrosis. Diabetes 2008;57:2470–9.

45. Shoghi KI, Finck BN, Schechtman KB, et al. In vivo metabolic phenotyping of myocardial substrate metabolism in rodents: differential efficacy of metformin and rosiglitazone monotherapy. Circ Cardiovasc Imaging 2009;2:373–81.

46. Baranowski M, Blachnio-Zabielska A, Zabielski P, et al. Pioglitazone induces lipid accumulation in the rat heart despite concomitant reduction in plasma free fatty acid availability. Arch Biochem Biophys 2008;477:86–91.

47. Cittadini A, Napoli R, Monti MG, et al. Metformin prevents the development of chronic heart failure in the SHHF rat model. Diabetes 2012;61(4):944–53.

48. Bajaj M, Baig R, Suraamornkul S, et al. Effects of pioglitazone on intramyocellular fat metabolism in patients with type 2 diabetes mellitus. J Clin Endocrinol Metab 2010;95:1916–23.

49. van der Meer RW, Rijzewijk LJ, de Jong HW, et al. Pioglitazone improves cardiac function and alters myocardial substrate metabolism without affecting cardiac triglyceride accumulation and high-energy phosphate metabolism in patients with well-controlled type 2 diabetes mellitus. Circulation 2009;119:2069–77.

50. Dargie HJ, Hildebrandt PR, Riegger GA, et al. A randomized, placebo-controlled trial assessing the effects of rosiglitazone on echocardiographic function and cardiac status in type 2 diabetic patients with New York Heart Association functional class I or II heart failure. J Am Coll Cardiol 2007; 49:1696–704.

51. St John Sutton M, Rendell M, Dandona P, et al. A comparison of the effects of rosiglitazone and glyburide on cardiovascular function and glycemic control in patients with type 2 diabetes. Diabetes Care 2002;25:2058–64.

52. Giles TD, Miller AB, Elkayam U, et al. Pioglitazone and heart failure: results from a controlled study in patients with type 2 diabetes mellitus and systolic dysfunction. J Card Fail 2008;14:445–52.

53. Nissen SE, Wolski K. Effect of rosiglitazone on the risk of myocardial infarction and death from cardiovascular causes. N Engl J Med 2007;356:2457–71.

54. Nissen SE, Wolski K. Rosiglitazone revisited: an updated meta-analysis of risk for myocardial infarction and cardiovascular mortality. Arch Intern Med 2010; 170:1191–201.

55. Singh S, Loke YK, Furberg CD. Long-term risk of cardiovascular events with rosiglitazone: a meta-analysis. JAMA 2007;298:1189–95.

56. Lincoff AM, Wolski K, Nicholls SJ, et al. Pioglitazone and risk of cardiovascular events in patients with type 2 diabetes mellitus: a meta-analysis of randomized trials. JAMA 2007;298:1180–8.

57. McEvoy B. Pioglitazone and rosiglitazone cardiovascular safety meta-analysis. Presented at Joint Meeting of the Endocrinologic and Metabolic Drugs Advisory Committee and the Drug Safety and Risk Management Advisory Committee. Gaithersburg, July 13-14, 2010. Available at: http://www.fda.gov/downloads/AdvisoryCommittees/CommitteesMeeting Materials/Drugs/EndocrinologicandMetabolicDrugs AdvisoryCommittee/UCM224739.pdf. Accessed January 23, 2011.

58. Lago RM, Singh PP, Nesto RW. Congestive heart failure and cardiovascular death in patients with prediabetes and type 2 diabetes given thiazolidinediones: a meta-analysis of randomised clinical trials. Lancet 2007;370:1129–36.

59. Graham DJ, Ouellet-Hellstrom R, MaCurdy TE, et al. Risk of acute myocardial infarction, stroke, heart failure, and death in elderly Medicare patients treated with rosiglitazone or pioglitazone. JAMA 2010;304:411–8.

60. Wertz DA, Chang CL, Sarawate CA, et al. Risk of cardiovascular events and all-cause mortality in patients treated with thiazolidinediones in a managed-care population. Circ Cardiovasc Qual Outcomes 2010;3:538–45.

61. Gallagher AM, Smeeth L, Seabroke S, et al. Risk of death and cardiovascular outcomes with thiazolidinediones: a study with the general practice research database and secondary care data. PLoS One 2011;6:e28157.

62. Zimmet P. Addressing the insulin resistance syndrome: a role for the thiazolidinediones. Trends Cardiovasc Med 2002;12:354–62.

63. Nesto RW, Bell D, Bonow RO, et al. Thiazolidinedione use, fluid retention, and congestive heart failure: a consensus statement from the American Heart Association and American Diabetes Association. Diabetes Care 2004;27:256–63.

64. Erdmann E, Wilcox RG. Weighing up the cardiovascular benefits of thiazolidinedione therapy: the impact of increased risk of heart failure. Eur Heart J 2008;29:12–20.

65. Karalliedde J, Buckingham R, Starkie M, et al. Effect of various diuretic treatments on rosiglitazone-induced fluid retention. J Am Soc Nephrol 2006;17:3482–90.

66. Dagenais GR, Gerstein HC, Holman R, et al. Effects of ramipril and rosiglitazone on cardiovascular and renal outcomes in people with impaired glucose tolerance or impaired fasting glucose: results of the Diabetes REduction Assessment with ramipril and rosiglitazone Medication (DREAM) trial. Diabetes Care 2008;31:1007–14.

67. Home PD, Pocock SJ, Beck-Nielsen H, et al. Rosiglitazone evaluated for cardiovascular outcomes–an interim analysis. N Engl J Med 2007;357:28–38.

68. Dormandy JA, Charbonnel B, Eckland DJ, et al. Secondary prevention of macrovascular events in patients with type 2 diabetes in the PROactive Study (PROspective pioglitAzone Clinical Trial In macroVascular Events): a randomised controlled trial. Lancet 2005;366:1279–89.

69. Simo R, Rodriguez A, Caveda E. Different effects of thiazolidinediones on cardiovascular risk in patients with type 2 diabetes mellitus: pioglitazone versus rosiglitazone. Curr Drug Saf 2010;5:234–44.

70. Kirpichnikov D, McFarlane SI, Sowers JR. Metformin: an update. Ann Intern Med 2002;137:25–33.

71. Effect of intensive blood-glucose control with metformin on complications in overweight patients with type 2 diabetes (UKPDS 34). UK Prospective Diabetes Study (UKPDS) Group. Lancet 1998;352:854–65.

72. Misbin R. The phantom of lactic acidosis due to metformin in patients with diabetes. Diabetes Care 2002;25:2244–8.

73. Salpeter SR, Greyber E, Pasternak GA, et al. Risk of fatal and nonfatal lactic acidosis with metformin use in type 2 diabetes mellitus: systematic review and meta-analysis. Arch Intern Med 2003;163:2594–602.

74. Lalau J, Race J. Lactic acidosis in metformin-treated patients: prognostic value of arterial lactate levels and plasma metformin concentrations. Drug Saf 1999;20:377–84.

75. Stades A, Heikens J, Erkeleens D, et al. Metformin and lactic acidosis: cause or coincidence? a review of case reports. J Intern Med 2004;255:179–87.

76. Emslie-Smith AM, Boyle DI, Evans JM, et al. Contraindications to metformin therapy in patients with type 2 diabetes–a population-based study of adherence to prescribing guidelines. Diabet Med 2001;18:483–8.

77. Masoudi FA, Inzucchi SE, Wang Y, et al. Thiazolidinediones, metformin, and outcomes in older patients with diabetes and heart failure: an observational study. Circulation 2005;111:583–90.

78. Eurich DT, McAlister FA, Blackburn DF, et al. Benefits and harms of antidiabetic agents in patients with diabetes and heart failure: systematic review. BMJ 2007;335:497.

79. Misbin RI. Evaluating the safety of diabetes drugs: perspective of a Food and Drug Administration insider. Diabetes Care 2005;28:2573–6.

80. Shah DD, Fonarow GC, Horwich TB. Metformin therapy and outcomes in patients with advanced systolic heart failure and diabetes. J Card Fail 2010;16:200–6.

81. MacDonald MR, Eurich DT, Majumdar SR, et al. Treatment of type 2 diabetes and outcomes in patients with heart failure: a nested case-control study from the U.K. General Practice Research Database. Diabetes Care 2010;33:1213–8.

82. Roussel R, Travert F, Pasquet B, et al. Metformin use and mortality among patients with diabetes and atherothrombosis. Arch Intern Med 2010;170:1892–9.

83. Aguilar D, Chan W, Bozkurt B, et al. Metformin use and mortality in ambulatory patients with diabetes and heart failure. Circ Heart Fail 2011;4:53–8.

84. Inzucchi SE, Masoudi FA, Wang Y, et al. Insulin-sensitizing antihyperglycemic drugs and mortality after acute myocardial infarction: insights from the National Heart Care Project. Diabetes Care 2005;28:1680–9.

85. Romero SP, Andrey JL, Garcia-Egido A, et al. Metformin therapy and prognosis of patients with heart failure and new-onset diabetes mellitus. A propensity-matched study in the community. Int J Cardiol 2011. [Epub ahead of print].

86. Shaw JS, Wilmot RL, Kilpatrick ES. Establishing pragmatic estimated GFR thresholds to guide metformin prescribing. Diabet Med 2007;24:1160–3.

87. Eurich DT, Tsuyuki RT, Majumdar SR, et al. Metformin treatment in diabetes and heart failure: when academic equipoise meets clinical reality. Trials 2009;10:12.

88. Mather KJ, Verma S, Anderson TJ. Improved endothelial function with metformin in type 2 diabetes mellitus. J Am Coll Cardiol 2001;37:1344–50.

89. Li SN, Wang X, Zeng QT, et al. Metformin inhibits nuclear factor kappaB activation and decreases

serum high-sensitivity C-reactive protein level in experimental atherogenesis of rabbits. Heart Vessels 2009;24:446–53.

90. Hou X, Song J, Li XN, et al. Metformin reduces intracellular reactive oxygen species levels by upregulating expression of the antioxidant thioredoxin via the AMPK-FOXO3 pathway. Biochem Biophys Res Commun 2010;396:199–205.

91. Ashrafian H, Frenneaux MP, Opie LH. Metabolic mechanisms in heart failure. Circulation 2007;116: 434–48.

92. Bertrand L, Ginion A, Beauloye C, et al. AMPK activation restores the stimulation of glucose uptake in an in vitro model of insulin-resistant cardiomyocytes via the activation of protein kinase B. Am J Physiol Heart Circ Physiol 2006;291:H239–50.

93. Wang XF, Zhang JY, Li L, et al. Metformin improves cardiac function in rats via activation of AMP-activated protein kinase. Clin Exp Pharmacol Physiol 2011;38:94–101.

94. Sasaki H, Asanuma H, Fujita M, et al. Metformin prevents progression of heart failure in dogs: role of AMP-activated protein kinase. Circulation 2009; 119:2568–77.

95. Gundewar S, Calvert JW, Jha S, et al. Activation of AMP-activated protein kinase by metformin improves left ventricular function and survival in heart failure. Circ Res 2009;104:403–11.

96. Davis BJ, Xie Z, Viollet B, et al. Activation of the AMP-activated kinase by antidiabetes drug metformin stimulates nitric oxide synthesis in vivo by promoting the association of heat shock protein 90 and endothelial nitric oxide synthase. Diabetes 2006;55:496–505.

97. Finck BN, Kelly DP. Peroxisome proliferator-activated receptor gamma coactivator-1 (PGC-1) regulatory cascade in cardiac physiology and disease. Circulation 2007;115:2540–8.

98. Hallsten K, Virtanen KA, Lonnqvist F, et al. Enhancement of insulin-stimulated myocardial glucose uptake in patients with type 2 diabetes treated with rosiglitazone. Diabet Med 2004;21:1280–7.

Diabetes Mellitus and Myocardial Mitochondrial Dysfunction: Bench to Bedside

Alexandra König, BS, Christoph Bode, MD,
Heiko Bugger, MD*

KEYWORDS

- Mitochondria • Diabetic cardiomyopathy • Diabetes • Antioxidants • Metabolic therapy

KEY POINTS

- Myocardial mitochondrial dysfunction is a pathophysiologic hallmark of diabetic cardiomyopathy, likely contributing to the increased risk for heart failure in diabetics.
- Underlying mechanisms of mitochondrial dysfunction in diabetic cardiomyopathy include altered energy metabolism, oxidative stress, impaired calcium handling, and altered myocardial insulin action.
- Potential treatment options to be explored include mitochondria-targeted antioxidant therapy, strategies using advantages of caloric restriction, and further development of mitochondrial drug delivery systems.

INTRODUCTION

Individuals with diabetes mellitus are at a significantly greater risk of developing cardiomyopathy and heart failure despite adjusting for concomitant comorbidities such as coronary artery disease or hypertension.[1] This increased risk has been attributed to a cardiac disease process, termed diabetic cardiomyopathy (DCM), defined as ventricular dysfunction in patients with diabetes in the absence of coronary artery disease and hypertension.[2] Diastolic dysfunction is considered a frequent, and also the earliest, clinical manifestation of DCM, sometimes accompanied by subtle systolic dysfunction and impaired cardiac reserve, but frequently associated with cardiac hypertrophy.[3–6] The pathophysiology of DCM is complex and involves various molecular mechanisms, including interstitial and perivascular fibrosis, increased advanced glycation end products (AGE) formation, oxidative stress, apoptosis, activation of the renin-angiotensin system, impaired calcium handling, lipotoxicity, altered cardiac energy metabolism, and impaired mitochondrial energetics.[7,8] Several of these alterations occur in mitochondria or negatively affect mitochondrial physiology, which includes mitochondrial adenosine triphosphate (ATP) production and may thereby contribute to cardiac energy depletion. Because maintaining cardiac contractility depends on continuous high-energy phosphate regeneration, maintaining mitochondrial function may represent a desirable therapeutic target in diabetics. This article presents evidence supporting mitochondrial dysfunction in DCM, briefly describes pathophysiologic mechanisms contributing to mitochondrial dysfunction, and discusses potential treatment strategies.

MITOCHONDRIAL DYSFUNCTION IN HUMANS AND ANIMALS WITH DIABETES

The most compelling evidence for mitochondrial dysfunction in human diabetic hearts was recently

Funding support: H.B. was supported by grants from the Deutsche Forschungsgemeinschaft (Bu 2126/2-1). Department of Cardiology and Angiology, University Hospital of Freiburg, Hugstetter Strasse 55, Freiburg 79106, Germany
* Corresponding author.
E-mail address: heiko.bugger@uniklinik-freiburg.de

Heart Failure Clin 8 (2012) 551–561
http://dx.doi.org/10.1016/j.hfc.2012.06.001

provided by Anderson and colleagues,[9] who showed impaired mitochondrial respiratory capacity in atrial tissue of patients with type 2 diabetes using the skinned fibers technique. The investigators also showed increased mitochondrial H_2O_2 emission, depletion of glutathione, increased levels of 4-hydroxynonenal (4-HNE)–modified proteins and 3-nitrotyrosine–modified proteins, and increased sensitivity to calcium-induced opening of the mitochondrial permeability transition pore.[9,10] Scheuermann-Freestone and colleagues[12] and Diamant and colleagues[13] showed decreased phosphocreatine (pCr)/ATP ratios in hearts of patients with type 2 diabetes using[11] P nuclear magnetic resonance (NMR) spectroscopy, which suggests impaired high-energy phosphate metabolism in these subjects.[12,13] Because the decrease of pCr/ATP ratios is associated with impaired mitochondrial function in heart failure,[14,15] the reduced pCr/ATP ratios in diabetics indirectly suggest impaired myocardial mitochondrial energetics in these patients. Peterson and colleagues[16] reported that, in young women with obesity and insulin resistance, increased body mass index (BMI) and impaired glucose tolerance is associated with increased myocardial oxygen consumption (Mvo$_2$), reduced cardiac efficiency (CE; the ratio of cardiac work to O_2 consumption), and increased fatty acid (FA) use. Similar observations have been made in rodent models of obesity and type 2 diabetes, in which increased Mvo$_2$, increased FA use, and decreased CE are associated with impaired respiratory capacity, and in which FA-induced reactive oxygen species (ROS)–mediated mitochondrial uncoupling has been proposed to underlie the reduction in cardiac efficiency.[17–19]

Substantial evidence has accumulated that myocardial mitochondrial dysfunction occurs in animal models of type 1 and type 2 diabetes. Thirty years ago, Kuo and colleagues[20] showed reduced state 3 respiration of mitochondria isolated from obese and type 2 diabetic db/db mouse hearts. Impairment in state 3 respiration, mitochondrial oxidative stress, and abnormal mitochondrial ultrastructure have been observed in various rodent models with different degrees of obesity, insulin resistance, and insulin-dependent and non–insulin-dependent diabetes (for detailed review, see Refs.[21–24]). Thus, although more studies on mitochondrial function in human diabetic myocardium are desirable, the evidence thus far, as well as the substantial evidence of mitochondrial dysfunction that has accumulated from rodent studies, strongly suggest that myocardial mitochondrial function is compromised in human DCM. To understand what potential treatment options may improve myocardial

mitochondrial dysfunction, it is necessary to review molecular mechanisms that may underlie mitochondrial dysfunction in diabetic hearts (summarized in **Fig. 1**).

MECHANISMS FOR MYOCARDIAL MITOCHONDRIAL DYSFUNCTION IN DIABETES

Altered Substrate Utilization and Mitochondrial Uncoupling

The normal heart generates ATP mainly from the mitochondrial oxidation of FA (60%–70% of ATP generated) and, to a lesser extent, from glucose, lactate, and other substrates (30%–40%). The diabetic heart uses more FA to generate ATP, and glucose use is further reduced.[16,19,25] Increased myocardial FA oxidation results from increased myocardial FA uptake, in large part a consequence of increased circulating FA and triglyceride concentrations in diabetics. In addition, increased FA uptake drives signaling via peroxisome proliferator–activated receptor α (PPARα), a transcription factor, which increases the expression of all genes involved in cardiac FA use.[26,27] Myocardial expression of PPARα and its target genes is increased in models of diabetes, and cardiomyocyte-specific overexpression of PPARα (myosin heavy chain [MHC]-PPARα) resulted in increased FA use and decreased glucose use, thus mimicking the metabolic phenotype of the diabetic heart.[25,28–31] Despite increased FA oxidation, accumulation of triglycerides, ceramides, and other reactive lipid intermediates occurs in diabetic hearts and may exert detrimental lipotoxic effects within the myocardium, including lipoapoptosis.[32,33]

In type 2 diabetes, increased myocardial FA delivery results in increased cardiac FA uptake and increased myocardial oxygen consumption without a concomitant increase in contractility, resulting in reduced cardiac efficiency (cardiac work/Mvo$_2$).[16,19,25] A current explanation for the pathogenesis of decreased cardiac efficiency in diabetic hearts is the concept of FA-induced mitochondrial uncoupling, which has been reviewed in detail elsewhere.[34] In brief, a series of experiments performed in the Abel laboratory[17,18] suggests that increased myocardial FA uptake and oxidation results in increased reducing equivalent delivery to the respiratory chain, which may increase mitochondrial ROS production. These ROS may directly activate uncoupling proteins (UCPs), which leads to increased proton flux from the intermembrane space into the matrix that bypasses the F_0F_1-ATPase, resulting in decreased coupling of ATP synthesis to oxygen consumption (ie, increased mitochondrial uncoupling). This

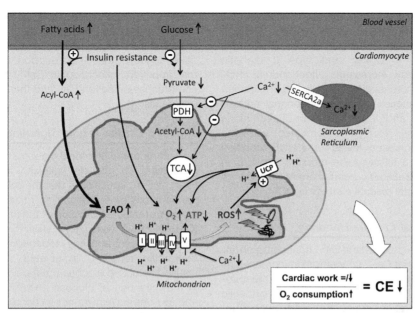

Fig. 1. Summary of mechanisms underlying myocardial mitochondrial dysfunction in type 2 diabetes. Increased delivery of FA to the heart may increase FA uptake and oxidation, resulting in increased reducing equivalent delivery to the respiratory chain and likely ROS production. ROS activate uncoupling proteins (UCPs), resulting in increased mitochondrial uncoupling, which leads to increased mitochondrial O_2 consumption and thereby to a further increase in FA oxidation. Because the increase in O_2 consumption results from mitochondrial uncoupling, ATP synthesis does not increase proportionally. Impaired intracellular Ca^{2+} handling results in decreased mitochondrial Ca^{2+} levels, thereby impairing activities of pyruvate dehydrogenase (PDH), tricarboxylic acid (TCA) cycle enzymes, and F_0F1-ATPase. Insulin resistance contributes to increased FA oxidation and reduced glucose uptake, impaired PDH and TCA cycle activity, and mitochondrial uncoupling. As a result of all mechanisms, myocardial O_2 consumption increases, but cardiac work either does not increase proportionally or is even decreased. Thus, cardiac efficiency (cardiac work/O_2 consumption) is impaired. CoA, coenzyme A; FAO, FA oxidation; SERCA2a, sarcoplasmic reticulum Ca(2+) ATPase 2a.

mitochondrial uncoupling reciprocally increases mitochondrial oxygen consumption and FA oxidation further and leads to cardiac energy depletion caused by inefficient ATP production, which may ultimately contribute to the development of contractile dysfunction. In addition, increased FA use in the diabetic heart may be energetically detrimental because FA use requires a higher oxygen cost to produce ATP compared with glucose use.[35]

Oxidative Stress

In diabetes, a substantial amount of ROS are generated within mitochondria, as opposed to cytosolic origins.[36] Mitochondrial oxidative stress may result from increased mitochondrial ROS production, either because of augmented delivery of electrons to the respiratory chain,[36,37] or from impaired electron transfer through the oxidative phosphorylation (OXPHOS) chain.[38] Decreased efficiency of mitochondrial ROS scavenger systems, which includes enzymes such as

manganese superoxide dismutase (MnSOD), catalase, or glutathione peroxidase, can also contribute to increased ROS accumulation. ROS can severely harm the cell by protein oxidation, by increasing reactive lipid peroxidation products, and by damaging mitochondrial DNA, which has been proposed to be particularly susceptible to oxidative damage.[39] In addition, superoxide can generate reactive nitrogen species from NO, leading to intracellular nitrosylation, for example protein tyrosine nitration.[31]

Because ROS have a short half-life, they are thought to cause damage close to their origin (ie, mitochondria can be both the origin and target of ROS). A proteomic approach by Turko and colleagues[31] revealed tyrosine nitration of several cardiac mitochondrial proteins in rats with alloxan-induced type 1 diabetes, and Lashin and colleagues[40] showed that increased mitochondrial 4-HNE accumulation impairs OXPHOS complex II activity in streptozotocin-diabetic rats. In OVE26 mice, transgenic overexpression of catalase or MnSOD normalized increased mitochondrial ROS production and restored impaired mitochondrial morphology, improved mitochondrial state 3 respiration, and normalized cardiomyocyte contractility.[41,42] Obese and type 2 diabetic rodents display increased mitochondrial H_2O_2 production, increased levels of lipid peroxidation products, induction of the mitochondrial antioxidant defense, and decreased levels of glutathione and coenzyme Q.[18,43–45] Combined with the finding of increased levels of 4-HNE–modified proteins and 3-nitrotyrosine–modified proteins in human type 2 diabetic hearts,[9] there is evidence of mitochondrial oxidative stress in DCM.

Mitochondrial Calcium Handling

After a cytosolic increase in Ca^{2+} concentration, intramitochondrial Ca^{2+} concentration increases as well, and there is growing evidence that the mitochondrial Ca^{2+} concentration can track cytosolic Ca^{2+} concentrations during the cardiac cycle.[46] Intramitochondrial Ca^{2+} increases the activity of several Ca^{2+}-sensitive metabolic enzymes (pyruvate dehydrogenase, isocitrate dehydrogenase, α-ketoglutarate dehydrogenase[47,48]), and is required for mitochondrial ATP production via the F_0F_1-ATPase.[49] Thus, Ca^{2+}-mediated activation of oxidative metabolism likely results in increased energy substrate oxidation and ATP production, and Ca^{2+} exchange between the cytosol and the mitochondria has therefore been suggested to provide a simple but elegant way to coordinate the rate of ATP production for cardiac contraction.

In streptozotocin-induced diabetes, the rate of Ca^{2+} uptake into rat heart mitochondria is low compared with normal rats and is accompanied by a reduction of α-ketoglutarate–supported mitochondrial state 3 respiration.[50,51] The lower mitochondrial concentrations of Ca^{2+} may be the consequence of smaller systolic transients in cytosolic Ca^{2+} concentration, possibly caused by reduced Ca^{2+} loading of the sarcoplasmic reticulum and various mechanisms that compromise activity of sarcoplasmic reticulum Ca(2+) ATPase 2a (SERCA2a) in these hearts.[52,53] Another possibility may be that mitochondria from type 1 diabetic hearts have depressed capacity to accumulate Ca^{2+}, because of an enhanced sensitivity to induction of mitochondrial permeability transition pore mitochondrial permeability transition pore (mPTP) opening.[54] This finding has been confirmed in patients with type 2 diabetes.[10] Type 2 diabetic ob/ob mice show reduced intracellular Ca^{2+} release on electrical stimulation, a slowed intracellular Ca^{2+} decay rate, and impaired mitochondrial Ca^{2+} handling.[55,56] In db/db mice, Ca^{2+} transients from isolated myocytes showed lower systolic and diastolic Ca^{2+} levels, the decay rate of Ca^{2+} transients was reduced, and increased Ca^{2+} leakage from the sarcoplasmic reticulum was observed.[57] Taken together, these data support the hypothesis that impaired mitochondrial Ca^{2+} handling may compromise mitochondrial, and therefore cardiac, energetics.

Impaired Cardiac Insulin Signaling

Rodent models with type 2 diabetes exhibit insulin resistance in multiple tissues, including the heart.[19,25] To specifically test the role of impaired cardiomyocyte insulin signaling, mice with a cardiomyocyte-restricted deletion of the insulin receptor (CIRKO mice) were generated.[58] CIRKO mice show a modest and age-dependent decrease in contractile function, associated with reduced insulin-stimulated glucose uptake and a decrease in the oxidation of glucose and FA as they age and as contractile dysfunction occurs.[58,59] CIRKO hearts show impaired mitochondrial respiration and ATP synthesis rates, reduced expression of genes encoding for OXPHOS subunits, as well as decreased mitochondrial levels of FA oxidation proteins, tricarboxylic acid (TCA) cycle proteins, and remodeling of the OXPHOS subunit composition.[59] In addition, CIRKO mice exhibit FA-induced ROS-mediated mitochondrial uncoupling, as observed in type 2 diabetic models, and the presence of mitochondrial defects caused by cardiac insulin resistance may predispose hearts to develop impaired cardiac efficiency following induction of diabetes.[60]

THERAPEUTIC STRATEGIES

Although significant evidence of defects in mitochondrial energetics in diabetic hearts has accumulated, the ultimate challenge is to develop effective and feasible therapeutic strategies to improve mitochondrial energetics in patients. Although the pathogenesis of mitochondrial dysfunction is multifactorial and likely involves more mechanisms than have been elucidated thus far, some of these mechanisms represent a substrate for therapeutic interventions and are discussed later.

Antioxidant Therapy

Genetic overexpression of mitochondrial antioxidant enzymes ameliorates detrimental effects of oxidative stress on mitochondria in diabetic hearts,[41,42] suggesting that increasing intramitochondrial ROS scavenging may be a promising therapeutic approach in diabetic hearts. In various diseases, natural antioxidants, such as vitamin E or coenzyme Q, have been used to treat animals and humans to ameliorate oxidative stress. With respect to DCM, α-tocopherol treatment reversed increased mitochondrial ROS production and uncoupling protein 2 (UCP2) expression in hearts of OLETF rats,[23] and vitamin E treatment modestly improved mitochondrial phosphorylation efficiency, possibly through a sparing effect on coenzyme Q 10 (CoQ10) or by increasing its biosynthesis.[24] The study of vitamin E treatment also showed that administration of CoQ10 and vitamin E did not result in a clear, direct enrichment of the compounds in the cardiac mitochondrial fraction.

To increase the efficiency of vitamin E and CoQ10, mitochondria-targeted derivatives of these molecules were developed by conjugating them to a lipophilic triphenylphosphonium (TPP) cation.[61] Mitochondria-targeted derivatives of α-tocopherol (MitoVitE) and ubiquinone (MitoQ) were rapidly and selectively accumulated within mitochondria and showed higher efficacy than untargeted compounds.[62–64] Following oral ingestion, MitoQ and MitoVitE enter the bloodstream, distribute to tissues in their intact active form, and accumulate several hundred-fold within mitochondria.[65]

In the heart, MitoQ treatment has been shown to reduce calcium-induced opening of the mPTP during hypoxia-reoxygenation,[66] and to prevent ROS-induced myocardial mitochondrial uncoupling in cocaine-treated rats.[67] Furthermore, MitoQ treatment prevented impairment in myocardial mitochondrial respiration and ATP synthesis during acute endotoxemia in rats,[68] and improved mitochondrial respiration rates, prevented mitochondrial swelling, lowered mitochondrial cytochrome c release, and improved left ventricle (LV) functional recovery in rat hearts following ischemia-reperfusion.[69] Antioxidants can also exert pro-oxidant effects in certain conditions, but Rodriguez-Cuenca and colleagues[70] recently showed that 28 weeks of oral administration of high-dose MitoQ to mice was safe and did not increase mitochondrial oxidative stress or affect endogenous mitochondrial antioxidant defense systems. Fewer studies have been published on the effects of MitoVitE, which showed moderate antioxidant effects in some, but not all, of the tissues investigated.[71–73] To our knowledge, studies investigating myocardial effects of MitoVitE are lacking. Thus, although no studies have examined the effect of MitoQ treatment on mitochondrial function in diabetic hearts, MitoQ may efficiently reduce mitochondrial oxidative stress, restore coupling of ATP synthesis to oxygen consumption, and improve mitochondrial function, and it therefore needs to be tested for

therapeutic purposes in diabetics. Phase II clinical trials using MitoQ have already been completed for treatment of other diseases.[74]

Many other mitochondria-targeted synthetic compounds with antioxidant effects have been generated, which has been reviewed elsewhere.[75,76] These include TPP-4-hydroxy-2,2, 6,6-tetramethylpiperidine-1-oxyl (Mito-TEMPOL), which effectively decreased lipid peroxidation in isolated energized mitochondria,[77] or SS-31, which is a small synthetic peptide with basic amino acid residues that allow 1000-fold to 5000-fold increased mitochondrial uptake. In angiotensin-induced hypertensive cardiomyopathy, reducing mitochondrial ROS levels by SS-31 treatment attenuated mitochondrial oxidative damage and upregulation of mitochondrial biogenesis, prevented apoptosis, and ameliorated angiotensin-induced cardiac hypertrophy, diastolic dysfunction, and fibrosis.[78] To our knowledge, none of these synthetic compounds has been tested in models of diabetic cardiomyopathy.

Caloric Restriction

For prevention and treatment of diabetes and its complications, the American Diabetes Association published nutrition recommendations that include diets with calorie restriction to reduce energy intake, which may increase weight loss, improve insulin sensitivity, and exert beneficial effects on the serum lipid profile.[79] Caloric restriction (CR) has been independently proved to increase lifespan and to lower cardiovascular risk.[11,80] The principle of CR can be broadly defined as restricting the diet of an organism to fewer calories (20%–50%) than ad libitum feeding without altering the levels of vitamins, minerals, and amino acids to include all essential nutrients. Lifelong CR in rhesus monkeys recently resulted in a 50% reduction in mortality caused by cardiovascular disease.[11] Studies suggest that caloric restriction may partially exert these effects by reducing mitochondrial ROS production.[81,82] In the heart, CR preserved mitochondrial function, attenuated mitochondrial H_2O_2 production, and decreased OXPHOS protein acetylation following ischemia-reperfusion.[83] A reversal of increased mitochondrial ROS production by CR was also observed in type 2 diabetic rats.[23]

CR also influences myocardial energy substrate metabolism. In obese subjects undergoing CR for 6 weeks, whole-body insulin sensitivity was increased and myocardial triglyceride content was decreased, although cardiac insulin sensitivity was unaffected during this short-term dietary intervention.[84] Hammer and colleagues[85] showed that prolonged caloric restriction in obese patients with type 2 diabetes decreased BMI and improved glucoregulation associated with decreased myocardial triglyceride content and improved diastolic heart function.

Effects of CR can be mimicked by resveratrol (Resv), a natural polyphenol that is contained in many common food components, such as peanuts, cranberries, blueberries, and grapes. Oral administration of large doses of Resv protects against the development of diet-induced insulin resistance in aged rodents fed a high-calorie diet,[86] and improves insulin resistance in patients with type 2 diabetes.[87] In glucose-treated mesangial cells, Resv efficiently reduced oxidative stress and maintained mitochondrial function.[88] In the heart, Resv protects cardiomyocytes from oxidative stress and cell death by improving mitochondrial function, reducing ROS, and increasing the expression of antioxidant enzymes. It improves cellular survival in doxorubicin-treated cardiomyocytes by stimulating a SIRT1-MnSOD pathway.[89,90] Resv may also prevent myocardial reperfusion injury by modulating mPTP opening, and may improve cardiac function in streptozotocin-diabetic rodents by enhancing SERCA2a expression.[91,92] The molecular mechanisms of Resv are probably multifactorial, but may include inhibition of cyclic adenosine monophosphate–degrading phosphodiesterases, such as phosphodiesterase 4, and activation of sirtuin 1 (SIRT1) and adenosine monophosphate–activated protein kinase (AMPK), which are known regulators of mitochondrial function and biogenesis.[93,94]

Thus, CR and/or Resv affect multiple mechanisms that directly or indirectly affect mitochondrial function in the heart, by modulating oxidative stress, calcium handling, lipotoxicity, and mPTP opening. Resv treatment may exert diverse beneficial effects on myocardial mitochondrial function in patients with diabetes. Although long-term commitment to CR may be challenging for some patients, Resv is a natural product that is well tolerated, easily absorbed, and therefore an ideal compound for further investigation.

Metabolic Modulation

Increased FA use in diabetic hearts is driven by increased serum levels of free FA and lipoprotein-containing triglyceride particles, which increase myocardial PPARα signaling. Several studies have attempted to reverse the substrate metabolic pattern by modulating myocardial delivery of FA and triglyceride. Systemic treatment with the PPARα agonist BM 17.0744 reduced plasma lipid and glucose concentrations,

improved systemic insulin sensitivity, lowered myocardial FA oxidation by 50%, and increased myocardial glucose use in db/db mice, but did not improve LV contractile function.[95] Three months of fenofibrate treatment of mice with diet-induced obesity, mild hyperglycemia, and hypertriglyceridemia increased myocardial glucose oxidation, decreased FA oxidation, and prevented reduction in cardiac power, which was only mildly reduced in untreated animals.[96] Systemic treatment with PPARγ agonists (so-called thiazolidinediones or glitazones) reduces peripheral insulin resistance by mechanisms that include lowering of serum FA levels because of promoting fat storage in adipose tissue. Treatment of db/db mice with rosiglitazone normalized plasma glucose and lipid concentrations, restored rates of cardiac glucose and FA oxidation, and improved cardiac efficiency.[97] In contrast, treatment of db/db mice with the PPARγ agonist 2-(2-(4-phenoxy-2-propylphenoxy)ethyl)-indole-5-acetic acid resulted in enhanced glucose oxidation and decreased palmitate oxidation, but did not improve contractile performance.[98] Glitazones have also been shown to impair mitochondrial complex I activity, mitochondrial state 3 respiration, and to increase ROS production in cell culture and skeletal muscle, and both fibrates and glitazones impair state 3 respiration in liver mitochondria and OXPHOS complex activities in heart mitochondria.[99–101] In addition, glitazone treatment increases fluid retention, which may exacerbate heart failure symptoms, and rosiglitazone treatment is associated with increased risk for myocardial infarction.[102,103] Thus, there are currently no convincing data supporting agonism of PPARα or PPARγ as a useful therapeutic approach in DCM.

Mitochondrial Drug Delivery Systems

A promising novel concept of mitochondrial therapy is the MITO-Porter system, developed by Yamada and colleagues.[104] Mito-Porter is a liposome-based carrier system for delivery of macromolecules into mitochondria via membrane fusion.[104] The mitochondrial matrix delivery efficiency was recently optimized by modifying the membrane fusion steps, now called Dual Function MITO-Porter (DF-Mito-Porter).[105] Yamada and Harashima[106] showed the successful delivery of DNase I into the mitochondrial matrix of HeLa cells, which was a 15-fold increased matrix delivery compared with the conventional Mito-Porter system. The system requires that the macromolecule of choice to be delivered to mitochondria can be successfully encapsulated. If possible, this system will allow the delivery of any protein, or even drug, to mitochondria and thus may provide a promising novel therapeutic option of mitochondria-specific treatment of any mitochondrial disease, including the diabetic heart.

SUMMARY

There is substantial evidence of mitochondrial dysfunction in diabetic hearts. Alterations in cardiac energy substrate metabolism and oxidative stress are major pathophysiologic mechanisms underlying these mitochondrial defects. There is currently no established treatment option for myocardial mitochondrial dysfunction in humans with diabetes, but studies in rodents indicate that preventing or treating mitochondrial dysfunction may have beneficial effects. This article presents several therapeutic options, some of which need to be tested in animal studies first, and some of which could potentially be ready for clinical trials, such as MitoQ. Considering the increasing prevalence of obesity and type 2 diabetes, and its accompanying cardiovascular complications, there is urgent need for more studies testing such novel treatment strategies. Therefore, modulating mitochondrial function may represent a novel approach to treating heart disease in the future.

REFERENCES

1. Kannel WB, McGee DL. Diabetes and cardiovascular disease. The Framingham study. JAMA 1979;241:2035.
2. Poornima IG, Parikh P, Shannon RP. Diabetic cardiomyopathy: the search for a unifying hypothesis. Circ Res 2006;98:596.
3. Aboukhoudir F, Rekik S. Left ventricular systolic function deterioration during dobutamine stress echocardiography as an early manifestation of diabetic cardiomyopathy and reversal by optimized therapeutic approach. Int J Cardiovasc Imaging 2011. [Epub ahead of print].
4. Devereux RB, Roman MJ, Paranicas M, et al. Impact of diabetes on cardiac structure and function: the Strong Heart Study. Circulation 2000;101:2271.
5. Fang ZY, Najos-Valencia O, Leano R, et al. Patients with early diabetic heart disease demonstrate a normal myocardial response to dobutamine. J Am Coll Cardiol 2003;42:446.
6. Poirier P, Bogaty P, Garneau C, et al. Diastolic dysfunction in normotensive men with well-controlled type 2 diabetes: importance of maneuvers in echocardiographic screening for preclinical diabetic cardiomyopathy. Diabetes Care 2001;24:5.
7. An D, Rodrigues B. Role of changes in cardiac metabolism in development of diabetic cardiomyopathy. Am J Physiol Heart Circ Physiol 2006;291:H1489.
8. Boudina S, Abel ED. Diabetic cardiomyopathy, causes and effects. Rev Endocr Metab Disord 2010;11:31.
9. Anderson EJ, Kypson AP, Rodriguez E, et al. Substrate-specific derangements in mitochondrial metabolism and redox balance in the atrium of the type 2 diabetic human heart. J Am Coll Cardiol 2009;54:1891.
10. Anderson EJ, Rodriguez E, Anderson CA, et al. Increased propensity for cell death in diabetic human heart is mediated by mitochondrial-dependent pathways. Am J Physiol Heart Circ Physiol 2011;300(1):H118–24.
11. Colman RJ, Anderson RM, Johnson SC, et al. Caloric restriction delays disease onset and mortality in rhesus monkeys. Science 2009;325:201.
12. Scheuermann-Freestone M, Madsen PL, Manners D, et al. Abnormal cardiac and skeletal muscle energy metabolism in patients with type 2 diabetes. Circulation 2003;107:3040.
13. Diamant M, Lamb HJ, Groeneveld Y, et al. Diastolic dysfunction is associated with altered myocardial metabolism in asymptomatic normotensive patients with well-controlled type 2 diabetes mellitus. J Am Coll Cardiol 2003;42:328.
14. Casademont J, Miro O. Electron transport chain defects in heart failure. Heart Fail Rev 2002;7:131.
15. Neubauer S, Horn M, Cramer M, et al. Myocardial phosphocreatine-to-ATP ratio is a predictor of mortality in patients with dilated cardiomyopathy. Circulation 1997;96:2190.
16. Peterson LR, Herrero P, Schechtman KB, et al. Effect of obesity and insulin resistance on myocardial substrate metabolism and efficiency in young women. Circulation 2004;109:2191.
17. Boudina S, Sena S, O'Neill BT, et al. Reduced mitochondrial oxidative capacity and increased mitochondrial uncoupling impair myocardial energetics in obesity. Circulation 2005;112:2686.
18. Boudina S, Sena S, Theobald H, et al. Mitochondrial energetics in the heart in obesity-related diabetes: direct evidence for increased uncoupled respiration and activation of uncoupling proteins. Diabetes 2007;56:2457.
19. Mazumder PK, O'Neill BT, Roberts MW, et al. Impaired cardiac efficiency and increased fatty acid oxidation in insulin-resistant ob/ob mouse hearts. Diabetes 2004;53:2366.
20. Kuo TH, Moore KH, Giacomelli F, et al. Defective oxidative metabolism of heart mitochondria from genetically diabetic mice. Diabetes 1983;32:781.
21. Bugger H, Abel ED. Rodent models of diabetic cardiomyopathy. Dis Model Mech 2009;2:454.

22. Howarth FC, Qureshi MA, Sobhy ZH, et al. Structural lesions and changing pattern of expression of genes encoding cardiac muscle proteins are associated with ventricular myocyte dysfunction in type 2 diabetic Goto-Kakizaki rats fed a high-fat diet. Exp Physiol 2011;96:765.

23. Minamiyama Y, Bito Y, Takemura S, et al. Calorie restriction improves cardiovascular risk factors via reduction of mitochondrial reactive oxygen species in type II diabetic rats. J Pharmacol Exp Ther 2007; 320:535.

24. Oliveira PJ, Seica R, Santos DL, et al. Vitamin E or coenzyme Q10 administration is not fully advantageous for heart mitochondrial function in diabetic goto kakizaki rats. Mitochondrion 2004;3:337.

25. Buchanan J, Mazumder PK, Hu P, et al. Reduced cardiac efficiency and altered substrate metabolism precedes the onset of hyperglycemia and contractile dysfunction in two mouse models of insulin resistance and obesity. Endocrinology 2005;146:5341.

26. Aoyama T, Peters JM, Iritani N, et al. Altered constitutive expression of fatty acid-metabolizing enzymes in mice lacking the peroxisome proliferator-activated receptor alpha (PPARalpha). J Biol Chem 1998;273:5678.

27. Campbell FM, Kozak R, Wagner A, et al. A role for peroxisome proliferator-activated receptor alpha (PPARalpha) in the control of cardiac malonyl-CoA levels: reduced fatty acid oxidation rates and increased glucose oxidation rates in the hearts of mice lacking PPARalpha are associated with higher concentrations of malonyl-CoA and reduced expression of malonyl-CoA decarboxylase. J Biol Chem 2002;277:4098.

28. Bugger H, Chen D, Riehle C, et al. Tissue-specific remodeling of the mitochondrial proteome in type 1 diabetic akita mice. Diabetes 2009;58:1986.

29. Finck BN, Lehman JJ, Leone TC, et al. The cardiac phenotype induced by PPARalpha overexpression mimics that caused by diabetes mellitus. J Clin Invest 2002;109:121.

30. Sharma S, Adrogue JV, Golfman L, et al. Intramyocardial lipid accumulation in the failing human heart resembles the lipotoxic rat heart. FASEB J 2004;18:1692.

31. Turko IV, Li L, Aulak KS, et al. Protein tyrosine nitration in the mitochondria from diabetic mouse heart. Implications to dysfunctional mitochondria in diabetes. J Biol Chem 2003;278:33972.

32. Chiu HC, Kovacs A, Ford DA, et al. A novel mouse model of lipotoxic cardiomyopathy. J Clin Invest 2001;107:813.

33. Zhou YT, Grayburn P, Karim A, et al. Lipotoxic heart disease in obese rats: implications for human obesity. Proc Natl Acad Sci U S A 2000; 97:1784.

34. Bugger H, Abel ED. Molecular mechanisms for myocardial mitochondrial dysfunction in the metabolic syndrome. Clin Sci (Lond) 2008; 114:195.

35. Morrow DA, Givertz MM. Modulation of myocardial energetics: emerging evidence for a therapeutic target in cardiovascular disease. Circulation 2005; 112:3218.

36. Nishikawa T, Edelstein D, Du XL, et al. Normalizing mitochondrial superoxide production blocks three pathways of hyperglycaemic damage. Nature 2000;404:787.

37. Yamagishi SI, Edelstein D, Du XL, et al. Leptin induces mitochondrial superoxide production and monocyte chemoattractant protein-1 expression in aortic endothelial cells by increasing fatty acid oxidation via protein kinase A. J Biol Chem 2001; 276:25096.

38. Esposito LA, Melov S, Panov A, et al. Mitochondrial disease in mouse results in increased oxidative stress. Proc Natl Acad Sci U S A 1999;96:4820.

39. Wallace DC. Mitochondrial genetics: a paradigm for aging and degenerative diseases? Science 1992;256:628.

40. Lashin OM, Szweda PA, Szweda LI, et al. Decreased complex II respiration and HNE-modified SDH subunit in diabetic heart. Free Radic Biol Med 2006;40:886.

41. Shen X, Zheng S, Metreveli NS, et al. Protection of cardiac mitochondria by overexpression of MnSOD reduces diabetic cardiomyopathy. Diabetes 2006; 55:798.

42. Ye G, Metreveli NS, Donthi RV, et al. Catalase protects cardiomyocyte function in models of type 1 and type 2 diabetes. Diabetes 2004;53: 1336.

43. Conti M, Renaud IM, Poirier B, et al. High levels of myocardial antioxidant defense in aging nondiabetic normotensive Zucker obese rats. Am J Physiol Regul Integr Comp Physiol 2004;286:R793.

44. Santos DL, Palmeira CM, Seica R, et al. Diabetes and mitochondrial oxidative stress: a study using heart mitochondria from the diabetic Goto-Kakizaki rat. Mol Cell Biochem 2003;246:163.

45. Vincent HK, Powers SK, Stewart DJ, et al. Obesity is associated with increased myocardial oxidative stress. Int J Obes Relat Metab Disord 1999;23:67.

46. Isenberg G, Han S, Schiefer A, et al. Changes in mitochondrial calcium concentration during the cardiac contraction cycle. Cardiovasc Res 1993; 27:1800.

47. Denton RM, Randle PJ, Martin BR. Stimulation by calcium ions of pyruvate dehydrogenase phosphate phosphatase. Biochem J 1972;128:161.

48. Nichols BJ, Denton RM. Towards the molecular basis for the regulation of mitochondrial

dehydrogenases by calcium ions. Mol Cell Biochem 1995;149–150:203.

49. Territo PR, Mootha VK, French SA, et al. Ca(2+) activation of heart mitochondrial oxidative phosphorylation: role of the F(0)/F(1)-ATPase. Am J Physiol Cell Physiol 2000;278:C423.

50. Flarsheim CE, Grupp IL, Matlib MA. Mitochondrial dysfunction accompanies diastolic dysfunction in diabetic rat heart. Am J Physiol 1996;271: H192.

51. Pierce GN, Dhalla NS. Heart mitochondrial function in chronic experimental diabetes in rats. Can J Cardiol 1985;1:48.

52. Belke DD, Dillmann WH. Altered cardiac calcium handling in diabetes. Curr Hypertens Rep 2004;6:424.

53. Bouchard RA, Bose D. Influence of experimental diabetes on sarcoplasmic reticulum function in rat ventricular muscle. Am J Physiol 1991;260: H341.

54. Oliveira PJ, Seica R, Coxito PM, et al. Enhanced permeability transition explains the reduced calcium uptake in cardiac mitochondria from streptozotocin-induced diabetic rats. FEBS Lett 2003;554:511.

55. Dong F, Zhang X, Yang X, et al. Impaired cardiac contractile function in ventricular myocytes from leptin-deficient ob/ob obese mice. J Endocrinol 2006;188:25.

56. Fauconnier J, Lanner JT, Zhang SJ, et al. Insulin and inositol 1,4,5-trisphosphate trigger abnormal cytosolic Ca2+ transients and reveal mitochondrial Ca2+ handling defects in cardiomyocytes of ob/ob mice. Diabetes 2005;54:2375.

57. Belke DD, Swanson EA, Dillmann WH. Decreased sarcoplasmic reticulum activity and contractility in diabetic db/db mouse heart. Diabetes 2004;53: 3201.

58. Belke DD, Betuing S, Tuttle MJ, et al. Insulin signaling coordinately regulates cardiac size, metabolism, and contractile protein isoform expression. J Clin Invest 2002;109:629.

59. Boudina S, Bugger H, Sena S, et al. Contribution of impaired myocardial insulin signaling to mitochondrial dysfunction and oxidative stress in the heart. Circulation 2009;119:1272.

60. Bugger H, Riehle C, Jaishy B, et al. Genetic loss of insulin receptors worsens cardiac efficiency in diabetes. J Mol Cell Cardiol 2012;52(5): 1019–26.

61. Smith RA, Porteous CM, Coulter CV, et al. Selective targeting of an antioxidant to mitochondria. Eur J Biochem 1999;263:709.

62. Jauslin ML, Meier T, Smith RA, et al. Mitochondria-targeted antioxidants protect Friedreich Ataxia fibroblasts from endogenous oxidative stress more effectively than untargeted antioxidants. FASEB J 2003;17:1972.

63. Kelso GF, Porteous CM, Coulter CV, et al. Selective targeting of a redox-active ubiquinone to mitochondria within cells: antioxidant and antiapoptotic properties. J Biol Chem 2001;276:4588.

64. Ross MF, Prime TA, Abakumova I, et al. Rapid and extensive uptake and activation of hydrophobic triphenylphosphonium cations within cells. Biochem J 2008;411:633.

65. Smith RA, Porteous CM, Gane AM, et al. Delivery of bioactive molecules to mitochondria in vivo. Proc Natl Acad Sci U S A 2003;100:5407.

66. Davidson SM, Yellon DM, Murphy MP, et al. Slow calcium waves and redox changes precede mitochondrial permeability transition pore opening in the intact heart during hypoxia and reoxygenation. Cardiovasc Res 2012;93:445.

67. Vergeade A, Mulder P, Vendeville-Dehaudt C, et al. Mitochondrial impairment contributes to cocaine-induced cardiac dysfunction: prevention by the targeted antioxidant MitoQ. Free Radic Biol Med 2010;49:748.

68. Supinski GS, Murphy MP, Callahan LA. MitoQ administration prevents endotoxin-induced cardiac dysfunction. Am J Physiol Regul Integr Comp Physiol 2009;297:R1095.

69. Adlam VJ, Harrison JC, Porteous CM, et al. Targeting an antioxidant to mitochondria decreases cardiac ischemia-reperfusion injury. FASEB J 2005;19:1088.

70. Rodriguez-Cuenca S, Cocheme HM, Logan A, et al. Consequences of long-term oral administration of the mitochondria-targeted antioxidant MitoQ to wild-type mice. Free Radic Biol Med 2010;48:161.

71. Dhanasekaran A, Kotamraju S, Kalivendi SV, et al. Supplementation of endothelial cells with mitochondria-targeted antioxidants inhibit peroxide-induced mitochondrial iron uptake, oxidative damage, and apoptosis. J Biol Chem 2004;279: 37575.

72. Mao G, Kraus GA, Kim I, et al. Effect of a mitochondria-targeted vitamin E derivative on mitochondrial alteration and systemic oxidative stress in mice. Br J Nutr 2011;106:87.

73. Mao G, Kraus GA, Kim I, et al. A mitochondria-targeted vitamin E derivative decreases hepatic oxidative stress and inhibits fat deposition in mice. J Nutr 2010;140:1425.

74. Gane EJ, Weilert F, Orr DW, et al. The mitochondria-targeted anti-oxidant mitoquinone decreases liver damage in a phase II study of hepatitis C patients. Liver Int 2010;30:1019.

75. Frantz MC, Wipf P. Mitochondria as a target in treatment. Environ Mol Mutagen 2010;51:462.

76. Sheu SS, Nauduri D, Anders MW. Targeting antioxidants to mitochondria: a new therapeutic direction. Biochim Biophys Acta 2006;1762:256.

77. Trnka J, Blaikie FH, Logan A, et al. Antioxidant properties of MitoTEMPOL and its hydroxylamine. Free Radic Res 2009;43:4.

78. Dai DF, Chen T, Szeto H, et al. Mitochondrial targeted antioxidant peptide ameliorates hypertensive cardiomyopathy. J Am Coll Cardiol 2011;58:73.

79. Bantle JP, Wylie-Rosett J, Albright AL, et al. Nutrition recommendations and interventions for diabetes: a position statement of the American Diabetes Association. Diabetes Care 2008;31(Suppl 1):S61.

80. Cohen HY, Miller C, Bitterman KJ, et al. Calorie restriction promotes mammalian cell survival by inducing the SIRT1 deacetylase. Science 2004; 305:390.

81. Colom B, Oliver J, Roca P, et al. Caloric restriction and gender modulate cardiac muscle mitochondrial H_2O_2 production and oxidative damage. Cardiovasc Res 2007;74:456.

82. Gredilla R, Sanz A, Lopez-Torres M, et al. Caloric restriction decreases mitochondrial free radical generation at complex I and lowers oxidative damage to mitochondrial DNA in the rat heart. FASEB J 2001;15:1589.

83. Shinmura K, Tamaki K, Sano M, et al. Caloric restriction primes mitochondria for ischemic stress by deacetylating specific mitochondrial proteins of the electron transport chain. Circ Res 2011;109:396.

84. Viljanen AP, Karmi A, Borra R, et al. Effect of caloric restriction on myocardial fatty acid uptake, left ventricular mass, and cardiac work in obese adults. Am J Cardiol 2009;103:1721.

85. Hammer S, Snel M, Lamb HJ, et al. Prolonged caloric restriction in obese patients with type 2 diabetes mellitus decreases myocardial triglyceride content and improves myocardial function. J Am Coll Cardiol 2008;52:1006.

86. Baur JA, Pearson KJ, Price NL, et al. Resveratrol improves health and survival of mice on a high-calorie diet. Nature 2006;444:337.

87. Brasnyo P, Molnar GA, Mohas M, et al. Resveratrol improves insulin sensitivity, reduces oxidative stress and activates the Akt pathway in type 2 diabetic patients. Br J Nutr 2011;106:383.

88. Xu Y, Nie L, Yin YG, et al. Resveratrol protects against hyperglycemia-induced oxidative damage to mitochondria by activating SIRT1 in rat mesangial cells. Toxicol Appl Pharmacol 2012;259(3): 395–401.

89. Danz ED, Skramsted J, Henry N, et al. Resveratrol prevents doxorubicin cardiotoxicity through mitochondrial stabilization and the Sirt1 pathway. Free Radic Biol Med 2009;46:1589.

90. Tatlidede E, Sehirli O, Velioglu-Ogunc A, et al. Resveratrol treatment protects against doxorubicin-induced cardiotoxicity by alleviating oxidative damage. Free Radic Res 2009;43:195.

91. Sulaiman M, Matta MJ, Sunderesan NR, et al. Resveratrol, an activator of SIRT1, upregulates sarcoplasmic calcium ATPase and improves cardiac function in diabetic cardiomyopathy. Am J Physiol Heart Circ Physiol 2010;298:H833.

92. Xi J, Wang H, Mueller RA, et al. Mechanism for resveratrol-induced cardioprotection against reperfusion injury involves glycogen synthase kinase 3beta and mitochondrial permeability transition pore. Eur J Pharmacol 2009;604:111.

93. Dolinsky VW, Dyck JR. Calorie restriction and resveratrol in cardiovascular health and disease. Biochim Biophys Acta 2011;1812:1477.

94. Lagouge M, Argmann C, Gerhart-Hines Z, et al. Resveratrol improves mitochondrial function and protects against metabolic disease by activating SIRT1 and PGC-1alpha. Cell 2006;127:1109.

95. Aasum E, Belke DD, Severson DL, et al. Cardiac function and metabolism in type 2 diabetic mice after treatment with BM 17.0744, a novel PPAR-alpha activator. Am J Physiol Heart Circ Physiol 2002;283:H949.

96. Aasum E, Khalid AM, Gudbrandsen OA, et al. Fenofibrate modulates cardiac and hepatic metabolism and increases ischemic tolerance in diet-induced obese mice. J Mol Cell Cardiol 2008;44:201.

97. How OJ, Larsen TS, Hafstad AD, et al. Rosiglitazone treatment improves cardiac efficiency in hearts from diabetic mice. Arch Physiol Biochem 2007;113:211.

98. Carley AN, Semeniuk LM, Shimoni Y, et al. Treatment of type 2 diabetic db/db mice with a novel PPARgamma agonist improves cardiac metabolism but not contractile function. Am J Physiol Endocrinol Metab 2004;286:E449.

99. Brunmair B, Staniek K, Gras F, et al. Thiazolidinediones, like metformin, inhibit respiratory complex I: a common mechanism contributing to their antidiabetic actions? Diabetes 2004;53:1052.

100. Nadanaciva S, Dykens JA, Bernal A, et al. Mitochondrial impairment by PPAR agonists and statins identified via immunocaptured OXPHOS complex activities and respiration. Toxicol Appl Pharmacol 2007;223:277.

101. Soller M, Drose S, Brandt U, et al. Mechanism of thiazolidinedione-dependent cell death in Jurkat T cells. Mol Pharmacol 2007;71:1535.

102. Nesto RW, Bell D, Bonow RO, et al. Thiazolidinedione use, fluid retention, and congestive heart failure: a consensus statement from the American Heart Association and American Diabetes Association. Diabetes Care 2004;27:256.

103. Nissen SE, Wolski K. Rosiglitazone revisited: an updated meta-analysis of risk for myocardial infarction and cardiovascular mortality. Arch Intern Med 2010;170:1191.

104. Yamada Y, Akita H, Kamiya H, et al. MITO-Porter: a liposome-based carrier system for delivery of macromolecules into mitochondria via membrane fusion. Biochim Biophys Acta 2008;1778:423.

105. Yamada Y, Furukawa R, Yasuzaki Y, et al. Dual function MITO-Porter, a nano carrier integrating both efficient cytoplasmic delivery and mitochondrial macromolecule delivery. Mol Ther 2011;19:1449.

106. Yamada Y, Harashima H. Delivery of bioactive molecules to the mitochondrial genome using a membrane-fusing, liposome-based carrier, DF-MITO-Porter. Biomaterials 2012;33:1589.

Postprandial Dysmetabolism and the Heart

Alan J. Garber, MD, PhD

KEYWORDS

- Postprandial dysmetabolism • Cardiovascular disease • Type 2 diabetes
- Impaired glucose tolerance • Endothelial function

KEY POINTS

- Postprandial dysmetabolism (ie, abnormal elevations in blood glucose and lipid levels after a meal) is associated with an increased risk of cardiovascular disease.
- Both postprandial hyperglycemia and postprandial hyperlipidemia have a direct detrimental effect on endothelial function that is more pronounced when both derangements coexist.
- Pharmacotherapies that specifically target postprandial hyperglycemia and/or postprandial hyperlipidemia have a beneficial effect on endothelial function, which may positively affect cardiovascular outcomes.

INTRODUCTION

Postprandial Dysmetabolism: Nature of the Problem

Postprandial dysmetabolism refers to abnormal elevations in blood glucose and lipid levels that occur after a meal.[1] In patients with type 2 diabetes (T2D), postprandial dysmetabolism is common, as hyperglycemia frequently coexists with dyslipidemia in both the fasting and postprandial stages.[2] However, postprandial dysmetabolism can also occur in the absence of overt T2D,[1] perhaps not surprisingly, as both components of this metabolic derangement are closely linked with insulin resistance,[3] which is recognized as the primary defect in T2D.[4] Indeed, insulin resistance, which can start many years before the onset of the disease, underlies the mildly elevated postprandial glucose (PPG) levels, known as impaired glucose tolerance (IGT), that precede overt diabetes. Initially, pancreatic β cells are able to compensate for the decreased sensitivity of peripheral tissues to insulin by increasing insulin secretion. However, β-cell function eventually deteriorates resulting in the increasingly elevated postprandial and fasting glucose levels that define T2D.[5] A lack of postprandial suppression of glucagon secretion, for which insulin resistance is partly responsible, is also apparent early in the natural history of T2D, leading to increased hepatic glucose output and further exacerbation of postprandial hyperglycemia.[6] In addition, insulin resistance has been linked independently with postprandial elevations in lipid levels.[7]

Patients with IGT and T2D are at increased risk for developing cardiovascular disease (CVD) compared with their normoglycemic counterparts[8–10]; however, traditional risk factors cannot explain fully the excess risk of CVD observed in these patients.[11] A growing body of evidence indicates that postprandial dysmetabolism may play a role in the development of atherosclerosis

Financial disclosures and conflicts of interest: Alan J. Garber, MD, PhD, has served as an advisor or consultant for: Boehringer Ingelheim Pharmaceuticals, Inc; LipoScience, Inc; Merck & Co, Inc; Novo Nordisk; OSI Pharmaceuticals, Inc; Takeda Pharmaceuticals North America, Inc; and as a speaker or a member of a speaker's bureau for: Merck & Co, Inc; Novo Nordisk; OSI Pharmaceuticals, Inc; Santarus, Inc.
Division of Diabetes, Endocrinology and Metabolism, Department of Medicine, Baylor College of Medicine, 1709 Dryden Road, Suite 1000, Houston, Tx 77030, USA
E-mail address: agarber@bcm.tmc.edu

through a detrimental effect on endothelial function, which is mediated by oxidative stress. Thus, postprandial dysmetabolism is now recognized as a risk factor for CVD that could account, at least in part, for the excess risk of CVD observed in patients with T2D.[12,13]

The aim of this review is to discuss:

- The evidence linking postprandial dysmetabolism with an increased risk of CVD
- The detrimental effect of postprandial dysmetabolism on the cardiovascular system
- The pharmacologic options available to address postprandial dysmetabolism

THE LINK BETWEEN POSTPRANDIAL DYSMETABOLISM AND CVD
Postprandial Hyperglycemia and Risk of CVD

An association between hyperglycemia and CVD has long been recognized.[14,15] This association extends below the diabetic threshold, as the CVD risk is already increased when blood glucose levels are only mildly elevated. For instance, both impaired fasting glucose (IFG) and IGT were associated with a significant increase in the relative risk (RR) for a cardiovascular event in a meta-analysis performed by Coutinho and colleagues[10] (n = 95,783). Of note, the risk was slightly greater with IGT than with IFG (RR = 1.58 vs 1.33), suggesting that postprandial hyperglycemia may play an important role in the development of macrovascular complications.

Indeed, several epidemiologic studies have shown postprandial hyperglycemia to be associated with increased CVD morbidity and mortality, in individuals both with or without overt T2D. In the Diabetes Epidemiology: Collaborative analysis Of Diagnostic criteria in Europe (DECODE) study (n = 25,364), 2-hour postload hyperglycemia, a surrogate for postprandial hyperglycemia, was associated with an increased risk of mortality for CVD regardless of fasting plasma glucose levels, and abnormalities in 2-hour plasma glucose were a better predictor of CVD and non-CVD mortality than fasting glucose alone.[16] Similarly, in the Funagata Diabetes Study in Japan (n = 2691), CVD mortality more than doubled in individuals with IGT or diabetes compared with their normoglycemic counterparts, whereas IFG did not have a significant effect (Fig. 1).[17]

More specifically, postprandial hyperglycemia has been linked to an increased risk in coronary artery disease (CAD)-related events, such as fatal and nonfatal ischemic heart disease, stroke, and CAD-related mortality. For instance, in the

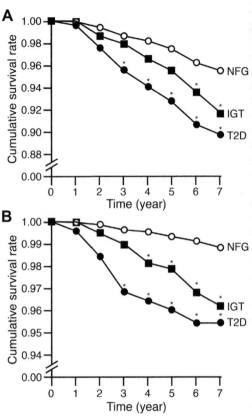

Fig. 1. Effect of impaired fasting glucose and type 2 diabetes on all-cause (A) and cardiovascular (B) mortality in the Funagata Diabetes Study. IGT, impaired fasting glucose; NFG, normal fasting glucose; T2D, type 2 diabetes. *P<.05. (Reproduced from Tominaga M, Eguchi H, Manaka H, et al. Impaired glucose tolerance is a risk factor for cardiovascular disease, but not impaired fasting glucose. The Funagata Diabetes Study. Diabetes Care 1999;22:920–4. Available at: http://care.diabetesjournals.org/content/22/6/920.long. ©1999, American Diabetes Association; with permission.)

Whitehall Study (n = 18,403), CAD-related mortality approximately doubled in individuals with IGT compared with normoglycemic individuals.[9] The Whitehall data are consistent with results from the Honolulu Heart Study (n = 8006), in which the rate of coronary heart disease was directly proportional to 1-hour glucose levels after a glucose challenge, with the risk doubling in those within the highest quintile of postchallenge glucose concentration compared with the lowest quintile.[18]

The increased risk of CAD associated with increasing blood glucose levels after an oral glucose challenge is not confined to men; results from the Bedford Survey (male: n = 285; female: n = 267) revealed that the odds ratio for death due to ischemic heart disease in individuals with a 2-hour postchallenge glucose level higher than 140 mg/dL (>5.6 mmol/L) was much greater in women than in men (5.16 vs 1.42, respectively).[19] Similarly, in the San Luigi Gonzaga Diabetes Study in individuals with T2D (male: n = 284; female: n = 145), PPG levels (but not fasting glucose or A1c) predicted cardiovascular events; compared with the first and second tertiles, hazard ratios in the third tertile of PPG levels were significantly greater in women than in men (5.54 vs 2.12, respectively).[20]

The risk of fatal stroke also increases with increasing glucose levels after an oral glucose tolerance test (OGTT). In the DECODE study, the RR of death from stroke increased by 21% in individuals with 2-hour plasma glucose concentration in the range of 140 to 198 mg/dL (7.8–11.0 mmol/L) compared with those who had levels below the lower end of this range.[16] Furthermore, in the Oslo study (n = 16,209 men), nonfasting glucose levels predicted fatal stroke in participants with or without diabetes, with a risk increase of 13% per 18 mg/dL (1 mmol/L) increase in blood glucose.[21]

Therefore, postprandial hyperglycemia is associated with increased CVD morbidity and mortality in individuals with or without T2D, and may be a better predictor of cardiovascular events than fasting plasma glucose, particularly in women.

Postprandial Dyslipidemia and Risk of CVD

Atherogenic dyslipidemia, characterized by elevated serum levels of very low-density lipoproteins (VLDL) and triglycerides and decreased levels of high-density lipoproteins (HDL), is frequently present in people with T2D and/or metabolic syndrome, and is an important cardiovascular risk factor.[22] Although elevated fasting triglyceride and HDL-cholesterol levels have both been associated with increased cardiovascular risk, several studies have shown postprandial triglyceride levels to be an independent and stronger predictor of risk than fasting HDL cholesterol.[23,24]

Indeed, postprandial hypertriglyceridemia, particularly in women, is associated with increased risk of cardiovascular mortality and cardiovascular events, such as myocardial infarction (MI) and stroke (**Table 1**).[25–30] For example, increasing nonfasting triglyceride serum levels have been linked to a significant increase in the RR for coronary deaths in women and a slight, but not significant, increase in men. In fact, women with nonfasting triglyceride serum levels above 310 mg/dL (3.5 mmol/L) have been shown to have an approximately 5-fold increase in the risk

of dying from coronary heart disease compared with women with triglyceride levels below 133 mg/dL (1.5 mmol/L).[25] Moreover, after adjusting for other common cardiovascular risk factors, nonfasting triglyceride levels (but not fasting triglyceride levels) have been strongly and independently associated with cardiovascular events.[26] In addition, increased nonfasting triglyceride levels significantly increased the risk of MI in both men and women, and of ischemic stroke in women (see **Table 1**).[28,29]

DIRECT EFFECT OF POSTPRANDIAL DYSMETABOLISM ON THE CARDIOVASCULAR SYSTEM

Given the link between both components of postprandial dysmetabolism and the increased risk of CVD, several studies have investigated the direct effect of these metabolic derangements on the cardiovascular system. Evidence indicates that both postprandial hyperglycemia and postprandial dyslipidemia can cause vascular damage by triggering endothelial dysfunction,[31–34] which is the initial step in the development of atherosclerosis and CVD.[35]

The most widely recognized abnormality of endothelial dysfunction is a reduction in the bioavailability of nitric oxide (NO), a signaling molecule released by the vascular endothelium with potent vasodilatory, anti-inflammatory, and anti-platelet effects.[36] As a result, several interrelated atherogenic changes take place, including impairment of endothelium-dependent vasodilation, hypercoagulation, and inflammation, with alterations in markers used to estimate endothelial function, which cannot be measured directly.

Both postprandial hyperglycemia and postprandial dyslipidemia independently have a detrimental effect on markers of endothelial dysfunction; interestingly, this effect worsens when both derangements coexist.[31–34,37–43]

Impact of Postprandial Hyperglycemia on the Cardiovascular System

Several studies have investigated the direct effect of postprandial hyperglycemia on markers of endothelial dysfunction. For example, Kawano and colleagues[31] measured flow-mediated vasodilation (FMD) of the brachial artery (a surrogate of endothelial function) in individuals with normal glucose tolerance (NGT) (n = 17), IGT (n = 24), or T2D (n = 17) at fasting, and after an OGTT. Compared with fasting values, FMD decreased significantly, and to similar levels, in individuals with IGT or with T2D, although FMD recovered more quickly in individuals with IGT compared

Table 1
Relative risk of cardiovascular outcomes with nonfasting triglyceride levels

Authors,[Ref.] Year	Population	Follow-Up	Outcome(s), No. of Event(s)	Adjusted Relative Risk (95% CI)
Tverdal et al,[30] 1989	37,546 men aged 35–49 y, without history of CVD or diabetes	9 y (mean)	Coronary death (n = 369)	1.1 (1.0–1.2)
Stensvold et al,[25] 1993	24,535 women aged 35–49 y, without history of CVD or diabetes	14.6 y (mean)	Coronary death (n = 108)	Men: 1.1 (1.0–1.2) Women: 1.6 (1.2–2.1)
Stampfer et al,[28] 1996	14,916 men without history of CVD (85% nonfasting)	7 y	MI, cases (n = 266) vs controls (n = 308)	1.4 (1.1–1.8)
Eberly et al,[27] 2003	2809 male participants without clinical evidence of CVD in the MRFIT study	25 y	8-y nonfatal or fatal CHD (n = 175) 25-y fatal CHD (n = 328)	1.6 (1.2–2.3) fasting 1.5 (1.0–2.1) nonfasting 1.2 (1.0–1.6) fasting 1.3 (1.0–1.6) nonfasting
Nordestgaard et al,[29] 2009	7587 women and 6394 men form the general population in Copenhagen (Denmark)	26 y (mean)	MI (n = 1793) Ischemic heart disease (n = 3479)	1.2 (1.1–1.4) women 1.0 (1.0–1.1) men 1.1 (1.0–1.2) women 1.0 (1.0–1.1) men
Bansal et al,[26] 2007	26,509 healthy USA women, 20,118 fasting, 6391 nonfasting (<8 h since last meal)	11.4 y (mean)	Cardiovascular events (n = 1001)	1.1 (0.9–1.3) fasting 1.7 (1.2–2.4) nonfasting 4.5 (2.0–10.2) 2–4 h since last meal

Abbreviations: CI, confidence interval; CHD, coronary heart disease; CVD, cardiovascular disease; MI, myocardial infarction; MRFIT, Multiple Risk Factor Intervention Trial.

Reproduced from Ansar S, Koska J, Reaven PD. Postprandial hyperlipidemia, endothelial dysfunction and cardiovascular risk: focus on incretins. Cardiovasc Diabetol 2011;10:61. Available at: http://www.cardiab.com/content/10/1/61. ©2011 licensee BioMed Central Ltd; with permission.

with those with T2D. Of note, there were no changes in serum triglyceride levels in any of the groups after the OGTT, suggesting that the changes observed in FMD can be attributed to hyperglycemia. In addition, an increase in plasma levels of thiobarbituric acid reactive substances (a marker of oxidative stress) was associated with decreasing FMD, suggesting that an increase in reactive oxygen species may play a role in suppressing vasodilation.

Postprandial hyperglycemia has also been shown to induce hypercoagulability through platelet activation and changes in several factors involved in the coagulation cascade. In individuals with T2D (n = 12), markers of platelet activation in vivo and in vitro were significantly increased by acute hyperglycemia, but not during euglycemia.[41] In addition, in individuals with or without

T2D, an oral glucose load significantly increased plasma fibrinopeptide A, prothrombin fragment 1+2, and Factor VII, and decreased the half-life of fibrinogen, indicating activation of the coagulation cascade.[39,40]

In another study, the acute effect of raising glucose levels on several markers of inflammation, namely the cytokines interleukin-6 (IL-6), tumor necrosis factor α (TNF-α), and interleukin-18 (IL-18), was investigated in individuals with NGT (n = 20) or IGT (n = 15).[37] Cytokines increased significantly and to similar levels in both the NGT and IGT groups, but remained elevated for longer in the IGT group. In the IGT group, a transient increase in glucose resulted in significantly greater increases in cytokine levels compared with those observed during the sustained elevation of a hyperglycemic clamp, suggesting that the consequences of hyperglycemic spikes (similar to those occurring in the postprandial state) may be more damaging than those of continuous hyperglycemia on markers of inflammation. Infusion of the antioxidant glutathione suppressed the elevation in plasma cytokines induced by glucose spikes in both the NGT and IGT groups, suggesting that the detrimental effect of hyperglycemia on inflammation is mediated by oxidative stress.

Postprandial hyperglycemia also increases levels of inflammation markers in individuals with T2D (n = 20), compared with normoglycemic individuals (n = 20). After a high-carbohydrate meal, individuals with T2D had significantly elevated levels of TNF-α, IL-6, intercellular adhesion molecule 1 (ICAM-1), and vascular cell adhesion molecule 1 (VCAM-1) compared with normoglycemic individuals in the control group (n = 20).[38] Of note, ingestion of vitamin E and ascorbic acid with the meal abolished the increase in these inflammation markers, supporting the hypothesis that an oxidative mechanism mediates hyperglycemia-induced inflammation.[38]

Impact of Postprandial Dyslipidemia on the Cardiovascular System

Postprandial dyslipidemia also has a detrimental effect on endothelial function, as determined by FMD of the brachial artery and markers of inflammation. Following a fat tolerance test, FMD decreased significantly compared with fasting values in normoglycemic individuals (n = 12) and, to a greater extent, in individuals with T2D (n = 12).[42] In individuals with T2D and normoglycemic individuals, deterioration in endothelial function inversely correlated with fasting HDL-cholesterol levels, and directly and positively correlated with the magnitude of postprandial hypertriglyceridemia. Postprandial lipidemia also increased oxidative stress postprandially in both groups, although the increase was greater in the T2D group.[42]

In addition, increases in carotid intima-media thickness (IMT), which can be used to quantitatively evaluate early atherosclerotic changes, have been associated with postprandial hypertriglyceridemia induced by a high-fat meal in individuals with T2D.[43] Carotid IMT increased significantly after meal ingestion in individuals with normal fasting triglyceride levels but elevated postprandial triglyceride levels; these increases were more pronounced in individuals with elevated fasting and postprandial triglyceride levels versus individuals with fasting and postprandial triglyceride levels within the normal ranges. Fasting LDL-cholesterol and PPG levels and, more strongly, postprandial triglyceride levels, all had a significant, independent, positive correlation with the observed increase in carotid IMT.[43]

Similarly, in individuals with (n = 20) or without (n = 20) T2D, postprandial hyperlipidemia induced by a high-fat meal significantly increased levels of several markers of inflammation, such as cytokines (TNF-α, IL-6) and adhesion molecules (ICAM-1 and VCAM-1), compared with fasting levels.[38] Furthermore, in normoglycemic individuals (n = 18) a high-fat meal significantly increased the levels of endothelial microparticles (a marker of endothelial damage) compared with the levels observed after an isocaloric low-fat meal. This increase in endothelial microparticles directly correlated with a postprandial elevation of serum triglycerides.[34]

Cumulative Effect of Postprandial Hyperglycemia and Postprandial Dyslipidemia on the Cardiovascular System

Postprandial hyperglycemia and postprandial dyslipidemia are both associated with endothelial dysfunction; however, given that they frequently coexist, it is difficult to establish whether each factor has a distinct role. To elucidate the individual contribution of hyperglycemia and dyslipidemia to the development of endothelial dysfunction, the effect of a high-fat load alone, a glucose load alone, or a combination of both on serum glycemic and lipid levels, and on several markers of inflammation was investigated in individuals with T2D (n = 30) or normoglycemic individuals (n = 20).[44]

First, serum glycemic and lipid levels were examined. After the high-fat load alone and high-fat load/glucose load combination, serum triglycerides significantly increased from preprandial values in the normoglycemic (from 1 to 3 hours) and in the T2D group (from 1 to 4 hours; ie, for longer than in normoglycemic individuals); serum triglyceride levels did not change significantly from preprandial values after the glucose load alone. Conversely, after the glucose load alone and the high-fat load/glucose load combination, glycemic levels significantly increased in normoglycemic individuals (at 1 hour) and in the T2D group (from 1 to 3 hours; ie, for longer than in normoglycemic individuals); glycemic levels did not change significantly from preprandial values after the high-fat load alone.

Second, markers of inflammation were assessed. Following the same timeline as serum triglyceride and glucose levels, serum levels of inflammation markers (ICAM-1, VCAM-1, and E-selectin) and a marker of oxidative stress (nitrotyrosine) significantly increased from baseline values after the high-fat load alone and after the glucose load alone. Of note, increases in inflammation markers were more pronounced after the high-fat load/glucose load combination, suggesting that postprandial hyperglycemia and hypertriglyceridemia have an independent and cumulative effect on markers of endothelial dysfunction, and that oxidative stress may be the common mediator of this phenomenon.[44]

THERAPEUTIC OPTIONS FOR THE MANAGEMENT OF POSTPRANDIAL DYSMETABOLISM: CLINICAL OUTCOMES

Evidence suggests that there is a link between post-prandial dysmetabolism, endothelial dysfunction, and CVD risk; therefore, pharmacotherapies that significantly improve postprandial hyperglycemia and/or postprandial dyslipidemia are likely to have a beneficial effect on endothelial function. As many pharmacotherapies also modify other cardio-vascular risk factors, such as fasting glucose and lipids, body weight, and blood pressure, a direct cause-effect relationship is difficult to establish; nevertheless, the results of several studies appear to indicate that this is the case.

For example, in a study in drug-naïve individuals with T2D (n = 175), treatment with repaglinide, a rapid and short-acting insulin secretagogue, re-sulted in significantly greater reductions in PPG peaks than treatment with glyburide, which has a slower and longer-acting effect on insulin secre-tion. Conversely, reductions in fasting plasma glucose were greater in the glyburide group, whereas A1c reductions were similar in both groups, and there were no significant changes from baseline in lipid profiles or blood pressure in either group. However, carotid IMT regression was observed with repaglinide treatment, but not with glyburide, whereby carotid IMT remained stable. Thus, at comparable A1c levels, amelioration of PPG peaks appears to be more effective in reversing athero-sclerotic changes than amelioration of fasting hyperglycemia.[45]

In another study in individuals with T2D (n = 23) and normoglycemic individuals (n = 10), the effect of insulin aspart versus soluble human insulin on postprandial glycemia and endothelial function (as-sessed by changes in FMD in the brachial artery) was investigated. As expected, insulin aspart, which is more rapidly absorbed than soluble human insulin, provided significantly greater reductions in postprandial hyperglycemia. Compared with nor-moglycemic individuals, FMD after the meal test significantly decreased in both insulin-treated groups; however, the magnitude of change was significantly greater in the soluble human insulin group than in the insulin aspart group. Changes in free fatty acids and triglycerides after the meal were comparable in both insulin-treated groups,

suggesting that improvements in endothelial func-tion can be achieved by controlling PPG.[46]

The most compelling evidence that therapies that improve postprandial hyperglycemia can also reduce the risk of CVD has been obtained with the α-glucosidase inhibitor acarbose, which directly reduces PPG by delaying the enzymatic breakdown of carbohydrates (and therefore their absorption) in the small intestine.[47] In the Study to Prevent Non-Insulin-Dependent Diabetes Mellitus (STOP-NIDDM) (n = 1429 individuals with IGT), the decrease in postprandial hyperglycemia observed with acarbose was associated with a significant RR reduction in cardiovascular events (49%) and MI (91%) compared with placebo.[48] Furthermore, in a substudy of the STOP-NIDDM trial, treatment with acarbose significantly reduced the progression of atherosclerosis, assessed through measurements of carotid IMT, when compared with placebo.[49] Moreover, treatment with acarbose was found to significantly reduce the risk for cardiovascular events (35%) and MI (64%) compared with placebo in a meta-analysis that included data from 2180 individuals with T2D (**Fig. 2**).[50] As well as improving glycemic control, acarbose treatment had a beneficial effect on other cardiovascular risk factors, such as triglyceride levels and blood pressure (believed to be secondary effects resulting from improved PPG regulation) and body weight,[49] all of which are likely to play a role in the reductions in cardiovascular risk observed with acarbose.

Early evidence suggests that incretin-based therapies, which are antihyperglycemic agents available for the treatment of T2D, may also improve cardiovascular outcomes.[50–56] The incretin hormones (such as glucagon-like peptide 1 [GLP-1] and glucose-dependent insulinotropic peptide) are released in the intestine after food ingestion; they slow gastric emptying, increase insulin secretion, and decrease hepatic glucose output in a glucose-dependent manner, thus regu-lating PPG levels. However, incretins have limited therapeutic potential, as they are rapidly degraded by the enzyme dipeptidyl-peptidase 4 (DPP-4). Long-acting GLP-1 receptor agonists resistant to degradation by DPP-4 (such as exenatide and lira-glutide) and DPP-4 inhibitors (such as sitagliptin, vildagliptin, saxagliptin, and linagliptin) have been developed to overcome their susceptibility to degradation while remaining pharmacologically active[57]; indeed, as the only drug class capable of simultaneously targeting insulin insufficiency and inappropriate hyperglucagonemia (2 key defects in the pathophysiology of T2D[58]), GLP-1 receptor agonists and DPP-4 inhibitors significantly improve glycemic control (A1c, fasting plasma glucose

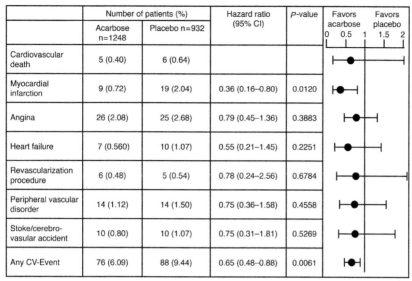

	Number of patients (%)		Hazard ratio (95% CI)	P-value	Favors acarbose	Favors placebo
	Acarbose n=1248	Placebo n=932				
Cardiovascular death	5 (0.40)	6 (0.64)				
Myocardial infarction	9 (0.72)	19 (2.04)	0.36 (0.16–0.80)	0.0120		
Angina	26 (2.08)	25 (2.68)	0.79 (0.45–1.36)	0.3883		
Heart failure	7 (0.560)	10 (1.07)	0.55 (0.21–1.45)	0.2251		
Revascularization procedure	6 (0.48)	5 (0.54)	0.78 (0.24–2.56)	0.6784		
Peripheral vascular disorder	14 (1.12)	14 (1.50)	0.75 (0.36–1.58)	0.4558		
Stoke/cerebro-vasular accident	10 (0.80)	10 (1.07)	0.75 (0.31–1.81)	0.5269		
Any CV-Event	76 (6.09)	88 (9.44)	0.65 (0.48–0.88)	0.0061		

Fig. 2. Effect of acarbose on the development of cardiovascular (CV) events: meta-analysis of 7 randomized, double-blind, placebo-controlled acarbose studies with a minimum treatment duration of 52 weeks. (*Reproduced from* Hanefeld M, Cagatay M, Petrowitsch T, et al. Acarbose reduces the risk for myocardial infarction in type 2 diabetic patients: meta-analysis of seven long-term studies. Eur Heart J 2004;25:10–6. Available at: http://stroke. ahajournals.org/content/35/5/1073.long. ©2004 Oxford University Press; with permission.)

levels, and PPG levels). In addition, GLP-1 receptor agonists are associated with significant reductions in body weight and systolic blood pressure, and modest improvements in lipid profiles, whereas DPP-4 inhibitors generally have neutral effects on these parameters.[59] Head-to-head studies have confirmed these differences between these 2 subclasses of incretin therapies.[60,61]

Moreover, the GLP-1 receptor agonist exenatide inhibits postprandial excursions of lipids and lipoproteins and postprandial glycemic excursions after a high-fat meal in individuals with IGT (n = 20) or recent-onset T2D (n = 15).[62] Endothelial function, assessed with peripheral arterial tonometry,

was significantly higher with exenatide than with placebo, with changes in postprandial triglycerides accounting for 64% of exenatide's effect on the endothelium. Neither PPG nor insulin concentrations were significantly associated with endothelial function in this study.[63]

Given the beneficial effect that incretin-based therapies, especially GLP-1 receptor agonists, have on many of the risk factors associated with CVD (including postprandial hyperglycemia and dyslipidemia), it seems plausible that they may have a beneficial effect on cardiovascular outcomes. Early data, based on combined analyses of clinical studies, are available for all

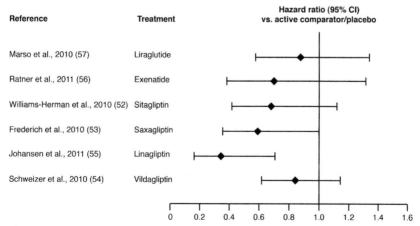

Reference	Treatment	Hazard ratio (95% CI) vs. active comparator/placebo
Marso et al., 2010 (57)	Liraglutide	
Ratner et al., 2011 (56)	Exenatide	
Williams-Herman et al., 2010 (52)	Sitagliptin	
Frederich et al., 2010 (53)	Saxagliptin	
Johansen et al., 2011 (55)	Linagliptin	
Schweizer et al., 2010 (54)	Vildagliptin	

Fig. 3. Effect of incretin-based therapies on major adverse cardiovascular events based on combined analyses of clinical studies. Hazard ratio with 95% confidence interval (CI).

Table 2
Summary of ongoing, long-term, cardiovascular outcome studies with available incretin-based therapies

Trial	Drug	Duration	Patients (n)
GLP-1 Receptor Agonists			
EXSCEL (Amylin Pharmaceuticals)	Exenatide once weekly	2010–2017	9500
LEADER (Novo Nordisk)	Liraglutide	2010–2016	9000
DPP-4 Inhibitors			
TECOS (Merck)	Sitagliptin	2008–2014	14000
SAVOR-TIMI 53 (AstraZeneca)	Saxagliptin	2010–2015	12000
CAROLINA (Boehringer Ingelheim)	Linagliptin	2010–2018	6000

approved incretin-based therapies. Except for linagliptin,[55] the number of cardiovascular events in clinical trials was too small to establish whether incretin-based therapies had a positive impact on these outcomes. However, compared with placebo and/or active comparators, incretin-based therapies were associated with a reduction (albeit not significant) in the risk of having a major cardiovascular adverse event (**Fig. 3**).[51–56] Nevertheless, only long-term outcome studies, specifically designed to test the effect of incretin-based therapies on cardiovascular outcomes, will be able to establish a benefit. Long-term outcome studies for all incretin-based therapies approved in the United States are ongoing (**Table 2**).[64–68]

Pharmacologic intervention that improves postprandial lipid levels has also been linked with improvements in endothelial function. In individuals with T2D (n = 30), increases in postprandial triglyceride levels, markers of inflammation (ICAM-1, VCAM-1, and E-selectin), and oxidative stress (nitrotyrosine) after a high-fat load, which did not substantially increase PPG levels, were significantly smaller after treatment with simvastatin compared with placebo.[44] Simvastatin also appeared to have a direct effect on markers of inflammation, as the postprandial increase in these markers was ameliorated with simvastatin versus placebo; this direct effect is likely mediated through reductions in oxidative stress, as nitrotyrosine levels were significantly reduced with simvastatin versus placebo.[44]

SUMMARY

Epidemiologic evidence suggests that both components of postprandial dysmetabolism are associated with an increased risk of CVD in individuals with or without T2D. To elucidate how postprandial dysmetabolism increases cardiovascular risk, numerous studies have investigated the direct effect

of postprandial hyperglycemia and/or postprandial dyslipidemia on the vascular system. The results of these studies revealed that both metabolic derangements are independently linked to deterioration in endothelial function and that their detrimental effect is more pronounced when postprandial hyperglycemia and postprandial dyslipidemia coexist. The deterioration in endothelial function is often associated with postprandial increases in reactive oxygen species, suggesting that oxidative stress is the mechanism of action by which postprandial dysmetabolism induces vascular damage. Therefore, it seems likely that intervention to effectively control postprandial glycemia and postprandial dyslipidemia will improve endothelial function and possibly affect cardiovascular outcomes; the results of various studies appear to indicate that this is the case. However, a direct cause-effect relationship cannot be established, as previous research was not specifically designed to test the effect of targeting postprandial dysmetabolism on the vascular system and cardiovascular outcomes. Future prospective, randomized controlled trials will be needed to establish whether postprandial dysmetabolism is an independent cardiovascular risk factor and whether intervention to control it improves cardiovascular outcomes.

ACKNOWLEDGMENTS

The author is grateful to Dr Angela Pozo Ramajo, of Watermeadow Medical (supported by Novo Nordisk Inc), for writing assistance.

REFERENCES

1. O'Keefe JH, Bell DSH. Postprandial hyperglycemia/hyperlipidemia (postprandial dysmetabolism) is a cardiovascular risk factor. Am J Cardiol 2007; 100:899–904.

2. Ceriello A. The post-prandial state and cardiovascular disease: relevance to diabetes mellitus. Diabetes Metab Res Rev 2000;16:125–32.

3. Yamagishi S, Matsui T, Ueda S, et al. Clinical utility of acarbose, an alpha-glucosidase inhibitor in cardiometabolic disorders. Curr Drug Metab 2009;10:159–63.

4. DeFronzo RA, Tripathy D. Skeletal muscle insulin resistance is the primary defect in type 2 diabetes. Diabetes Care 2009;32(Suppl 2):S157–63.

5. Ramlo-Halsted BA, Edelman SV. The natural history of type 2 diabetes: practical points to consider in developing prevention and treatment strategies. Clin Diabetes 2000;18:80–4.

6. Dunning BE, Gerich JE. The role of alpha-cell dysregulation in fasting and postprandial hyperglycemia in type 2 diabetes and therapeutic implications. Endocr Rev 2007;28:253–83.

7. Annuzzi G, De Natale C, Iovine C, et al. Insulin resistance is independently associated with postprandial alterations of triglyceride-rich lipoproteins in type 2 diabetes mellitus. Arterioscler Thromb Vasc Biol 2004;24:2397–402.

8. Haffner SM, Lehto S, Rönnemaa T, et al. Mortality from coronary heart disease in subjects with type 2 diabetes and in nondiabetic subjects with and without prior myocardial infarction. N Engl J Med 1998;339:229–34.

9. Fuller JH, Shipley MJ, Rose G, et al. Coronary-heart-disease risk and impaired glucose tolerance. The Whitehall study. Lancet 1980;1:1373–6.

10. Coutinho M, Gerstein HC, Wang Y, et al. The relationship between glucose and incident cardiovascular events. A metaregression analysis of published data from 20 studies of 95,783 individuals followed for 12.4 years. Diabetes Care 1999;22:233–40.

11. Laakso M. Hyperglycemia as a risk factor for cardiovascular disease in type 2 diabetes. Prim Care 1999;26:829–39.

12. Bell DS, O'Keefe JH, Jellinger P. Postprandial dysmetabolism: the missing link between diabetes and cardiovascular events? Endocr Pract 2008;14:112–24.

13. Tushuizen ME, Diamant M, Heine RJ. Postprandial dysmetabolism and cardiovascular disease in type 2 diabetes. Postgrad Med J 2005;81:1–6.

14. Klein R. Hyperglycemia and microvascular and macrovascular disease in diabetes. Diabetes Care 1995;18:258–68.

15. Stratton IM, Adler AI, Neil HA, et al. Association of glycaemia with macrovascular and microvascular complications of type 2 diabetes (UKPDS 35): prospective observational study. BMJ 2000;321(7258):405–12.

16. DECODE Study Group. Glucose tolerance and mortality: comparison of WHO and American Diabetes Association diagnostic criteria. Lancet 1999;354:617–21. Available at: http://www.thelancet.com/journals/lancet/article/PIIS0140-6736(98)12131-1/fulltext. Accessed February 1, 2012.

17. Tominaga M, Eguchi H, Manaka H, et al. Impaired glucose tolerance is a risk factor for cardiovascular disease, but not impaired fasting glucose. The Funagata Diabetes Study. Diabetes Care 1999;22:920–4. Available at: http://care.diabetesjournals.org/content/22/6/920.long. Accessed February 1, 2012.

18. Donahue RP, Abbott RD, Reed DM, et al. Postchallenge glucose concentration and coronary heart disease in men of Japanese ancestry. Honolulu Heart Program. Diabetes 1987;36:689–92.

19. Jarrett RJ, McCartney P, Keen H. The Bedford survey: ten year mortality rates in newly diagnosed diabetics, borderline diabetics and normoglycaemic controls and risk indices for coronary heart disease in borderline diabetics. Diabetologia 1982;22:79–84.

20. Cavalot F, Petrelli A, Traversa M, et al. Postprandial blood glucose is a stronger predictor of cardiovascular events than fasting blood glucose in type 2 diabetes mellitus, particularly in women: lessons from the San Luigi Gonzaga Diabetes Study. J Clin Endocrinol Metab 2006;91:813–9.

21. Håheim LL, Holme I, Hjermann I, et al. Nonfasting serum glucose and the risk of fatal stroke in diabetic and non-diabetic subjects. 18-year follow-up of the Oslo Study. Stroke 1995;26:774–7.

22. UK Prospective Diabetes Study Group. Plasma lipids and lipoproteins at diagnosis of NIDDM by age and sex. Diabetes Care 1997;20:1683–7.

23. Patsch JR, Miesenböck G, Hopferwieser T, et al. Relation of triglyceride metabolism and coronary artery disease. Studies in the postprandial state. Arterioscler Thromb 1992;12:1336–45.

24. Ansar S, Koska J, Reaven PD. Postprandial hyperlipidemia, endothelial dysfunction and cardiovascular risk: focus on incretins. Cardiovasc Diabetol 2011;10:61. Available at: http://www.cardiab.com/content/10/1/61. Accessed February 1, 2012.

25. Stensvold I, Tverdal A, Urdal P, et al. Non-fasting serum triglyceride concentration and mortality from coronary heart disease and any cause in middle aged Norwegian women. BMJ 1993;307(6913):1318–22.

26. Bansal S, Buring JE, Rifai N, et al. Fasting compared with non-fasting triglycerides and risk of cardiovascular events in women. JAMA 2007;298:309–16.

27. Eberly LE, Stamler J, Neaton JD, Multiple Risk Factor Intervention Trial Research Group. Relation of triglyceride levels, fasting and nonfasting, to fatal and nonfatal coronary heart disease. Arch Intern Med 2003;163:1077–83.

28. Stampfer MJ, Krauss RM, Ma J, et al. A prospective study of triglyceride level, low-density lipoprotein particle diameter, and risk of myocardial infarction. JAMA 1996;276:882–8.

29. Nordestgaard BG, Langsted A, Freiberg JJ. Nonfasting hyperlipidemia and cardiovascular disease. Curr Drug Targets 2009;10:328–35. Available at: http://www.benthamdirect.org/pages/content.php?CDT/2009/00000010/00000004/0004J.SGM. Accessed February 1, 2012.

30. Tverdal A, Foss OP, Leren P, et al. Serum triglycerides as an independent risk factor for death from coronary heart disease in middle-aged Norwegian men. Am J Epidemiol 1989;129(3):458–65.

31. Kawano H, Motoyama T, Hirashima O, et al. Hyperglycemia rapidly suppresses flow-mediated endothelium-dependent vasodilation of brachial artery. J Am Coll Cardiol 1999;34:146–54. Available at: http://www.sciencedirect.com/science/article/pii/S073510 9799001680. Accessed February 1, 2012.

32. Ceriello A, Falleti E, Motz E, et al. Hyperglycemia-induced circulating ICAM-1 increase in diabetes mellitus: the possible role of oxidative stress. Horm Metab Res 1998;30:146–9.

33. Moers A, Fenselau S, Schrezenmeir J. Chylomicrons induce E-selectin and VCAM-1 expression in endothelial cells. Exp Clin Endocrinol Diabetes 1997;105(Suppl 2):35–7.

34. Ferreira AC, Peter AA, Mendez AJ, et al. Postprandial hypertriglyceridemia increases circulating levels of endothelial cell microparticles. Circulation 2004;110:3599–603.

35. Widlansky ME, Gokce N, Keaney JF Jr, et al. The clinical implications of endothelial dysfunction. J Am Coll Cardiol 2003;42:1149–60. Available at: http://www.sciencedirect.com/science/article/pii/S0 73510970300994X. Accessed February 1, 2012.

36. Zeitler PS, Nadeau KJ. Insulin resistance. Childhood precursors and adult disease. Totowa (NJ): Humana Press; 2008. p. 180–1.

37. Esposito K, Nappo F, Marfella R, et al. Inflammatory cytokine concentrations are acutely increased by hyperglycemia in humans. Circulation 2002;106:2067–72.

38. Nappo F, Esposito K, Cioffi M, et al. Postprandial endothelial function in healthy subjects and in type 2 diabetic patients: role of fat and carbohydrates meals. J Am Coll Cardiol 2002;39:1145–50.

39. Ceriello A. Coagulation activation in diabetes mellitus: the role of hyperglycemia and therapeutic prospects. Diabetologia 1993;36:1119–25.

40. Ceriello A, Giacomello R, Stel G, et al. Hyperglycemia-induced thrombin formation in diabetes. The possible role of oxidative stress. Diabetes 1995;44:924–8.

41. Gresele P, Guglielmini G, De Angelis M, et al. Acute, short-term hyperglycemia enhances shear stress-induced platelet activation in patients with type II diabetes mellitus. J Am Coll Cardiol 2003;41:1013–20.

42. Anderson RA, Evans ML, Ellis GR, et al. The relationships between post-prandial lipaemia, endothelial function and oxidative stress in healthy individuals and patients with type 2 diabetes. Atherosclerosis 2001;154:475–83. Available at: http://www.atherosclerosis-journal.com/article/S0021-9150(00)00 499-8/abstract. Accessed February 1, 2012.

43. Teno S, Uto Y, Nagashima H, et al. Association of postprandial hypertriglyceridemia and carotid intima-media thickness in patients with type 2 diabetes. Diabetes Care 2000;23:1401–6.

44. Ceriello A, Quagliaro L, Piconi L, et al. Effect of postprandial hypertriglyceridemia and hyperglycemia on circulating adhesion molecules and oxidative stress generation and the possible role of simvastatin treatment. Diabetes 2004;53:701–10.

45. Esposito K, Giugliano D, Nappo F, et al. Campanian Postprandial Hyperglycemia Study Group. Regression of carotid atherosclerosis by control of postprandial hyperglycemia in type 2 diabetes mellitus. Circulation 2004;110:214–9. Available at: http://circ.ahajournals.org/content/110/2/214.long. Accessed February 1, 2012.

46. Ceriello A, Cavarape A, Martinelli L, et al. The postprandial state in Type 2 diabetes and endothelial dysfunction: effects of insulin aspart. Diabet Med 2004;21:171–5.

47. Bischoff H. Pharmacology of alpha-glucosidase inhibition. Eur J Clin Invest 1994;24(Suppl 3):3–10.

48. Chiasson JL, Josse RG, Gomis R, et al, STOP-NIDDM Trial Research Group. Acarbose treatment and the risk of cardiovascular disease and hypertension in patients with impaired glucose tolerance. JAMA 2003;290:486–94. Available at: http://jama.ama-assn.org/content/290/4/486.long. Accessed February 1, 2012.

49. Hanefeld M, Chiasson JL, Koehler C, et al. Acarbose slows progression of intima-media thickness of the carotid arteries in subjects with impaired glucose tolerance. Stroke 2004;35:1073–8.

50. Hanefeld M, Cagatay M, Petrowitsch T, et al. Acarbose reduces the risk for myocardial infarction in type 2 diabetic patients: meta-analysis of seven long-term studies. Eur Heart J 2004;25:10–6. Available at: http://stroke.ahajournals.org/content/35/5/1073.long. Accessed February 1, 2012.

51. Marso SP, Moses A, Zychma MJ, et al. Cardiovascular safety of liraglutide: a pooled analysis from phase II and III liraglutide clinical development studies [abstract]. Circulation 2010;122:A16904.

52. Williams-Herman D, Engel SS, Round E, et al. Safety and tolerability of sitagliptin in clinical studies: a pooled analysis of data from 10,246 patients with type 2 diabetes. BMC Endocr Disord 2010;10:7.

53. Frederich R, Alexander JH, Fiedorek FT, et al. A systematic assessment of cardiovascular outcomes in the saxagliptin drug development program for type 2 diabetes. Postgrad Med 2010;122:16–27.

54. Schweizer A, Dejager S, Foley JE, et al. Assessing the cardio-cerebrovascular safety of vildagliptin: meta-analysis of adjudicated events from a large Phase III type 2 diabetes population. Diabetes Obes Metab 2010;12:485–94.

55. Johansen OE, Neubacher D, Von Eynatten M, et al. Cardiovascular risk with linagliptin in patients with

type 2 diabetes: a pre-specified, prospective, and adjudicated meta-analysis from a large phase III program. Presented at American Diabetes Association Annual Meeting 2011, San Diego. Available at: http://professional.diabetes.org/Abstracts_Display.aspx?TYP=1&CID=88732. Accessed February 1, 2012.

56. Ratner R, Han J, Nicewarner D, et al. Cardiovascular safety of exenatide BID: an integrated analysis from controlled clinical trials in participants with type 2 diabetes. Cardiovasc Diabetol 2011;10:22.

57. Drucker DJ, Nauck MA. The incretin system: glucagon-like peptide-1 receptor agonists and dipeptidyl peptidase-4 inhibitors in type 2 diabetes. Lancet 2006;368:1696–705.

58. Hansen M, Hare KJ, Holst JJ, et al. Inhibition of glucagon secretion by GLP-1 agonists and DPP4 inhibitors. J Clin Metab Diabetes 2011;2:7–13.

59. Drab SR. Incretin-based therapies for type 2 diabetes mellitus: current status and future prospects. Pharmacotherapy 2010;30:609–24.

60. Pratley RE, Nauck M, Bailey T, et al. Liraglutide versus sitagliptin for patients with type 2 diabetes who did not have adequate glycaemic control with metformin: a 26-week, randomised, parallel-group, open-label trial. Lancet 2010;375:1447–56.

61. Bergenstal RM, Wysham C, Macconell L, et al. Efficacy and safety of exenatide once weekly versus sitagliptin or pioglitazone as an adjunct to metformin for treatment of type 2 diabetes (DURATION-2): a randomised trial. Lancet 2010;376:431–9.

62. Schwartz EA, Koska J, Mullin MP, et al. Exenatide suppresses postprandial elevations in lipids and lipoproteins in individuals with impaired glucose tolerance and recent onset type 2 diabetes mellitus. Atherosclerosis 2010;212:217–22. Available at: http://www.atherosclerosis-journal.com/article/S0021-9150(10)00406-5/abstract. Accessed February 1, 2012.

63. Koska J, Schwartz EA, Mullin MP, et al. Improvement of postprandial endothelial function after a single dose of exenatide in individuals with impaired

glucose tolerance and recent-onset type 2 diabetes. Diabetes Care 2010;33:1028–30. Available at: http://care.diabetesjournals.org/content/33/5/1028.long. Accessed February 1, 2012.

64. Amylin Pharmaceuticals. Exenatide Study of Cardiovascular Event Lowering Trial (EXSCEL): a trial to evaluate cardiovascular outcomes after treatment with exenatide once weekly in patients with type 2 diabetes mellitus. Available at: http://clinicaltrials.gov/ct2/show/NCT01144338. Accessed February 1, 2012.

65. Novo Nordisk. Liraglutide effect and action in diabetes: evaluation of cardiovascular outcome results—a long term evaluation (LEADER™). Available at: http://clinicaltrials.gov/ct2/show/NCT01179048?term=Liraglutide+LEADER&rank=1. Accessed February 1, 2012.

66. Merck & Co, Inc. TECOS: a randomized, placebo controlled clinical trial to evaluate cardiovascular outcomes after treatment with sitagliptin in patients with type 2 diabetes mellitus and inadequate glycemic control. Available at: http://clinicaltrials.gov/ct2/show/NCT00790205?term=TECOS+sitagliptin&rank=1. Accessed February 1, 2012.

67. AstraZeneca. A multicentre, randomised, double-blind, placebo-controlled phase IV trial to evaluate the effect of saxagliptin on the incidence of cardiovascular death, myocardial infarction or ischaemic stroke in patients with type 2 diabetes (SAVOR-TIMI 53). Available at: http://clinicaltrials.gov/ct2/show/NCT01107886?term=SAVOR-TIMI+53+saxagliptin&rank=1. Accessed February 1, 2012.

68. Boehringer Ingelheim Pharmaceuticals. A multicentre, international, randomised, parallel group, double blind study to evaluate cardiovascular safety of linagliptin versus glimepiride in patients with type 2 diabetes mellitus at high cardiovascular risk (CAROLINA). Available at: http://clinicaltrials.gov/ct2/show/NCT01243424?term=CAROLINA+linagliptin&rank=1. Accessed February 1, 2012.

Insulin Resistance and Atherosclerosis

Vasudevan A. Raghavan, MBBS, MD, MRCP (UK)[a,b,*]

KEYWORDS

- Insulin resistance • Atherosclerosis • Cardiovascular disease

KEY POINTS

- Overweight/obesity is associated with ectopic steatosis and progressive insulin resistance in various organs such as the liver, skeletal muscle, and adipose tissue.
- Atherogenic dyslipidemia, hyperinsulinemia, and hyperglycemia lead to endothelial dysfunction and atherosclerosis through multiple metabolic pathways.
- Insulin resistance is associated with activation of proinflammatory signals that promote atherosclerosis.
- Stress on the endoplasmic reticulum has more recently been identified as an important pathway that contributes to insulin resistance.

INTRODUCTION

Easy and affordable availability of calorie-dense food substrates and increasing adoption of a sedentary lifestyle without regular exercise has resulted in an increase in the incidence and prevalence of obesity worldwide. A major consequence is the increase in the number of those with diabetes mellitus (DM), which is projected to reach about 300 million people worldwide by 2020.[1]

DM is a group of metabolic diseases characterized by hyperglycemia resulting from defects in insulin secretion, insulin action, or both. The vast majority of DM cases belong to 2 etiopathogenetic categories commonly referred to as type 1 diabetes mellitus (T1DM) and type 2 diabetes mellitus (T2DM). In T1DM, the cause is an absolute deficiency of insulin secretion, and at-risk individuals can often be identified by serologic testing of autoimmune markers of pancreatic islet-cell damage and also by genetic markers. In T2DM, by far the more prevalent variety, the cause is a combination of resistance to insulin action and an inadequate compensatory insulin secretory response. In the latter category a clinically asymptomatic period, during which the patient experiences a degree of hyperglycemia sufficient to cause pathologic and functional changes in various target tissues, may be present for a long time before DM is detected. During this asymptomatic period, it is possible to demonstrate an abnormality in carbohydrate metabolism by measurement of plasma fasting glucose or after a challenge with an oral glucose load.[2]

PATHWAYS OF INSULIN RESISTANCE

Insulin resistance (IR) represents an altered and suboptimal biological response to normal insulin concentrations. Although the definition encompasses several biological actions of insulin in the body, it typically refers to a state in which a given concentration of insulin is associated with a subnormal glucose response.[3] Through its highly integrated actions on carbohydrate, protein, and lipid metabolism, insulin exerts a significant effect on the regulation of glucose homeostasis, most apparent in its effects in 3 tissues: liver, muscle, and adipose tissue. Insulin's actions are initiated by interaction with a specific transmembrane protein receptor, encoded by a single gene composed of 22 exons located on

[a] Division of Endocrinology, Department of Internal Medicine, Texas A&M Health Sciences Center and College of Medicine, Temple, TX 76508, USA; [b] Cardiometabolic, Lipid Clinic and Medical Weight Management Services, Scott and White, Center for Diagnostic Medicine, 1605 South, 31st Street, Temple, TX 76508, USA
* Center for Diagnostic Medicine, Suite M1209, 1605 South 31st Street, Temple, TX 76508.
E-mail address: raghavan@medicine.tamhsc.edu

Heart Failure Clin 8 (2012) 575–587
http://dx.doi.org/10.1016/j.hfc.2012.06.014
1551-7136/12/$ – see front matter © 2012 Elsevier Inc. All rights reserved

chromosome 19.[4] Detailed insulin effects, insulin receptor interaction, and mechanisms of IR are beyond the scope of this review and are discussed elsewhere in detail,[3] but it appears that 2 major postreceptor signaling pathways convey the insulin signal downstream.[5,6] One pathway involving the phosphorylation of insulin receptor substrate (IRS)-1 and -2 and activation of phosphatidylinositol-3-kinase (hereafter referred to as the PI3K pathway) appears to be necessary for mediating metabolic effects of insulin.[7,8] The second signaling pathway appears to involve the phosphorylation of Shc and activation of Ras, Raf, MEK, and mitogen-activated protein (MAP) kinases (Erk1 and Erk2) (hereafter referred to as the MAPK pathway). In contrast to the PI3K pathway, activation of the MAPK pathway contributes solely to the nuclear and mitogenic effects of insulin and plays no role in mediating the metabolic actions of insulin.[9,10]

Subsequent reports by the groups of Jiang and Cusi[11,12] have established the concept of "selective insulin resistance." Jiang and colleagues[11] compared insulin signaling via the PI3K and MAPK pathways in vascular tissue of lean and obese Zucker rats using both in vivo and ex vivo studies. These investigators demonstrated a significant decrease in the ability of insulin to stimulate the phosphorylation of IRS-1, the association of the p85 regulatory subunit of PI3K with IRS-1, the activity of PI3K, and the phosphorylation of Akt (a downstream serine kinase of the PI3K pathway) in the vasculature of obese insulin-resistant rats. By contrast, the stimulatory effect of insulin on MAPK remained intact in these animals. Cusi and colleagues[12] studied the 2 pathways of insulin signaling in human muscle biopsy samples obtained from patients with T2DM, obese nondiabetic individuals, and lean control subjects before and after euglycemic-hyperinsulinemic clamp. Insulin stimulation of the PI3K pathway was dramatically reduced in obese nondiabetic individuals and virtually absent in T2DM patients. By contrast, insulin stimulation of the MAPK pathway was normal in obese and diabetic subjects. Subsequent studies[13,14] have similarly established that IR has differential effects on these 2 pathways. As IR often is associated with hyperinsulinemia, especially earlier in the natural course of DM, it follows that the mitogenic-pathway effects of insulin are amplified in T2DM and, indeed, prediabetes/other insulin-resistant states (**Fig. 1**).

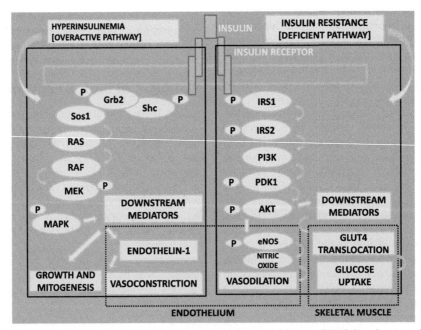

Fig. 1. Insulin resistance (IR) is selective to the phosphatidylinositol-3-kinase (PI3K) (predominantly metabolic) effects of insulin. Hyperinsulinemia, a common concomitant of IR, results in exaggerated mitogen-activated protein kinase (nuclear and mitogenic) effects of insulin. Akt, protein kinase B; eNOS, endothelial nitric oxide synthase; ET-1, endothelin 1; GLUT4, Glucose transporter 4; Grb2, growth factor receptor-binding protein 2; IRS, insulin receptor substrate; MAPK, mitogen activated protein kinase; MEK, MAPK and extracellular signal-regulated kinase (ERK) kinase; NO, nitric oxide; PDK1, 3-phospho-inositide dependent protein kinase-1; PI3K, Phosphoinosital 3 kinase; RAF, v-raf-1 murine leukemia viral oncogene homolog 1 [several isoforms]; RAS, rat sarcoma [small GTPases]; SHC, Src homology 2 domain-containing; SOS-son of sevenless.

ATHEROSCLEROSIS

Ross and Glomset[15] proposed more than 3 decades ago a proliferative model for atherosclerosis, whereby endothelial denuding injury led to platelet aggregation, release of platelet-derived growth factor, and proliferation of smooth muscle cells in the arterial intima, thereby forming the nidus of the atherosclerotic plaque and updating Virchow's centuries-old concept of a "response to injury" model (initially proposed in 1856), which envisaged atherosclerosis merely as a passive deposition of lipid debris in arterial wall. This simplistic concept has since evolved, largely as a consequence of the advances in cell biology techniques, and current thinking is that atherosclerosis is indeed a complex process invoking endothelial dysfunction, vascular smooth muscle dysfunction, immune dysfunction, and inflammation.[16,17]

Atherosclerosis is perhaps initiated by endothelial dysfunction in the presence of structural alterations such as the absence of a confluent luminal elastin layer and the exposure of proteoglycans,[2] which cause apolipoprotein-B (apoB)-enriched particles such as low-density lipoprotein (LDL) to accumulate in the subendothelial space. Elevated levels of circulating LDL cholesterol promote atherosclerosis and cardiovascular disease (CVD).[18] ApoB100 binding to negatively charged extracellular matrix proteoglycans leads to intimal retention of LDL particles, where they are vulnerable to oxidative modification by reactive oxygen species and enzymes such as myeloperoxidase or lipoxygenases released from inflammatory cells. Oxidized LDL (oxLDL) promotes expression of adhesion molecules and the secretion of chemokines by endothelial cells, which in conjunction with platelet-derived chemokines drive immune cell infiltration into the intima. Early lesions ("fatty-streak") consist of T cells and monocyte-derived macrophage-like foam cells loaded with lipids. Accrual of dying cells and other cellular debris along with cholesterol crystals form a necrotic core. Fibroatheromatous plaques are covered by a fibrous cap composed of collagen and smooth muscle cells (SMCs), which are replaced by macrophages in the thinning inflamed caps that are prone to rupture. The "shoulder" regions are heavily infiltrated by T cells and mast cells, which produce enzymes and proinflammatory mediators, contributing to adventitial inflammation of advanced plaques.[19] The pathogenesis of atherosclerosis is discussed in greater detail elsewhere.[20]

IR is associated with cellular processes that in fact can facilitate atherosclerosis (Fig. 2). The pathophysiologic processes involved in the initiation and progression of early atherosclerotic lesions are somewhat different from those associated with the formation of clinically dangerous plaques[21,22], and distinguishing the effects of IR and hyperglycemia on these processes is important. As alluded to earlier, early- to mid-stage atherogenesis involves the subendothelial retention of apoB-containing lipoproteins, activation of endothelial cells, recruitment of monocytes and other inflammatory cells, cholesterol loading of lesional cells, and migration of SMCs to the intima. By contrast, advanced plaque progression is influenced primarily by processes that promote plaque necrosis and thinning of a collagenous "scar" overlying the lesion, called the fibrous cap. The objective of this review is to describe how IR and hyperglycemia promote atherogenesis and plaque progression. It should be noted that IR and hyperglycemia are likely to have additive or synergistic proatherogenic effects in the setting of T2DM. For example, glucotoxicity may contribute to IR, and treatment of hyperglycemia in T2DM has been shown to improve IR in some tissues.[23]

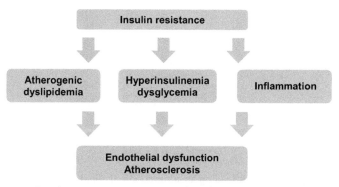

Fig. 2. Insulin resistance–related processes are associated with endothelial dysfunction and promotion of atherosclerosis.

INSULIN RESISTANCE, ATHEROGENIC DYSLIPIDEMIA, AND ATHEROSCLEROSIS

Altered metabolism of triglyceride-rich lipoproteins (TGRLP) is an integral part of the metabolic milieu in insulin-resistant states. **Fig. 3** illustrates the lipid pathways that operate in IR states. Insulin is an anabolic hormone, and normally causes synthesis of nonesterified fatty acids (NEFA) or free fatty acid (FFA) to coalesce into triacylglycerol. In obesity-associated states where IR is an early pathophysiologic abnormality, excessive fat breakdown leads to increased delivery of FFA to the liver. This process leads to increased hepatic synthesis and secretion of triglyceride packaged within the very low-density lipoprotein (VLDL). Impaired clearance of VLDL and intestinally derived chylomicrons leads to prolonged plasma retention of these particles as partially lipolyzed remnant particles. These remnants, which include cholesterol-enriched intermediate-density lipoproteins (IDLs), are particularly atherogenic in humans and in several animal models.[24,25] Increased hepatic production and/or slow plasma clearance of large VLDL also results in increased production of precursors of small dense LDL (sdLDL) particles. As many as 7 distinct LDL subspecies that differ in their metabolic behavior and pathologic roles have been identified.[26] Plasma VLDL levels correlate with increased density and decreased size of LDL.[27,28] In addition, LDL size and density are inversely related to plasma levels of high-density lipoprotein (HDL), especially the HDL$_2$ subclass.[29] sdLDL particles arise from the intravascular processing of specific larger VLDL precursors through

a series of steps, including lipolysis.[26] Further triglyceride enrichment of the lipolytic products through the action of cholesteryl ester transfer protein (CETP), together with hydrolysis of triglyceride and phospholipids by hepatic lipase, leads to increased production of small dense LDL particles.[24,25] It also appears that the plasma-retention time for these particles is prolonged on account of their reduced affinity for LDL receptors.[26] HDL particles are heterogeneous, and multiple subclasses differing in diameter and density have been identified, ranging from the small dense HDL$_{3c}$, HDL$_{3b}$, and HDL$_{3a}$ to the larger HDL$_{2a}$ and HDL$_{2b}$.[30] The reasons for the reduction in plasma HDL concentration associated with T2DM and IR are multifactorial, but a major factor appears to be increased transfer of cholesterol from HDL to TGRLP, with reciprocal transfer of triglyceride to HDL. Triglyceride-rich HDL particles are hydrolyzed by hepatic lipase and, as a result, are rapidly catabolized and cleared from plasma.[31] Typically the reduced HDL levels in plasma of patients with T2DM are manifest as reductions in the HDL$_{2b}$ subspecies and relative or absolute increases in smaller denser HDL$_{3b}$ and HDL$_{3c}$.

Increased atherogenicity of sdLDL appears to be related to several properties, including reduced LDL receptor affinity,[32,33] greater propensity for transport into the subendothelial space,[34] increased binding to arterial wall proteoglycans,[35] and susceptibility to oxidative modifications.[36–38] These in vitro findings corroborate the concept that sdLDL contributes to arterial damage in patients with the atherogenic dyslipidemia seen in insulin-resistant states.

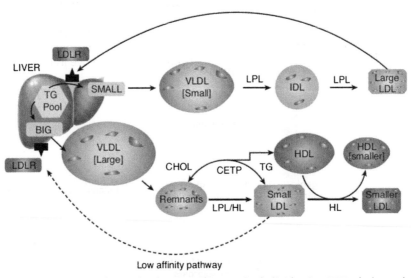

Low affinity pathway

Fig. 3. Insulin resistance: lipid pathways leading to atherogenic dyslipidemia. CETP, cholesteryl ester transfer protein; CHOL, cholesterol; HL, hepatic lipase; IDL-intermediate density lipoprotein; LDL, low density lipoprotein; LDLR, low density lipoprotein receptor; LPL, lipoprotein lipase; TG, triglyceride; VLDL, very low density lipoprotein.

HYPERGLYCEMIA AND ATHEROSCLEROSIS: POSSIBLE MECHANISMS

Epidemiologic evidence supports an association between glycemic control and CVD risk.[39] The United Kingdom Prospective Diabetes Study (UKPDS) provided additional insights into the relationship between glycemic control and CVD in patients with T2DM, indicating a linear relationship between hemoglobin A_{1c} (HbA$_{1c}$) and CVD end points, particularly myocardial infarction.[40] However, the relationship between HbA$_{1c}$ and microvascular complications is stronger than that for macrovascular outcomes such as myocardial infarction, stroke, and so forth, raising the question as to whether glucose plays a greater role in the pathogenesis of microvascular than in macrovascular outcomes in DM. Similar relationships between hyperglycemia and CVD outcomes have been demonstrated in T1DM, but the association appears to be less pronounced.[41]

It has been proposed that glucose might act directly or indirectly via the generation of advanced glycation end products (AGEs) or reactive oxygen species. Advanced glycated end products are a class of chemical by-products that result from the combination of protein and sugar (usually glucose) and are increasingly recognized as a mediator of hyperglycemia-induced cytopathology. Hyperglycemia inside the cell increases diacylglycerol (DAG) levels, a critical activating cofactor for the classic isoforms of protein kinase C, β, δ, and α.[42–45] Protein kinase C (PKC) activation leads to a variety of genetic effects, schematically shown in **Fig. 4**. The vasodilator nitric oxide (NO) levels are low because endothelial NO synthase (eNOS) expression is diminished, whereas the vasoconstrictor endothelin-1 expression is increased. Transforming growth factor β (TGF-β) and plasminogen activator inhibitor 1 (PAI-1) are also increased. At the bottom of the figure, the rows of blue boxes list the pathologic effects that may result from the abnormalities in the white boxes above.[45–49] Also illuminating are several studies demonstrating that inhibition of PKC prevented early renal and retinal complications of DM.[46,49,50] PKC activation has been linked to increased inflammation via increased nuclear factor κB (NF-κB) activation,[51,52] which in turn leads to the expression of several proinflammatory genes, including adhesion molecules that facilitate monocyte adhesion to endothelial cells.[51] This process eventually triggers the pathway by which foam cells may form. Glucose alone can affect monocyte/macrophage activation in vitro.

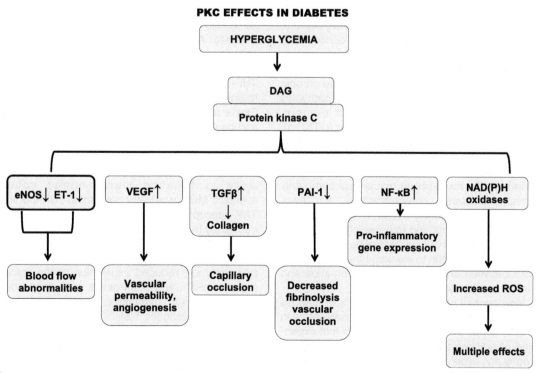

PKC EFFECTS IN DIABETES

Fig. 4. Effects of protein kinase C in diabetes mellitus. eNOS, endothelial nitric oxide synthase; ET-1, endothelin 1; NAD(P)H, reduced nicotinamide adenine dinucleotide phosphate; NFκB, nuclear factor kappa beta; PAI-1, Plasminogen Activator Inhibitor Type 1; ROS, reactive oxygen species; TGFβ, transforming growth factor beta; VEGF, Vascular Endothelial growth factor.

Monocytes exposed to high glucose concentration show increased expression of interleukin (IL)-1β, and IL-6[53] resulting in induction of PKC, activation of NF-κB, and robust release of superoxide, which could play a role in glucose-mediated oxidative stress.[53] Glucose auto-oxidation results in the generation of several reactive oxygen species such as the superoxide anion, and can facilitate LDL oxidation in vitro.[54] Cell-surface scavenger receptors on arterial macrophages take up modified lipoproteins including oxLDL that have become oxidized as a result of glucose-mediated oxidative stress[54,55] or modified by AGEs.[55] Moreover, AGE-modified albumin can inhibit scavenger receptor B1 (SR-B1)-mediated efflux of cholesterol to HDL.[56] AGE proteins in the circulation may also interfere with the functions of SR-B1 in reverse cholesterol transport by inhibiting the selective uptake of HDL-cholesteryl ester, as well as cholesterol efflux from peripheral cells to HDL. Thus, hyperglycemia affects alterations in the delivery and removal of lipid from macrophages by lipoproteins and other proteins.

INSULIN RESISTANCE, INFLAMMATION, AND ENDOTHELIAL DYSFUNCTION

Although epidemiologic evidence suggesting a correlation between inflammation and IR has existed for more than half a century, it has become abundantly clear that obesity and the concomitant development of inflammation are major components of IR. Studies of human obesity and IR have revealed a clear association between the chronic activation of proinflammatory signaling pathways and decreased insulin sensitivity. For example, elevated levels of tumor necrosis factor α (TNF-α), IL-6, and IL-8 have all been reported in various diabetic and insulin-resistant states.[57–61] The inflammatory marker C-reactive protein (CRP), a nonspecific acute-phase reactant, is commonly elevated in states characterized by IR.[62] Also, experiments in naturally occurring rodent models of obesity, knockout and transgenic mice, as well as detailed studies of insulin signaling at the molecular level have begun to elucidate the mechanistic links between obesity-induced inflammation and insulin-resistant states.

How accrual of pathologic amounts of adipose tissue initiates systemic inflammation has not been precisely elucidated. One theory holds that expansion of adipose tissue leads to adipocyte hypertrophy and hyperplasia, eventually outstripping the local oxygen supply and leading to hypoxia and activation of cellular stress pathways.[63] This process causes cell-autonomous inflammation, and the release of cytokines and other proinflammatory signals. Adipokines such as resistin, leptin, and adiponectin perhaps also affect inflammation and insulin sensitivity. Locally secreted chemokines attract proinflammatory macrophages into the adipose tissue, where they form crown-like structures around large dead or dying adipocytes. These tissue macrophages then release cytokines that further perpetuate inflammation involving neighboring adipocytes, thereby exacerbating inflammation and IR. Hepatic inflammation from steatosis occurs in obesity whereby hepatocyte stress pathway responses may be triggered (reviewed in the article by Bugianesi and colleagues elsewhere in this issue), resulting in hepatocyte-autonomous inflammation. Activation of Kupffer cells (liver-resident macrophage-like cells), releasing locally acting cytokines, can potentially exacerbate inflammation and hepatic IR. In addition, overnutrition is often accompanied by elevations in tissue and circulating FFA concentrations, and saturated FFAs can directly activate proinflammatory responses in vascular endothelial cells, adipocytes, and myeloid-derived cells.[64] A state of systemic inflammation then ensues.

TNF-α is a proinflammatory cytokine secreted predominantly by monocytes and macrophages, and has varied biological effects on lipid metabolism, coagulation, and endothelial function. Activation of the TNF receptor results in stimulation of NF-κB signaling via inhibitor of NF-κB kinase subunit β (IKKβ). A landmark study by Hotamisligil and colleagues[65] showed that adipose tissue isolated from different obese rodent models overexpressed TNF-α. This group also showed that immunoneutralization of TNF-α in obese fa/fa rats ameliorated IR.[65] Similar correlations between TNF-α levels, obesity, and insulin IR were soon demonstrated in humans.[61] Corresponding in vitro experiments demonstrated that by activating IKKβ, TNF-α stimulation leads to serine phosphorylation of IRS-1, attenuating its ability to transduce insulin-mediated cellular events.[66] Mice genetically deficient in TNF-α or the TNF-α receptor 1 gene (TNFR1) do not develop IR caused by high-fat feeding or obesity.[67]

TNF-α can also affect insulin signaling independent of IRS-1. TNF-α–treated cultured 3T3-L1 adipocytes show reduced expression of the insulin receptor, IRS1, and Glut4 genes, as well as a decrease in insulin-stimulated glucose uptake.[68] Ruan and colleagues[69] also showed that TNF-α induced a decrease in many 3T3-L1 adipocyte genes, including GLUT4, hormone-sensitive lipase (HSL), long-chain fatty acyl coenzyme-A synthetase, adiponectin, the transcription factor CCAAT/ enhancer binding protein α (C/EBP), and the nuclear receptors peroxisome proliferator-activated receptor γ (PPARγ) and retinoic acid x receptor

(RXR). As many of these genes have direct and indirect effects on glucose homeostasis, changes in adipocyte expression of these genes will likely contribute to IR.[69]

c-Jun N-terminal kinase 1 (JNK1) (encoded by MAPK8) also contributes to the development of IR in obese and diabetic states. Hirosumi and colleagues[70] found elevated JNK activity in liver, adipose tissue, and skeletal muscle of obese insulin-resistant mice, and knockout of JNK1 (JNK1$^{-/-}$) resulted in the amelioration of IR in mice fed a high-fat diet. At the cellular level, these investigators also showed that JNK1 knockout led to decreased IRS-1 phospho-Ser307 in liver. Of importance, deletion of JNK1 also caused resistance to the development of obesity, so the improved insulin sensitivity in these animals could be a result of decreased adiposity and/or decreased JNK1 activity in insulin target cells. The role of JNK2 has also been assessed, and seems to play a significant role in the development of obesity-induced IR. Recent data suggest that JNK2 can be involved in metabolic regulation when JNK1 is absent, because JNK1$^{+/-}$JNK2$^{-/-}$ mice phenocopy JNK1$^{-/-}$ mice in their reduced adiposity and improved insulin sensitivity.[71] It appears that functional in vivo interactions between these isoforms may contribute to the regulation of insulin action.

Salicylate and its derivative acetylsalicylic acid (aspirin) have been used to treat symptoms of T2DM for a very long time. At higher doses they are effective in reducing blood sugar levels, but adverse effects such as gastrointestinal bleeding and tinnitus have precluded their widespread use for this purpose.[72] These compounds are weak inhibitors of IKKβ, thus preventing IRS-1 serine307 phosphorylation with some insulin-sensitizing effects.[73] Kim and colleagues[74] showed that lipid infusion causes acute IR in rodents and that pretreatment of lipid-infused rats with salicylates improves glucose use in skeletal muscle, as measured during hyperinsulinemic-euglycemic clamp studies. These investigators also performed lipid infusions in IKKβ heterozygous knockout mice (IKKβ$^{+/-}$) and reported similar improvements in insulin sensitivity when compared with wild-type controls.[74] Yuan and colleagues[75] showed that TNF-α treatment of 3T3L1 adipocytes induces IR, an effect that could be prevented by pretreatment of cells with aspirin. A parallel experiment was performed in adipocytes using okadaic acid to activate IKKβ independent of TNF-α stimulation, and again, aspirin prevented okadaic acid–induced IR. In vivo studies of aspirin-treated obese rats and mice have shown that salicylate pretreatment protects them from IR.[75] Mice with a liver-specific

constitutively active IKKβ transgene (LIKK) developed hyperglycemia and decreased hepatic insulin sensitivity, with mild secondary systemic IR in skeletal muscle. There was liver expression of the proinflammatory markers IL-6, IL-1β, and TNF-α similar to that found in the liver of obese mice. In rescue experiments, LIKK mice treated with sodium salicylate or IL-6 neutralizing antibodies had markedly improved insulin sensitivity. In addition, mice expressing the liver-specific IκBα super-repressor transgene (LISR), which prevents the activation of IKKβ, protected both LIKK and obese mice from hepatic IR. Another important finding in this study was the elevated expression of the macrophage-specific markers, Emr1 (also known as F4/80) and Cd68, in the livers of LIKK and obese mice. Coexpression of LISR and LIKK in compound transgenic mice reduced both IR and the expression of these same macrophage markers. These data indicate that hepatic inflammation caused by a high-fat diet is mediated by both hepatocytes and Kupffer cells (liver macrophages).[76] These studies illustrate the role of IKKβ in the development of obesity and inflammation-induced IR.

As alluded to earlier, NO is an endogenous signaling molecule produced by NOS and acts as a signal transduction molecule for several physiologic processes such as vasodilation. It is also involved in many pathophysiologic states such as IR. Several IR inducers such as FFAs, proinflammatory cytokines, and oxidative stress activate the expression of Nos2, the gene that encodes inducible NOS (iNOS).[77] NO reduces Akt activity by causing S-nitrosylation of a specific cysteine residue.[78] Increased iNOS activity also results in the degradation of IRS-1 in cultured skeletal muscle cells.[77] Nos2 knockout mice are protected from obesity-induced skeletal muscle IR, and this is associated with improved PI3K-Akt activity.[79] It appears that Nos2 is also required for the development of sepsis-induced skeletal muscle IR, perhaps also mediated by the S-nitrosylation of the insulin receptor IRS-1 and Akt.[80,81] These studies suggest that increased iNOS activity may play a direct role in the pathogenesis of IR.

IL-10 is a cytokine produced by macrophages and lymphocytes that exerts anti-inflammatory activity by inhibiting TNF-α–induced NF-κB through reduction in IKK activity and inhibition of NF-κB DNA binding activity.[82] It has been shown in human subjects that IR is more prevalent in subjects with reduced serum levels of IL-10.[83] Consistent with the concept that IL-10 may have insulin-sensitizing effects is the laboratory evidence that mice treated with IL-10 did not become insulin resistant when treated with either IL-6 or lipid infusions.[83] Lumeng and colleagues[84] showed that IL-10–treated 3T3L1 adipocytes are protected from TNF-α–induced cellular IR. Recombinant IL-10 therapy for conditions such as psoriasis have raised hopes that immunomodulation of IL-10 activity can be a potential treatment of IR.[85]

THE ROLE OF THE MACROPHAGE IN PROMOTING ATHEROSCLEROSIS IN INSULIN-RESISTANT STATES

An important discovery in obesity-induced inflammation and IR was the finding that bone marrow–derived macrophages are present in adipose tissue of obese mice and humans.[86,87] Weisberg and colleagues[86] compared adipose tissue RNA profiles for various mouse models of obesity and found that a subset of genes, though not typically expressed in adipocytes, were confirmed through immunohistochemistry to be resident in adipose tissue and macrophage derived. The percentage of macrophages in a given adipose tissue depot positively correlated with adiposity and adipocyte size. Weisberg and colleagues also found that adipose tissue macrophages were responsible for nearly all adipose tissue TNF-α expression and a significant portion of Nos2 and IL-6 expression. The investigators quantified the infiltration of macrophages in subcutaneous adipose tissue from obese human subjects and reported that as much as 50% of the total cell content consists of macrophages, compared with 10% in lean controls.[86] Xu and colleagues[87] reported similar findings and showed that thiazolidinedione (TZD) treatment could repress the expression of macrophage-specific genes, providing an additional mechanism by which TZD treatment improves insulin sensitivity.

A study by Arkan and colleagues[88] showed that inhibition of the macrophage inflammatory pathway protects mice from obesity-induced IR. In this study, the investigators generated both a myeloid-specific deletion of IKKβ (IKKβ$^{\Delta mye}$) and liver-specific deletion of IKKβ (IKKβ$^{\Delta hep}$). IKKβ$^{\Delta hep}$ mice were found to be protected from hepatic IR induced by a high-fat diet, but that this was a tissue-autonomous effect because these mice still developed IR in muscle and fat. There was a significant reduction in the expression of inflammatory markers in the liver, suggesting that inactivation of inflammation can prevent IR induced by a high-fat diet. Also, tissue-specific deletion of IKKβ in myeloid cells (IKKβ$^{\Delta mye}$ mice) led to improvement in insulin sensitivity, with globally improved insulin action in muscle, liver, and fat. As such, these results showed that inactivation of myeloid IKKβ activity prevented systemic IR,

most likely by blocking local paracrine interaction between resident macrophages and insulin target tissues.

Monocyte chemoattractant protein 1 (MCP-1), also known as chemokine ligand 2 (Ccl2), and its cognate receptor chemokine receptor 2 (Ccr2), are also major components of IR in obese mice. MCP-1 is a chemokine secreted primarily by macrophages and endothelial cells that promotes the recruitment of monocytes to inflamed tissues. Ccr2 is expressed in monocytes but also in the lung, spleen, and thymus.[89] Weisberg and colleagues[90] found that obesity-matched Ccr2$^{-/-}$ mice displayed reduced adipose tissue macrophage infiltration, reduced hepatic steatosis, decreased inflammatory profiles, and improved systemic insulin sensitivity. Ccr2 deficiency also attenuated high-fat diet–induced weight gain by causing a reduction in caloric intake, highlighting the possible involvement of Ccr2 in the control of eating behavior. Also, treatment of obese mice with a pharmacologic antagonist of Ccr2 led to decreased adipose tissue macrophage infiltration and improved insulin sensitivity.[90] Complementary studies on MCP-1 have shown that its expression is increased in obese mice, suggesting that changes in Mcp1 levels promote the recruitment of macrophages to adipose tissue, which then causes inflammation and IR. Studies on transgenic mice that overexpress MCP-1 under the control of the adipose tissue-specific AP2 promoter found that MCP-1 overexpression is associated with macrophage infiltration and IR.[91,92] Kanda and colleagues[92] also showed that the onset of these abnormalities in obese mice could be prevented by genetic deletion of MCP-1. MCP-1 may also have a role in energy metabolism. Unlike other studies, Inouye and colleagues[93] showed that MCP-1 knockout mice fed a high-fat diet developed hyperinsulinemia and increased adiposity independent of adipose tissue macrophage levels, which were unchanged. Differences in experimental approaches as well as the complexity/redundancy of chemokine signaling may have accounted for these conflicting conclusions. In all, most evidence suggests that the MCP-1/Ccr2 axis could provide an important mechanistic link between obesity, adipose tissue inflammation, and IR.

ENDOPLASMIC RETICULUM STRESS

Another potential cause of inflammation in obesity is so-called endoplasmic reticulum (ER) stress. This idea is based on the premise that nutrient excess causes mechanical stress, excess lipid accumulation and protein synthesis, and abnormal energy metabolism, all of which lead to an overburdened ER. This "hypersynthetic" state in the ER interrupts the normal folding of proteins and activates the so-called unfolded protein response (UPR), thereby triggering stress-response pathways. The role of the UPR is both to alleviate the ER stress and, paradoxically, to activate apoptosis, depending on the nature and severity of the stressor.[94] Özcan and colleagues[95] showed that in cultured liver cells, ER stress induction is associated with IR via JNK-mediated serine phosphorylation of IRS-1. This study also demonstrated that obese mice deficient for one allele of X-box binding protein-1 (XBP1), a transcription factor that promotes expression of molecular chaperones in response to ER stress, are more severely insulin resistant compared with obese controls. These mice exhibit ER stress, increased JNK activity, and IRS-1 serine phosphorylation. This group also showed that reduction of ER stress by oral administration of active chemical chaperones improved glucose homeostasis in obese mice.[96] A recent study[97] found that fetuin-A levels were increased in those who suffered from DM and nonalcoholic fatty liver disease (NAFLD). In this study, a total of 180 age-matched and sex-matched subjects with normal glucose tolerance, NAFLD alone, newly diagnosed diabetes mellitus (NDDM) alone, and those with both NDDM and NAFLD were recruited. The levels of fetuin-A were significantly increased in NDDM with NAFLD compared with subjects who had NDDM alone or NAFLD alone. The investigators further used HepG2 cells to investigate the regulation of fetuin-A. Treatment with ER stress activator, thapsigargin, increased the expression of fetuin-A mRNA and protein in a time-dependent and dose-dependent manner. Pretreatment with the ER stress inhibitor 4-phenylbutyrate reversed high glucose or palmitate-induced fetuin-A expression, and treatment with 4-phenylbutyrate in both streptozotocin-induced and high-fat diet–induced diabetic mice not only decreased hepatic fetuin-A levels but also improved hyperglycemia. ER stress induced by high glucose and palmitate increased the expression of fetuin-A, and further contributed to the development of IR.[97]

However, the ER stress–insulin signaling relationship seems more nuanced, as suggested by another recent study.[98] These investigators sought to distinguish the adaptive and deleterious effects of lipid-induced ER stress on hepatic insulin action. Exposure of human hepatoma HepG2 cells or mouse primary hepatocytes to the saturated fatty acid palmitate enhanced ER stress in a dose-dependent manner. Exposure of HepG2 cells to prolonged mild ER stress activation induced by low levels of thapsigargin, tunicamycin, or palmitate augmented insulin-stimulated Akt phosphorylation, with subsequent attenuation of the acute stress response to high-level palmitate challenge. By contrast, exposure of HepG2 cells or hepatocytes to severe ER stress induced by high levels of palmitate was associated with reduced insulin-stimulated Akt phosphorylation and glycogen synthesis, as well as increased expression of glucose-6-phosphatase. Attenuation of ER stress using chemical chaperones (trimethylamine N-oxide or tauroursodeoxycholic acid) partially protected against the lipid-induced changes in insulin signaling. These findings in liver cells suggested that mild ER stress associated with chronic low-level palmitate exposure induced an adaptive UPR that enhances insulin signaling and protects against the effects of high-level palmitate. However, in the absence of chronic adaptation, severe ER stress induced by high-level palmitate exposure induces deleterious UPR signaling that contributes to IR and metabolic dysregulation.

SUMMARY

IR is a complex metabolic defect that most likely has several causes dependent on the individual's genetic substrate and the underlying pathophysiologic state. Atherogenic dyslipidemia, hyperinsulinemia, dysglycemia, inflammation associated with obesity, and ectopic steatosis in liver and skeletal muscle all collude to facilitate endothelial dysfunction and predispose to the initiation and propagation of atherosclerosis. With regard to the relationship between IR and atherosclerosis, a fascinating array of cellular and metabolic defects have been demonstrated in elegantly conducted laboratory studies and human studies, yet more research is needed to define ways by which human intervention can fundamentally alter the metabolic and vascular milieu and slow the pace of atherosclerosis, and thus favorably affect CVD outcomes. Underscoring this need is the fact that a majority of diabetic patients die from CVD, and to date, aggressive management of the various risk factors does not seem to abrogate the so-called residual risk. Lifestyle methods leading to a reduction in body weight has salutary effects on IR and CVD outcomes, and remains a mainstay in the therapeutic armamentarium of a physician seeking to improve IR.

REFERENCES

1. Muoio DM, Newgard CB. Mechanisms of disease: molecular and metabolic mechanisms of insulin resistance and beta-cell failure in type 2 diabetes. Nat Rev Mol Cell Biol 2008;9(3):193–205.

2. Diagnosis and classification of diabetes mellitus. Diabetes Care 2012;35(Suppl 1):S64–71.

3. Moller DE, Flier JS. Insulin resistance—mechanisms, syndromes, and implications. N Engl J Med 1991; 325(13):938–48.

4. Seino S, Seino M, Nishi S, et al. Structure of the human insulin receptor gene and characterization of its promoter. Proc Natl Acad Sci U S A 1989; 86(1):114–8.

5. Cheatham B, Kahn CR. Insulin action and the insulin signaling network. Endocr Rev 1995;16(2):117–42.

6. White MF. The IRS-signalling system: a network of docking proteins that mediate insulin action. Mol Cell Biochem 1998;182(1–2):3–11.

7. Shepherd PR, Kahn BB. Glucose transporters and insulin action—implications for insulin resistance and diabetes mellitus. N Engl J Med 1999;341(4): 248–57.

8. Shulman GI. Cellular mechanisms of insulin resistance in humans. Am J Cardiol 1999;84(1A):3J–10J.

9. Sasaoka T, Rose DW, Jhun BH, et al. Evidence for a functional role of Shc proteins in mitogenic signaling induced by insulin, insulin-like growth factor-1, and epidermal growth factor. J Biol Chem 1994;269(18):13689–94.

10. Sasaoka T, Ishiki M, Sawa T, et al. Comparison of the insulin and insulin-like growth factor 1 mitogenic intracellular signaling pathways. Endocrinology 1996;137(10):4427–34.

11. Jiang ZY, Lin YW, Clemont A, et al. Characterization of selective resistance to insulin signaling in the vasculature of obese Zucker (fa/fa) rats. J Clin Invest 1999;104(4):447–57.

12. Cusi K, Maezono K, Osman A, et al. Insulin resistance differentially affects the PI 3-kinase- and MAP kinase-mediated signaling in human muscle. J Clin Invest 2000;105(3):311–20.

13. Zecchin HG, Bezerra RM, Carvalheira JB, et al. Insulin signalling pathways in aorta and muscle from two animal models of insulin resistance—the obese middle-aged and the spontaneously hypertensive rats. Diabetologia 2003;46(4):479–91.

14. Law RE, Meehan WP, Xi XP, et al. Troglitazone inhibits vascular smooth muscle cell growth and intimal hyperplasia. J Clin Invest 1996;98(8):1897–905.

15. Ross R, Glomset JA. The pathogenesis of atherosclerosis (first of two parts). N Engl J Med 1976; 295(7):369–77.

16. Libby P, Hansson GK. Involvement of the immune system in human atherogenesis: current knowledge and unanswered questions. Lab Invest 1991;64(1): 5–15.

17. Hansson GK, Libby P. The immune response in atherosclerosis: a double-edged sword. Nat Rev Immunol 2006;6(7):508–19.

18. Hansson GK, Hermansson A. The immune system in atherosclerosis. Nat Immunol 2011;12(3):204–12.

19. Yla-Herttuala S, Bentzon JF, Daemen M, et al. Stabilisation of atherosclerotic plaques. Position paper of the European Society of Cardiology (ESC) working group on atherosclerosis and vascular biology. Thromb Haemost 2011;106(1):1–19.

20. Weber C, Noels H. Atherosclerosis: current pathogenesis and therapeutic options. Nat Med 2011; 17(11):1410–22.

21. Lusis AJ. Atherosclerosis. Nature 2000;407(6801): 233–41.

22. Tabas I. Macrophage death and defective inflammation resolution in atherosclerosis. Nat Rev Immunol 2010;10(1):36–46.

23. Henry RR. Glucose control and insulin resistance in non-insulin-dependent diabetes mellitus. Ann Intern Med 1996;124(1 Pt 2):97–103.

24. Krauss RM. Triglycerides and atherogenic lipoproteins: rationale for lipid management. Am J Med 1998;105(1A):58S–62S.

25. Krauss RM. Atherogenicity of triglyceride-rich lipoproteins. Am J Cardiol 1998;81(4A):13B–7B.

26. Berneis KK, Krauss RM. Metabolic origins and clinical significance of LDL heterogeneity. J Lipid Res 2002;43(9):1363–79.

27. McNamara JR, Jenner JL, Li Z, et al. Change in LDL particle size is associated with change in plasma triglyceride concentration. Arterioscler Thromb 1992;12(11):1284–90.

28. McNamara JR, Campos H, Ordovas JM, et al. Effect of gender, age, and lipid status on low density lipoprotein subfraction distribution. Results from the Framingham Offspring Study. Arteriosclerosis 1987; 7(5):483–90.

29. Krauss RM, Williams PT, Lindgren FT, et al. Coordinate changes in levels of human serum low and high density lipoprotein subclasses in healthy men. Arteriosclerosis 1988;8(2):155–62.

30. Blanche PJ, Gong EL, Forte TM, et al. Characterization of human high-density lipoproteins by gradient gel electrophoresis. Biochim Biophys Acta 1981; 665(3):408–19.

31. Hopkins GJ, Barter PJ. Role of triglyceride-rich lipoproteins and hepatic lipase in determining the particle size and composition of high density lipoproteins. J Lipid Res 1986;27(12):1265–77.

32. Campos H, Arnold KS, Balestra ME, et al. Differences in receptor binding of LDL subfractions. Arterioscler Thromb Vasc Biol 1996;16(6):794–801.

33. Pascot A, Lemieux I, Prud'homme D, et al. Reduced HDL particle size as an additional feature of the atherogenic dyslipidemia of abdominal obesity. J Lipid Res 2001;42(12):2007–14.

34. Bjornheden T, Babyi A, Bondjers G, et al. Accumulation of lipoprotein fractions and subfractions in the arterial wall, determined in an in vitro perfusion system. Atherosclerosis 1996;123(1–2): 43–56.

35. Anber V, Griffin BA, McConnell M, et al. Influence of plasma lipid and LDL-subfraction profile on the interaction between low density lipoprotein with human arterial wall proteoglycans. Atherosclerosis 1996; 124(2):261–71.

36. Chait A, Brazg RL, Tribble DL, et al. Susceptibility of small, dense, low-density lipoproteins to oxidative modification in subjects with the atherogenic lipoprotein phenotype, pattern B. Am J Med 1993; 94(4):350–6.

37. de Graaf J, Hak-Lemmers HL, Hectors MP, et al. Enhanced susceptibility to in vitro oxidation of the dense low density lipoprotein subfraction in healthy subjects. Arterioscler Thromb 1991;11(2):298–306.

38. Tribble DL, Holl LG, Wood PD, et al. Variations in oxidative susceptibility among six low density lipoprotein subfractions of differing density and particle size. Atherosclerosis 1992;93(3):189–99.

39. Kannel WB, McGee DL. Diabetes and glucose tolerance as risk factors for cardiovascular disease: the Framingham study. Diabetes Care 1979;2(2):120–6.

40. Turner RC, Millns H, Neil HA, et al. Risk factors for coronary artery disease in non-insulin dependent diabetes mellitus: United Kingdom Prospective Diabetes Study (UKPDS: 23). BMJ 1998;316(7134):823–8.

41. Prince CT, Becker DJ, Costacou T, et al. Changes in glycaemic control and risk of coronary artery disease in type 1 diabetes mellitus: findings from the Pittsburgh Epidemiology of Diabetes Complications Study (EDC). Diabetologia 2007;50(11):2280–8.

42. Koya D, King GL. Protein kinase C activation and the development of diabetic complications. Diabetes 1998;47(6):859–66.

43. Derubertis FR, Craven PA. Activation of protein kinase C in glomerular cells in diabetes. Mechanisms and potential links to the pathogenesis of diabetic glomerulopathy. Diabetes 1994;43(1):1–8.

44. Xia P, Inoguchi T, Kern TS, et al. Characterization of the mechanism for the chronic activation of diacylglycerol-protein kinase C pathway in diabetes and hypergalactosemia. Diabetes 1994;43(9):1122–9.

45. Koya D, Jirousek MR, Lin YW, et al. Characterization of protein kinase C beta isoform activation on the gene expression of transforming growth factor-beta, extracellular matrix components, and prostanoids in the glomeruli of diabetic rats. J Clin Invest 1997;100(1):115–26.

46. Ishii H, Jirousek MR, Koya D, et al. Amelioration of vascular dysfunctions in diabetic rats by an oral PKC beta inhibitor. Science 1996;272(5262):728–31.

47. Kuboki K, Jiang ZY, Takahara N, et al. Regulation of endothelial constitutive nitric oxide synthase gene expression in endothelial cells and in vivo: a specific vascular action of insulin. Circulation 2000;101(6): 676–81.

48. Studer RK, Craven PA, DeRubertis FR. Role for protein kinase C in the mediation of increased fibronectin accumulation by mesangial cells grown in high-glucose medium. Diabetes 1993; 42(1):118–26.

49. Feener EP, Xia P, Inoguchi T, et al. Role of protein kinase C in glucose- and angiotensin II-induced plasminogen activator inhibitor expression. Contrib Nephrol 1996;118:180–7.

50. Koya D, Haneda M, Nakagawa H, et al. Amelioration of accelerated diabetic mesangial expansion by treatment with a PKC beta inhibitor in diabetic db/db mice, a rodent model for type 2 diabetes. FASEB J 2000; 14(3):439–47.

51. Piga R, Naito Y, Kokura S, et al. Short-term high glucose exposure induces monocyte-endothelial cells adhesion and transmigration by increasing VCAM-1 and MCP-1 expression in human aortic endothelial cells. Atherosclerosis 2007;193(2):328–34.

52. Yan SD, Schmidt AM, Anderson GM, et al. Enhanced cellular oxidant stress by the interaction of advanced glycation end products with their receptors/binding proteins. J Biol Chem 1994; 269(13):9889–97.

53. Dasu MR, Devaraj S, Jialal I. High glucose induces IL-1beta expression in human monocytes: mechanistic insights. Am J Physiol Endocrinol Metab 2007;293(1):E337–46.

54. Kawamura M, Heinecke JW, Chait A. Pathophysiological concentrations of glucose promote oxidative modification of low density lipoprotein by a superoxide-dependent pathway. J Clin Invest 1994; 94(2):771–8.

55. Miyazaki A, Nakayama H, Horiuchi S. Scavenger receptors that recognize advanced glycation end products. Trends Cardiovasc Med 2002;12(6): 258–62.

56. Ohgami N, Miyazaki A, Sakai M, et al. Advanced glycation end products (AGE) inhibit scavenger receptor class B type I-mediated reverse cholesterol transport: a new crossroad of AGE to cholesterol metabolism. J Atheroscler Thromb 2003;10(1): 1–6.

57. Roytblat L, Rachinsky M, Fisher A, et al. Raised interleukin-6 levels in obese patients. Obes Res 2000;8(9):673–5.

58. Straczkowski M, Dzienis-Straczkowska S, Stepien A, et al. Plasma interleukin-8 concentrations are increased in obese subjects and related to fat mass and tumor necrosis factor-alpha system. J Clin Endocrinol Metab 2002;87(10):4602–6.

59. Hotamisligil GS, Spiegelman BM. Tumor necrosis factor alpha: a key component of the obesity-diabetes link. Diabetes 1994;43(11):1271–8.

60. Sartipy P, Loskutoff DJ. Monocyte chemoattractant protein 1 in obesity and insulin resistance. Proc Natl Acad Sci U S A 2003;100(12):7265–70.

61. Hotamisligil GS, Arner P, Caro JF, et al. Increased adipose tissue expression of tumor necrosis

factor-alpha in human obesity and insulin resistance. J Clin Invest 1995;95(5):2409–15.

62. Visser M, Bouter LM, McQuillan GM, et al. Elevated C-reactive protein levels in overweight and obese adults. JAMA 1999;282(22):2131–5.

63. de Luca C, Olefsky JM. Inflammation and insulin resistance. FEBS Lett 2008;582(1):97–105.

64. Kim F, Tysseling KA, Rice J, et al. Free fatty acid impairment of nitric oxide production in endothelial cells is mediated by IKKbeta. Arterioscler Thromb Vasc Biol 2005;25(5):989–94.

65. Hotamisligil GS, Shargill NS, Spiegelman BM. Adipose expression of tumor necrosis factor-alpha: direct role in obesity-linked insulin resistance. Science 1993;259(5091):87–91.

66. Hotamisligil GS, Peraldi P, Budavari A, et al. IRS-1-mediated inhibition of insulin receptor tyrosine kinase activity in TNF-alpha- and obesity-induced insulin resistance. Science 1996; 271(5249):665–8.

67. Uysal KT, Wiesbrock SM, Marino MW, et al. Protection from obesity-induced insulin resistance in mice lacking TNF-alpha function. Nature 1997; 389(6651):610–4.

68. Stephens JM, Lee J, Pilch PF. Tumor necrosis factor-alpha-induced insulin resistance in 3T3-L1 adipocytes is accompanied by a loss of insulin receptor substrate-1 and GLUT4 expression without a loss of insulin receptor-mediated signal transduction. J Biol Chem 1997;272(2):971–6.

69. Ruan H, Hacohen N, Golub TR, et al. Tumor necrosis factor-alpha suppresses adipocyte-specific genes and activates expression of preadipocyte genes in 3T3-L1 adipocytes: nuclear factor-kappaB activation by TNF-alpha is obligatory. Diabetes 2002;51(5): 1319–36.

70. Hirosumi J, Tuncman G, Chang L, et al. A central role for JNK in obesity and insulin resistance. Nature 2002;420(6913):333–6.

71. Tuncman G, Hirosumi J, Solinas G, et al. Functional in vivo interactions between JNK1 and JNK2 isoforms in obesity and insulin resistance. Proc Natl Acad Sci U S A 2006;103(28):10741–6.

72. Williamson RT. On the treatment of glycosuria and diabetes mellitus with sodium salicylate. Br Med J 1901;1(2100):760–2.

73. Yin MJ, Yamamoto Y, Gaynor RB. The anti-inflammatory agents aspirin and salicylate inhibit the activity of I(kappa)B kinase-beta. Nature 1998; 396(6706):77–80.

74. Kim JK, Kim YJ, Fillmore JJ, et al. Prevention of fat-induced insulin resistance by salicylate. J Clin Invest 2001;108(3):437–46.

75. Yuan M, Konstantopoulos N, Lee J, et al. Reversal of obesity- and diet-induced insulin resistance with salicylates or targeted disruption of IKKbeta. Science 2001;293(5535):1673–7.

76. Cai D, Yuan M, Frantz DF, et al. Local and systemic insulin resistance resulting from hepatic activation of IKK-beta and NF-kappaB. Nat Med 2005;11(2):183–90.

77. Sugita H, Fujimoto M, Yasukawa T, et al. Inducible nitric-oxide synthase and NO donor induce insulin receptor substrate-1 degradation in skeletal muscle cells. J Biol Chem 2005;280(14):14203–11.

78. Yasukawa T, Tokunaga E, Ota H, et al. S-nitrosylation-dependent inactivation of Akt/protein kinase B in insulin resistance. J Biol Chem 2005;280(9): 7511–8.

79. Perreault M, Marette A. Targeted disruption of inducible nitric oxide synthase protects against obesity-linked insulin resistance in muscle. Nat Med 2001; 7(10):1138–43.

80. Carvalho-Filho MA, Ueno M, Carvalheira JB, et al. Targeted disruption of iNOS prevents LPS-induced S-nitrosylation of IRbeta/IRS-1 and Akt and insulin resistance in muscle of mice. Am J Physiol Endocrinol Metab 2006;291(3):E476–82.

81. Carvalho-Filho MA, Ueno M, Hirabara SM, et al. S-nitrosylation of the insulin receptor, insulin receptor substrate 1, and protein kinase B/Akt: a novel mechanism of insulin resistance. Diabetes 2005;54(4):959–67.

82. Schottelius AJ, Mayo MW, Sartor RB, et al. Interleukin-10 signaling blocks inhibitor of kappaB kinase activity and nuclear factor kappaB DNA binding. J Biol Chem 1999;274(45):31868–74.

83. van Exel E, Gussekloo J, de Craen AJ, et al. Low production capacity of interleukin-10 associates with the metabolic syndrome and type 2 diabetes: the Leiden 85-Plus Study. Diabetes 2002;51(4): 1088–92.

84. Lumeng CN, Bodzin JL, Saltiel AR. Obesity induces a phenotypic switch in adipose tissue macrophage polarization. J Clin Invest 2007;117(1):175–84.

85. Asadullah K, Sterry W, Volk HD. Interleukin-10 therapy—review of a new approach. Pharmacol Rev 2003;55(2):241–69.

86. Weisberg SP, McCann D, Desai M, et al. Obesity is associated with macrophage accumulation in adipose tissue. J Clin Invest 2003;112(12):1796–808.

87. Xu H, Barnes GT, Yang Q, et al. Chronic inflammation in fat plays a crucial role in the development of obesity-related insulin resistance. J Clin Invest 2003;112(12):1821–30.

88. Arkan MC, Hevener AL, Greten FR, et al. IKK-beta links inflammation to obesity-induced insulin resistance. Nat Med 2005;11(2):191–8.

89. Kurihara T, Bravo R. Cloning and functional expression of mCCR2, a murine receptor for the C-C chemokines JE and FIC. J Biol Chem 1996;271(20): 11603–7.

90. Weisberg SP, Hunter D, Huber R, et al. CCR2 modulates inflammatory and metabolic effects of high-fat feeding. J Clin Invest 2006;116(1):115–24.

91. Kamei N, Tobe K, Suzuki R, et al. Overexpression of monocyte chemoattractant protein-1 in adipose tissues causes macrophage recruitment and insulin resistance. J Biol Chem 2006;281(36):26602–14.

92. Kanda H, Tateya S, Tamori Y, et al. MCP-1 contributes to macrophage infiltration into adipose tissue, insulin resistance, and hepatic steatosis in obesity. J Clin Invest 2006;116(6):1494–505.

93. Inouye KE, Shi H, Howard JK, et al. Absence of CC chemokine ligand 2 does not limit obesity-associated infiltration of macrophages into adipose tissue. Diabetes 2007;56(9):2242–50.

94. Rutkowski DT, Kaufman RJ. That which does not kill me makes me stronger: adapting to chronic ER stress. Trends Biochem Sci 2007;32(10):469–76.

95. Özcan U, Cao Q, Yilmaz E, et al. Endoplasmic reticulum stress links obesity, insulin action, and type 2 diabetes. Science 2004;306(5695):457–61.

96. Özcan U, Yilmaz E, Özcan L, et al. Chemical chaperones reduce ER stress and restore glucose homeostasis in a mouse model of type 2 diabetes. Science 2006;313(5790):1137–40.

97. Ou HY, Wu HT, Hung HC, et al. Endoplasmic reticulum stress induces the expression of fetuin-A to develop insulin resistance. Endocrinology 2012;153(7):2974–84.

98. Achard CS, Laybutt DR. Lipid-induced endoplasmic reticulum stress in liver cells results in two distinct outcomes: adaptation with enhanced insulin signaling or insulin resistance. Endocrinology 2012;153(5):2164–77.

Role of Lipotoxicity in Endothelial Dysfunction

Jeong-a Kim, PhD[a,b], Monica Montagnani, MD, PhD[c],
Sruti Chandrasekran, MD[d], Michael J. Quon, MD, PhD[d,*]

KEYWORDS

- Lipotoxicity - Endothelial dysfunction - Metabolic disorders - Cardiovascular disease

KEY POINTS

- Lipotoxicity is caused by abnormally high levels of triacylglycerol, nonesterified fatty acid (NEFA), and cholesterol that lead to pathophysiologic conditions in metabolic and cardiovascular (CV) tissues.
- Lipotoxicity-mediated endothelial dysfunction affects tissues, including cardiac muscle, neurons, kidney, skeletal muscle, pancreatic β-cells, and liver.
- The mechanisms underlying lipotoxicity include oxidative stress, inflammation, mitochondrial dysfunction, and endoplasmic reticulum (ER) stress as well as cell death.
- Treatment with exercise, diet, or pharmacologic agents directly or indirectly reduces lipids in the plasma to ameliorate endothelial dysfunction as well as pathophysiologic conditions in metabolic and CV tissues.

INTRODUCTION

CV disease is the leading cause of death in the United States. Reciprocal relationships between endothelial dysfunction and insulin resistance tightly link metabolic diseases, including obesity and diabetes, with their CV complications.[1] Obesity and diabetes per se increase the risk of CV morbidity and mortality at least 3-fold.[2]

Vascular endothelium plays an important role in maintaining vascular homeostasis and actively participates in the delivery of hormones, nutrients, and oxygen to metabolic target tissues. These functions are regulated by secretion of endothelium-dependent relaxing factors, endothelium-dependent hyperpolarizing factors, and endothelium-dependent contracting factors.[3] Imbalance among these factors contributes to endothelial dysfunction that

is associated with cardiac dysfunction, coronary artery disease, hypertension, diabetes, and neurologic disorders, leading to increased mortality and morbidity.[1,4] Excess circulating lipids (hyperlipidemia) caused by both overnutrition and disordered metabolism are important independent cause of both endothelial dysfunction and insulin resistance. High levels of lipids, including triglycerides (TGs), NEFAs, and low-density lipoprotein cholesterol (LDL-C) damage vascular tissues and their functions. This is known as lipotoxicity.[5-7] Lipotoxicity may be defined as pathologic changes at the cellular and organ levels that results from excess lipids in the circulation or in tissues.

Endothelial dysfunction caused by lipotoxicity is mediated through several diverse mechanisms that include increased oxidative stress and proinflammatory responses. The effect of lipotoxicity

[a] Division of Endocrinology, Diabetes, and Metabolism, Department of Medicine, UAB Comprehensive Diabetes Center, University of Alabama at Birmingham, 1808 7th Avenue South, BDB 777, Birmingham, AL 35294-0012, USA; [b] Department of Cell Biology, University of Alabama at Birmingham, 1808 7th Avenue South, BDB 777, Birmingham, AL 35294, USA; [c] Department of Biomedical Sciences and Human Oncology, Pharmacology Section, University "Aldo Moro" at Bari, Policlinico, Piazza G. Cesare, 11, 70124 Bari, Italy; [d] Department of Medicine, Division of Endocrinology, Diabetes & Nutrition, University of Maryland at Baltimore, 660 West Redwood Street, HH 495, Baltimore, MD 21201, USA
* Corresponding author.
E-mail address: quonm@medicine.umaryland.edu

Heart Failure Clin 8 (2012) 589–607
http://dx.doi.org/10.1016/j.hfc.2012.06.012
1551-7136/12/$ – see front matter © 2012 Elsevier Inc. All rights reserved.

on endothelial dysfunction is magnified even further in patients with obesity, metabolic syndrome, and diabetes.[1,8,9] This article discusses

1. Lipotoxic effects in vascular endothelium
2. Molecular mechanisms underlying the pathophysiology of endothelial dysfunction from lipotoxicity
3. Lifestyle intervention and therapeutic approaches that may oppose lipotoxicity-induced endothelial dysfunction and its CV and metabolic complications.

HYPERLIPIDEMIA AND ENDOTHELIAL DYSFUNCTION
Triglycerides

An elevated serum TG level is a risk factor for coronary heart disease.[10,11] Lipoprotein-associated TGs circulate in the plasma as very low-density lipoproteins or chylomicrons. Insulin receptor substrate-1 (IRS-1) knockout mice, a nonobese animal model of insulin resistance, have impairments in endothelium-dependent vascular relaxation and hypertriglyceridemia (HTG) with low activity of lipoprotein lipase (LPL).[12] This suggests that insulin resistance may play an important role in hypertriglyceridemia and endothelial dysfunction that may accelerate the progression of atherosclerosis. Through genome-wide association studies, Johansen and colleagues[13] identified common variants in APOA5, Glucokinase regulator, LPL, and APOB that are associated with HTG. Mutations of lipoproteins, LPL and glycosylphosphatidylinositol-anchored high-density lipoprotein–binding protein 1 (GP1HBP1) are associated with HTG.[14,15] LPL hydrolyzes TGs into glycerol and free fatty acids (FFAs). GP1HBP1 is necessary for TG hydrolysis.[16] In addition to genetic variations, diet, lack of exercise, and various medications affect HTG.[17] Lipodystrophy, Cushing syndrome, and medications, including β-blockers and tamoxifen, induce HTG.[18] A meta-analysis of population-based prospective studies shows that plasma TG level is a risk factor for CV disease independent of high-density lipoprotein (HDL).[19] The TG level associated with postprandial lipemia suppresses flow-mediated dilation in patients with hypothyroidism.[20] Flow-mediated dilation is negatively correlated with TG and thiobarbituric acid reactive substances level in the plasma. Thus, endothelial dysfunction after an oral fat challenge in these patients is due to HTG and reactive oxygen species.[20] A clinical study with 109 patients who had coronary heart disease during statin therapy compared ezetimibe add-on therapy to placebo. Endothelial function was assessed after 3 months. Flow-mediated dilation in patients treated with ezetimibe is improved and blood TG level is significantly reduced.[21] Ezetimibe improves postprandial hyperlipidemia and endothelial dysfunction.[22] In a previous report, the intima-media thickness of patients who received combination therapy of ezetimibe and simvastatin is not different from that in the patients treated with simvastatin only despite significant lowering effect of low-density lipoprotein (LDL), as shown in the Ezetimibe and Simvastatin in Hypercholesterolemia Enhances Atherosclerosis Regression trial.[23] This suggests that TG level independent of LDL may lead to endothelial dysfunction that contributes to development of atherosclerosis. TG increases inflammatory responses by activation of leukocytes.[24–26] Intramuscular TG content is also associated with insulin resistance in skeletal muscle[27,28] and endothelial dysfunction.[29] Accumulation of TG in the heart is associated with heart failure in animals and humans.[30,31] Thus, intracellular and plasma level of TG is associated with impairment of glucose tolerance and insulin resistance as well as CV dysfunction.

Nonesterified Fatty Acids

Increased plasma NEFAs and accelerated rates of lipolysis are characteristics of type 2 diabetes mellitus and obesity.[32–34] Acute elevation of plasma fatty acids leads to impairment of glucose uptake,[35] inhibition of hepatic gluconeogenesis,[36,37] and endothelial dysfunction.[38,39] Inhibition of lipolysis by using acipimox, a niacin derivative, improves glucose tolerance, insulin sensitivity, insulin-stimulated capillary recruitment, and acetylcholine-stimulated vasodilation.[40,41] Likewise, intralipid plus heparin impairs 20% of methacholine, but not single-nucleotide polymorphism–stimulated, vasodilation in lean healthy human subjects.[39] This suggests that fasting NEFA impairs glucose metabolism as well as endothelial function. NEFA levels independently predict all-cause and CV mortality in subjects with angiographic coronary artery disease.[42] Some other studies, however,[43,44] show fasting NEFA levels were not correlated with obesity when normalized to fat mass.[45] NEFA is liberated from adipose tissue under starvation conditions by hydrolysis of TG. Elevated fasting NEFA level is associated with obesity.[46] After a meal, dietary fat is hydrolyzed by LPL to NEFA and glycerol that are taken up by adipose tissue and re-esterified intracellularly. Some NEFA escapes, however, in a process called spillover.[47] A recent study shows that rates of delivery of NEFA were reduced in obese men compared with lean subjects when normalized to fat mass. The reduced lipid trafficking into adipose tissue leads to ectopic fat deposition.[48] Thus, postprandial fat content is determined by dietary fat, 40% to 50% of which may be from spillover.[48] Both fasting and postprandial NEFAs interact with glucose metabolism; NEFA level may be a predictor for CV disease that is associated with obesity and diabetes.

Cholesterol

Non-HDL cholesterol contributes to impairment of nitric oxide (NO) bioavailability due to increased production of reactive oxygen species and inhibition of endothelial NO synthase (eNOS) activity that leads to endothelial dysfunction and atherosclerosis.[49–51] Patients with high cholesterol have impaired endothelium-dependent vasodilation but not endothelial independent vasodilation.[50] This suggests that elevated cholesterol levels impair vascular function, which contributes to atherosclerosis. Plasma LDL levels in patients with type 2 diabetes mellitus are similar to those of nondiabetics, but LDL catabolism is significantly reduced.[52] Insulin treatment in type 2 diabetes mellitus and lipid lowering by diet or pharmacologic treatments, including statins, restores catabolism of LDL[52,53] and improves endothelial function.[54] Oxidized LDL (ox-LDL)/LDL-C ratio in type 2 diabetes mellitus is reduced by insulin therapy.[55] Ox-LDL displaces eNOS from caveolae to impair eNOS activity stimulated by acetylcholine.[56] Ox-LDL–mediated inhibition of eNOS is restored by HDL.[57] Ox-LDL is taken up by macrophages to promote foam cell formation and reduces cholesterol efflux and reverse cholesterol transport.[58,59] These processes contribute to atherosclerosis and CV diseases. A decreased HDL level is associated with obesity and HTG, insulin resistance and diabetes that may be due to increased HDL catabolism.[60–62] In a more recent study, HDL isolated from patients with CAD fails to activate eNOS and does not have anti-inflammatory and endothelial repair activity when compared with HDL isolated from healthy subjects.[63] HDL isolated from patients with type 2 diabetes mellitus is not able to reverse the ox-LDL–mediated inhibition of endothelium-dependent vasorelaxation.[64] This suggests not all HDL is beneficial. Thus, deregulated cholesterol metabolism affects endothelial function and blood flow that contributes to atherosclerosis and CV events.

LIPOTOXICITY IN TISSUES
Cardiomyopathy

Obesity, insulin resistance, and diabetes are associated with cardiomyopathy that leads to premature morbidity and mortality. Obesity-mediated endothelial dysfunction, dysregulated autonomic regulation, and altered hormonal profiles contribute to the impairment of cardiac function.[65–67] Obese people have 2 to 3 times higher risk for developing heart failure than normal weight people.[68] Excess lipid intake or dyslipidemia causes ectopic lipid accumulation in cardiomyocytes. This results in cell death, increased ER stress, mitochondrial dysfunction, accumulation of ceramide, and increased exposure to reactive oxygen species.[69] Accumulation of TG in myocytes results in alternative substrate metabolism. Thus, cardiac energy metabolism is shifted toward more O_2 consumption and lower ATP production that leads to cardiac dysfunction. Ceramide metabolized from FFA is a major mediator of lipotoxicity that is blocked by myriocin or by stimulation of sphingomyelinase.[69,70] Dietary fat determines lipid profiles in the plasma and tissues and causes various pathophysiologic conditions. In recent studies, a diet with high fat/low carbohydrate is more preventive in progression of heart failure than a diet with low fat/high carbohydrate.[71–75] A diet high in polyunsaturated fatty acid reduces coronary heart disease, whereas a diet with high cholesterol increases coronary heart disease.[76–79] Studies using various high fat diet and rodent models are well described in a recent review.[75] More studies regarding recommendations for optimal diet to patients with cardiomyopathy are necessary.

Nephropathy

Nephrotic subjects tend to develop CV disease associated with metabolic disorders and vascular complications. Diabetic nephropathy is a major risk factor for CV disease and increases morbidity and mortality.[80] Diabetic nephropathy progresses in 5 stages: glomerular hyperfiltration, incipient nephropathy, microalbuminuria, overt proteinuria, and end-stage renal disease.[81] Endothelial dysfunction precedes manifestation of microalbuminuria and is an independent risk factor for CV disease and diabetic nephropathy.[82,83] Hypercholesterolemia decreases NO availability, which leads to activation of podocyte and renal injury.[84,85] The common lipid abnormalities found in chronic kidney disease patients are HTG, reduced HDL, and increased lipoprotein (a).[86] Lipoprotein (a) level is a risk factor for CVD and is associated with glomerular filtration rate.[87] Decreased catabolism of very low-density lipoproteins, chylomicrons, and their remnants leads to accumulation in the plasma. Increased ApoC(III), a potent inhibitor of LPL, leads to increased serum

TG.[88] Proposed mechanisms include increased reabsorption of lipids, including, fatty acids, phospholipids, and cholesterol, that stimulates tubulointerstitial inflammation and tissue injury.[89,90] Accumulation of oxidized lipoproteins, especially ox-LDL, causes inflammation in glomerular mesangium that contributes to recruitment of macrophages.[91,92] Diabetic nephropathy can contribute to dyslipidemia and lipid-lowering therapies that can improve endothelial function may have beneficial effects on both renal and CV functions.

Neuropathy

Patients with diabetic neuropathy have peripheral nerve disorders with symptoms of pain, numbness, weakness, and difficulties with balance.[93,94] It is characterized as axonopathy with distal predominance, with axons failing to regenerate.[95] Both myelinated and unmyelinated fibers undergo axonal change, leading to axonopathy.[95] Impaired autonomic nerve functions inducing a reduction of blood flow contributes to alterations in the microvasculature, leading to diabetic nephropathy and retinopathy.[96,97] Impairment of vascular function is associated with diabetic neuropathy and CV disease.[98,99] Loss of autonomic control is associated with impairment of ventricular function independently from endothelial dysfunction.[100] Accumulation of sorbitol, oxidized lipid, and poly (ADP-ribose) polymerase (PARP) and activation of lipoxygenase in peripheral nerve are observed in a high-fat diet rodent model.[101] FFA causes toxicity in cultured neuronal and Schwann cell lines.[102] Elevated FFAs due to increased lipolysis in adipocytes may increase secretion of inflammatory cytokines affecting peripheral nerve inflammation. Neuronal cells express receptors for ox-LDL and glycated LDL, including ox-LDL receptor 1, scavenger receptors, receptor for advanced glycation end products, and Toll-like receptors (TLRs).[103,104] This suggests that ox-LDL and glycated LDL can injure neuronal cells through stimulation of inflammatory response and oxidative stress.[103] Dysregulated lipids directly and indirectly impair neuronal function through mediators, including inflammatory cytokines and active oxygen/nitrogen species produced by other tissues that contribute to neuropathy.

MOLECULAR MECHANISMS

Lipid-mediated toxicities contribute to functional abnormalities in various tissues, including vascular endothelium, cardiac, and renal tissues. The proposed mechanisms are

- Oxidative stress
- Inflammation
- Mitochondrial dysfunction
- ER stress
- Cell death

These mechanisms are interlinked and contribute to complex pathophysiology.

Oxidative Stress

Increased lipids in the plasma, ectopic lipid accumulation, and intracellular lipid droplets cause oxidative stress.[27,105] Reactive oxygen and nitrogen species react with proteins, lipid, and carbohydrates to modify structure and function of cellular components.[106,107] Lipids affect cellular redox status through metabolic pathways. Vascular endothelium is an important redox-sensitive tissue because it transports various metabolites between tissues. Nicotinamide adenine dinucleotide phosphate-oxidase (NAD(P)H oxidase) creates oxidative stress by producing superoxide that can be converted to hydrogen peroxide and reacts with NO.[108–110] This reaction determines bioavailability of NO, a major determinant of endothelial dysfunction.[109] In the Zucker fatty rat, plasma FFA and TG levels are higher than lean controls causing impairment of acetylcholine-stimulated vasodilation.[111] Treatment of primary vascular endothelial cells with palmitate stimulates production of superoxide and increased expression of NAD(P)H oxidase subunits.[109,111] Inhibition of NADP oxidase activity with apocynin or dipenyleneiodine or by knockdown of NAD(P)H oxidase (NOX) 4 (a NOX subunit) suppresses production of superoxide or expression of NAD(P)H oxidase subunits. These data suggest that saturated fatty acids stimulate production of reactive oxygen species that leads to reduction of NO, bioavailability, and subsequent endothelial dysfunction. In addition to increased expression of NAD(P)H oxidase subunits, diacylglycerol stimulates activation of protein kinase C, a kinase that phosphorylates p47phox. Phosphorylation of p47phox is important for the activation of NAD(P)H oxidase and assembly of multiple NAD(P)H oxidase subunits to form an NAD(P)H oxidase holoenzyme.[112,113] Another mechanism to increase oxidative stress requires mitochondrial dysfunction. The mitochondrial respiratory chain (mainly complex I and III) produces superoxide when fatty acids are oxidized.[114,115] Fatty acids are metabolized by β-oxidation to produce NADH (Nicotinamide adenin dinucleotide) and $FADH_2$ (Flavin adenin dinucleotide) that enter the electron transport chain. This generates ATP by oxidative phosphorylation in mitochondria, where oxygen serves as an electron acceptor. During this process, a proton gradient is formed across the mitochondrial membrane where addition of a single electron to oxygen generates superoxide.[114,116,117] Accumulated protons leak from the intermembrane space to the matrix, resulting in reduced proton motive force that generates heat instead of ATP. This is called uncoupling. Uncoupling protein 2 knockout mice have increased diet-induced atherosclerosis, endothelial dysfunction, and decreased antioxidative capacity.[118] Additionally, uncoupling of eNOS and stimulation of xanthine oxidase produces superoxide.[119–121] Increased reactive oxygen species increases lipid peroxidation and oxidized cholesterol and reduces NO availability to promote vascular insulin resistance and endothelial dysfunction.

Inflammation

Obesity and type 2 diabetes mellitus are characterized by a chronic proinflammatory state.[122,123] Increased plasma or intracellular lipid contents cause proinflammatory responses. Inflammation is closely linked to atherosclerosis, a major sequelae of dyslipidemia-mediated endothelial dysfunction.[124] NEFA stimulates TLRs 2/4 that activate Ikappa B kinase (IKKβ)/nuclear factor (NF)-κB and c-Jun N-terminal kinase (JNK)/activator protein-1, pathways leading to increased expression of other cytokines and cell adhesion molecules, including tumor necrosis factor (TNF)-α, interleukin (IL)-1β, intercellular adhesion molecule, vascular cell adhesion molecule, and E-selectin in endothelial cells.[125] NEFA-mediated proinflammatory signaling inhibits insulin signaling that leads to impairment of glucose tolerance, vascular insulin resistance, and lipogenesis.[125–127] Activation of TLRs by NEFA occurs in macrophages to facilitate atherogenic processes that exacerbate pathophysiology in metabolic and CV tissues.[128] NEFA activates bone morphogenic proteins 2 and 4 that contribute to vascular calcification and differentiation of smooth muscle cells associated with vascular stiffness.[109,129] Ox-LDL also acts as a ligand for TLRs to stimulate proinflammatory responses.[130] The mechanisms for inflammatory signaling to inhibit insulin signaling are increased serine phosphorylation of IRS-1 and IRS-2, facilitated degradation of IRS-1 and IRS-2, and ceramide production.[131] Increased serine phosphorylation of IRS-1 and IRS-2 leads to inhibition of interaction with insulin receptor, plasma membrane, and phosphatidylinositol 3-kinases that are linked to reduced activation of Akt and impairment of eNOS activation.[132–135] This mechanism contributes to impairment of glucose uptake and blood flow in skeletal muscle.[38,119,136] Activation of TLRs by NEFA or LPS increases ceramide production that

contributes to inhibition of insulin-stimulated phosphorylation of Akt as well as facilitation of apoptosis.[131,137]

Mitochondrial Dysfunction

Mitochondria are intracellular organelles that oxidize fatty acid. Electron transfer from NAD(P)H to NAD(P)$^+$ couples with production of ATP, an energy source for movement and cellular enzymatic process.[117] When metabolic stress conditions occur, cells adapt by increasing mitochondrial biogenesis.[138,139] More mitochondria may compensate for increased cellular energy needs. eNOS and NO play important roles in mitochondrial biogenesis through AMP-activated protein kinase (AMPK)/nuclear respiratory factor 1/peroxisome proliferator-activated receptor (PPAR) γ coactivator 1α (PGC1α)–mediated mechanisms.[140,141] Maladaptation of this process leads to mitochondrial dysfunction and decreased ATP production. Thus, mitochondrial dysfunction is associated with decreased fat oxidation and accumulation of intramuscular lipids.[142] Mitochondria also play important roles in apoptosis (discussed later).

ER Stress

Obesity and type 2 diabetes mellitus cause increased ER stress in animal models and humans.[143–146] ER stress is involved in both impairment of energy metabolism and inflammation.[147] The lipid peroxidation product, 4-hydroxy-trans-2 nonenal (HNE), increases ER stress. Treatment of endothelial cells with phenylbutric acid or taurine-conjugated ursodeoxycholic reduces HNE-induced leukocyte rolling and adhesion.[148] ER stress leads to unfolded protein responses (UPRs) by (1) increasing expression of molecular chaperones, (2) facilitating degradation of proteins, and (3) inhibiting protein synthesis.[147] Molecules in the ER, including ATF6, IRE-1α/XBP-1, and p-PERK/p-eIF2α, are involved in UPRs to protect cells from stress conditions. When UPR is insufficient to protect cells from ER stress, cells are subjected to pathologic conditions, including inflammation, apoptosis, and lipid accumulation, that promote atherogenesis.[144,149–152] Activation of JNK is a well-known mechanism underlying obesity-induced insulin resistance and ER stress.[143,144,153] JNK directly phosphorylates IRS-1 at serine 307, leading to inhibition of insulin signaling pathways that contribute to inflammatory responses, impairment of glucose tolerance, and endothelial dysfunction.[125,154–156]

Apoptosis

Excess lipids increase ceramide, reactive oxygen species, lipid peroxidation, and membrane destabilization that lead to cell death through apoptosis. Inhibition of ceramide synthesis by myriocin reverses high fat/high cholesterol–mediated endothelial dysfunction and atherosclerosis.[157] Antiapoptotic molecules, including Bcl2 and Bax, are phosphorylated by Akt. This action is inhibited by ceramide to cause apoptosis.[158,159] Ceramide increases iNOS expression through NF-κB, leading to production of peroxinitrite that is toxic to cells.[160,161] Ox-LDL promotes endothelial cell death and atherosclerosis. This is opposed by HDL and ApoA.[162,163] Endothelial dysfunction and subsequent reduction of NO inhibits caspase activity by nitrosylation.[164,165] Thus, tissue damage by lipotoxicity is a major mechanism underlying the pathophysiology caused by dyslipidemia and diabetes.

ROLE OF EXERCISE IN OPPOSING LIPOTOXICITY AND ENDOTHELIAL DYSFUNCTION

Exercise plays a pivotal role in improving lipotoxicity and endothelial dysfunction.[166,167] Increased lipid accumulation with intramyocellular TGs in obese individuals with limited physical activity leads to reduced β-oxidation. Activation of peroxidation pathways predisposes to insulin resistance and its complications.[168] Intermediates of peroxidation pathways (thiobarbituric acid derivative, 4-hydroxynonenol, and malondialdehyde) may lead to increased levels of TNF-α and other proinflammatory factors that mediate insulin resistance and endothelial dysfunction.[168] Exercise and endurance training help increase turnover of stored excess lipids by increasing β-oxidation and reducing peroxidation pathways. In one study, even low-intensity exercise of 2 h/wk for 3 months had a positive impact on opposing lipotoxicity and increasing total fat oxidation.[169] Exercise has beneficial effects not only on skeletal muscle lipotoxicity but also on cardiac muscle. Two weeks of intensive swimming by mice led to an increase in diacylglycerol acyltransferase expression with greater TG uptake and oxidation in cardiac muscle. This was accompanied by decreased plasma cholesterol, TG, FFA, ceramide, and diacylglycerol. Lipid uptake genes, CD36 and LPL; PDK4 (Pyruvate dehydrogenase kinas, isozyme4), a regulator of glucose oxidation and acyl coenzyme A oxidase; PPAR α mRNA; and mRNA for PGC1α (a regulator of mitochondrial biogenesis) increased with 2 weeks of physical activity. Adipose TG lipase, the enzyme that initiates intracellular TG lipolysis, was induced with exercise.[170] The other benefits of exercise to oppose lipotoxicity include increased expression of superoxide dismutase.[171,172]

Oxidative enzyme activity in skeletal muscle improves with moderate intensity physical activity in previously sedentary men and women with 4 months of physical activity and moderate weight loss. Exercise improves enzymatic activity of the mitochondrial electron transport chain and increased surface area of the inner mitochondrial membrane with increased cardiolipin levels leading to mitochondrial biogenesis.[173]

AMPK is a fuel-sensing enzyme that is activated in response to exercise. It is also expressed in adipose tissue, liver, and other organs in response to exercise in intensity-dependent matter. Even low-intensity exercise, when prolonged, can also increase expression of AMPK. AMPK activity causes increased glucose uptake in muscle, promotes fatty acid oxidation, exerts anti-inflammatory and anti-fibrinolytic actions, raises HDL cholesterol, and decreases protein synthesis in skeletal muscle. AMPK also has central actions to decrease food intake in response to leptin action in the hypothalamus.[174] Hypothalamic insulin and leptin sensitivity is also improved by anti-inflammatory effect of cytokines, IL-6 and IL-10, that are positively influenced by exercise.[175] Other beneficial effects of exercise include increase in GLUT4 expression[176] and effects on muscle glycogen synthase activity. These actions of exercise oppose lipotoxicity and translate into improved CV outcomes.

The effect of exercise to oppose endothelial dysfunction is mediated, in part, by increased bioavailability of NO in the vasculature.[177] Regular physical activity improves blood glucose control and can prevent or delay type 2 diabetes mellitus, along with beneficial effects on blood pressure, lipids, CV morbidity, mortality, and quality of life. The American College of Sports Medicine and the American Diabetes Association recommend combined aerobic and resistance training exercise and aerobic activity of moderate intensity, 40% to 60% of $\dot{V}$ O_2max, 3 days a week, with no more than 2 consecutive days between bouts of physical activity.[178]

PHARMACOLOGIC TREATMENTS

Endothelial function is an important predictor of clinical outcomes, especially in populations with high CV risk. Therefore, targeting established and modifiable risk factors for lipotoxicity and endothelial dysfunction is a rational primary strategy for preventing CV complications associated with dyslipidemias and insulin-resistance. Combined therapy with statins or PPAR agonists and renin-angiotensin-aldosterone system (RAAS) blockade has additive beneficial effects on endothelial dysfunction, dyslipidemia, and insulin resistance compared with monotherapy in patients with CV risk factors that are mediated through both distinct and interrelated mechanisms.[179] In addition to primary prevention based on caloric restriction, weight loss, physical exercise, and smoking cessation, pharmacotherapies, including insulin sensitizers, hypolipidemic agents, and/or inhibitors of the renin-angiotensin system, effectively modify risk factors to result in beneficial effects on both metabolic and vascular homeostasis. A combinatorial therapeutic strategy aimed at improving circulating lipid profile, lowering oxidative stress, and attenuating inflammation by distinct cellular mechanisms may be helpful in improving the risk/benefit profile of pharmacotherapy for endothelial dysfunction.

Statins

Statins comprise either natural or synthetic compounds (**Box 1**) acting as 3-hydroxy-3-methylglutaryl coenzyme A (HMG-CoA) reductase inhibitors. HMG-CoA reductase converts HMG-CoA to mevalonic acid in the cholesterol biosynthetic pathway, the rate-limiting step in cholesterol synthesis. By inhibiting HGM-CoA reductase activity, statins decrease hepatic sterol synthesis. This decreases hepatocellular cholesterol. Hepatocytes respond to decreased intracellular cholesterol concentration by increasing synthesis of LDL receptors to enhance hepatic LDL reuptake from the circulation. The net result is an increased fractional catabolism of LDL that reduces serum LDL-C concentration and total cholesterol.[180] Several large randomized controlled trials have unequivocally demonstrated that inhibition of HMG-CoA reductase with subsequent of lowering LDL-C has large beneficial impacts on CV risk.[181–183]

In addition to LDL lowering, statins have several pleiotropic effects associated with improvements in markers of vascular disease risk, including

- Inflammation
- Plaque stability
- Endothelial function[184–188]

Direct actions of statins to affect Rho/Rho kinase pathways in human leukocytes have been reported.[189,190] Several other in vitro and in vivo studies have suggested that statins exert physiologic effects independent from LDL cholesterol lowering. For example, beneficial vascular effects of statins may depend on their ability to modulate levels of C-reactive protein (CRP). CRP induces synthesis of cytokines, cell adhesion molecules, and tissue factor in monocytes and endothelial cells[188,191] and upregulates angiotensin II type 1

> **Box 1**
> **Statins**
>
> *Natural compounds*
> - Lovastatin
> - Simvastatin
> - Pravastatin
>
> *Synthetic compounds*
> - Atorvastatin
> - Fluvastatin
> - Rosuvastatin

(AT1) receptors in vascular smooth muscle cells.[192] Therapy with statins decreases IL-1β–induced plasma CRP levels independently of cholesterol lowering in transgenic mice expressing human CRP.[193] These direct anti-inflammatory effects in vivo occur at the transcriptional level and have been confirmed in cultured human liver slices and in human hepatoma cells.[193] Improved endothelial function in response to statins may also result from prevention of NO oxidation and upregulation of eNOS expression,[194,195] partly by eNOS mRNA stabilization.[196]

Additional mechanisms by which statins exert their beneficial effects on endothelial function may involve eNOS coupling and vascular bioavailability of BH4 (tetrahydrobiopterin), a critical cofactor that is required to maintain eNOS enzymatic coupling activity.[197,198] This effect has been attributed to statin-mediated upregulation of GTPCH I (guanosine triphosphate cyclohydrolase), the rate-limiting enzyme in BH4 biosynthesis, initially demonstrated in cultured human endothelial cells.[199] Improved endothelial function in response to statin therapy has also been linked to increased NO and reduced peroxynitrite and O_2^- generation in cell culture[198,200,201] as well as in animal models.[202] Clinical evidence supports the concept that improved endothelial function with treatment with statins is associated with early reduction of systemic oxidative stress,[203] partly as a result of reduction in NOX activity in the arterial wall.[204] In addition, statins are known to downregulate AT1 receptor density,[205] and this may result in a direct NOX inhibitory action through blockade of Rac isoprenylation.

PPAR Agonists

The nuclear receptor transcription factors, PPARs, including PPARα, PPARγ, and PPARβ/δ isotypes, are each encoded by separate genes. PPARs are established drug targets for treating dyslipidemia and diabetes.[206] PPARα agonists (fenofibrate, gemfibrozil, ciprofibrate, and clofibrate), PPARγ agonists (pioglitazone and rosiglitazone),[207] and dual or pan agonists (bezafibrate, muraglitazar, ragaglitazar, tesaglitazar, and aleglitazar)[208] have both metabolic and CV actions.

Fibrates

Although peroxisome proliferation does not occur in humans, fibrate drugs, which lower TGs and raise HDL, were found to do so via PPARα activation.[209] Subsequent studies established that PPARα activation induces expression of LPL that releases fatty acids from TGs and represses apolipoprotein ApoC(III), an endogenous LPL inhibitor. PPARα increases expression of CD36, which participates in fatty acid uptake, and fatty acid binding proteins involved in fatty acid delivery. PPARα also regulates multiple enzymes involved in β-oxidation of fatty acids. PPARα activation also induces expression of APOA1, a major constituent of HDL. Fibrate therapy may help limit inflammatory responses induced by FFA in vascular and inflammatory cells. In endothelial cells, PPARα activated by synthetic agonists or LPL-mediated release of natural ligands inhibits adhesion molecule expression.[210,211] Additional effects include suppression of monocyte-macrophage migration[212] and monocyte chemoattractant protein-1 and reduced inflammatory markers, including CRP, lipoprotein-associated phospholipase A_2, IL-6, fibrinogen, and TNF-α.[213] PPARα activation also limits inflammation in vascular smooth muscle cells that may indirectly influence atherosclerosis. PPARα activation represses inflammation by inhibiting key proximal inflammatory mediators, including NF-κB and activator protein-1. In vascular smooth muscle cells, PPARα also limits cellular proliferation by targeting the cyclin-dependent kinase inhibitor and tumor suppressor, p16^{InK4a}, resulting in inhibition of retinoblastoma protein phosphorylation, decreased G_1 phase to S phase transition, and less intimal hyperplasia in vivo. In macrophages, activation of PPARα decreases coagulation proteins and promotes cholesterol efflux,[214] conferring additional protection from atherosclerosis.[215] In addition, fibrates may decrease angiotensin II–mediated oxidative stress and inflammation in the vascular wall.[216] Furthermore, fibrates may improve endothelial function indirectly via increased adiponectin levels and improved insulin sensitivity and flow-mediated vasodilation.[217]

Despite increasing in vitro evidence of vascular protective properties, fibrates have shown controversial results in the clinical setting: in the Veterans Affairs High-Density Lipoprotein Intervention Trial,

gemfibrozil was shown to exert a statistically significant 22% relative risk reduction in CV events in a subgroup of patients with established heart disease and concomitant glucose intolerance or high fasting plasma insulin level.[218,219] A subsequent study, the Fenofibrate Intervention and Event Lowering in Diabetes trial, did not find any significant difference in the primary endpoint between groups, although treatment with fenofibrate was associated with reduced secondary CV endpoints.[220] The Action to Control Cardiovascular Risk in Diabetes, lipid arm, study reported that combining a statin and fenofibrate was no better in decreasing CV events than a statin alone.[221] As suggested in other fibrate trials, however, a benefit was seen in the subgroup with more significantly elevated TG levels and lower HDL levels.[222] The absence of trials focusing on patients with more significantly elevated TGs and lower HDL levels where fibrates may be most helpful, may help to resolve this issue.

Thiazolidinediones

Synthetic PPARγ receptor agonists ameliorate lipotoxicity by multiple mechanisms. These include a decrease of circulating NEFAs by inhibition of lipolysis,[223,224] reduction of muscle long-chain fatty acyl coenzyme A levels,[225,226] and a redistribution of fat and changes in body composition.[5] Thiazolidinediones (TZDs) also ameliorate lipotoxicity and endothelial dysfunction via effects mediated through increased plasma adiponectin levels[227] and subsequent adiponectin-mediated antiatherogenic effects.[228,229] More recently, beneficial effects of TZDs have been related to their ability to ameliorate mitochondrial lipotoxicity, a condition characterized by reduced expression of multiple nuclear genes that encode enzymes involved in oxidative metabolism, such as PGC1,[34] a master regulator of mitochondrial biogenesis.[230] Treatment with TZDs upregulates PGC1α and PGC1β mRNA expression in association with increased expression of pyruvate dehydrogenase alpha 1 and other mitochondrial oxidative phosphorylation genes.[231] In addition to effects on lipid metabolism, TZDs may directly regulate multiple target genes relevant to inflammation and atherosclerosis.[232] In vascular tissues, PPARγ regulates production of endothelial mediators, including NO,[233] and modulates expression of genes involved in cell adhesion,[234] inflammation,[235] oxidative stress,[236] and vasoconstriction.[237,238] In macrophages, PPARγ anti-inflammatory actions play a protective role in atherosclerosis.[214] In the vascular compartment, PPARγ ligands reduce AT1 receptor mRNA and protein expression,[239] with decreases in reactive oxygen species and NADP oxidase activity as well as responsiveness to angiotensin II. These beneficial cellular and molecular properties of TZDs are not always supported by results from clinical trials. For example, effects of pioglitazone on CV events were investigated in PROactive, a large prospective study designed to test possible glucose-independent CV benefits in patients undergoing TZDs therapy.[240] Although only a nonstatistically significant trend toward benefit was seen with pioglitazone for multiple primary endpoints (10% risk reduction), a 16% reduction was found when more standard, objective secondary endpoints, such as myocardial infarction, stroke, and CV mortality, were evaluated.[240] In addition, pioglitazone decreased plaque volume in human coronaries[241] and carotid intima-media thickness.[242] It is possible that these improvements may be related to pioglitazone-mediated increases in HDL.[243,244] The effects of rosiglitazone on CV disease have been more controversial, partly because no large prospective study on CV outcomes was undertaken with this agent. Several meta-analyses of rosiglitazone data, including one by its manufacturer, suggest a possible increased risk of CV events, although the magnitude of this risk has been debated.[245–247] Potential insight into the different clinical responses of PPARγ agonists may come from their structure/activity relationship: as a consequence of their specific binding to the large PPARγ/retinoid X receptor nuclear complex, TZDs may have differing transcriptional effects resulting in differences in accessory molecule recruitment and/or release.[247] For instance, pioglitazone lowers TGs, whereas rosiglitazone does not.[248]

Dual PPAR Agonists

There is significant interest in designing molecules that target 2 or more PPAR isoforms to combine insulin-sensitizing properties with TG-lowering/HDL-raising effects. Dual or pan PPAR ligands include compounds such as tesaglitazar, muraglitazar, and aleglitazar.[249] Muraglitazar prevents the onset of diabetes and its complications in db/db mice[250] and reduces hemoglobin A_{1C} and improves lipid profiles in diabetic patients.[251] Another dual PPAR modulator, tesaglitazar, reduces atherosclerosis in mice with LDL receptor deficiency,[252] improves metabolic abnormalities and renal function, decreases blood pressure, and prevents glomerular and interstitial lesions in obese Zucker rats[253] and db/db mice.[254] Tesaglitazar suppresses both hyperglycemia and dyslipidemia in diabetic patients.[255] Chiglitazar improves impaired insulin and glucose tolerance and decreases plasma TG, total cholesterol, NEFAs,

and LDL-C levels in animal models of obesity.[256] Despite promising animal studies and positive clinical intervention trials, use and testing of several dual/pan PPAR modulators in humans have been discontinued because of severe side effects, including renal failure, fibrosarcomas, urinary cancer, and anemia. Aleglitazar is the only dual-PPARα/γ agonist currently in late-stage development.[206,257] A large prospective CV trial among patients with diabetes and acute coronary syndromes is under way with aleglitazar (clinicaltrials.gov NCT01042769).

RAAS Inhibitors

In addition to well-known actions in the vasculature, the RAAS plays an important role in skeletal muscle, liver, and adipose tissue that may interfere with insulin action and lipid control. High FFA levels and increased LDL and low HDL cholesterol levels may cause further dysregulation of the RAAS and contribute to endothelial dysfunction and atherosclerosis due to dyslipidemia and lipotoxicity. Consequently, pharmacologic treatments to block RAAS activity may benefit both vascular and metabolic physiology. Angiotensin receptor blockers and angiotensin-converting enzyme inhibitors are agents that directly affect the RAAS, either by blocking the binding of angiotensin II to the AT1 receptor or decreasing the production of angiotensin II, respectively.[258] Several large-scale clinical trials have demonstrated that the use of angiotensin receptor blockers or angiotenin-converting enzyme inhibitors can significantly reduce the incidence of glucose intolerance, dyslipidemia, and atherosclerotic lesions in hypertensive patients and/or patients with other symptoms of the metabolic syndrome.[259–265]

SUMMARY

Lipotoxicity, caused in large part by overnutrition, directly leads to endothelial dysfunction. Excess lipids in both the circulation and at the tissue level contribute to endothelial dysfunction that underlies much of the pathophysiology of both metabolic disease, including obesity and diabetes and their CV complications. Direct lipotoxic effects on other organs as well as secondary insults from endothelial dysfunction synergize to cause substantial morbidity and mortality. Lifestyle interventions, including reduced calorie intake, diet, and exercise as well as a variety of pharmacologic interventions targeting various mechanisms underlying lipotoxicity in vascular endothelium significantly modify metabolic and CV risk.

REFERENCES

1. Kim JA, Montagnani M, Koh KK, et al. Reciprocal relationships between insulin resistance and endothelial dysfunction: molecular and pathophysiological mechanisms. Circulation 2006; 113(15):1888–904.

2. Marks JB, Raskin P. Cardiovascular risk in diabetes: a brief review. J Diabet Complications 2000;14(2):108–15.

3. Rubanyi GM. Endothelium-derived relaxing and contracting factors. J Cell Biochem 1991;46(1): 27–36.

4. Aggoun Y. Obesity, metabolic syndrome, and cardiovascular disease. Pediatr Res 2007;61(6): 653–9.

5. DeFronzo RA. Insulin resistance, lipotoxicity, type 2 diabetes and atherosclerosis: the missing links. The Claude Bernard lecture 2009. Diabetologia 2010;53(7):1270–87.

6. van de Weijer T, Schrauwen-Hinderling VB, Schrauwen P. Lipotoxicity in type 2 diabetic cardiomyopathy. Cardiovasc Res 2011;92(1):10–8.

7. Duncan JG. Lipotoxicity: what is the fate of fatty acids? J Lipid Res 2008;49(7):1375–6.

8. Steinberg HO, Chaker H, Leaming R, et al. Obesity/insulin resistance is associated with endothelial dysfunction. Implications for the syndrome of insulin resistance. J Clin Invest 1996;97(11):2601–10.

9. Berg AH, Scherer PE. Adipose tissue, inflammation, and cardiovascular disease. Circ Res 2005; 96(9):939–49.

10. Nordestgaard BG, Benn M, Schnohr P, et al. Nonfasting triglycerides and risk of myocardial infarction, ischemic heart disease, and death in men and women. JAMA 2007;298(3):299–308.

11. Sarwar N, Danesh J, Eiriksdottir G, et al. Triglycerides and the risk of coronary heart disease: 10,158 incident cases among 262,525 participants in 29 Western prospective studies. Circulation 2007; 115(4):450–8.

12. Abe H, Yamada N, Kamata K, et al. Hypertension, hypertriglyceridemia, and impaired endothelium-dependent vascular relaxation in mice lacking insulin receptor substrate-1. J Clin Invest 1998; 101(8):1784–8.

13. Johansen CT, Wang J, Lanktree MB, et al. Excess of rare variants in genes identified by genome-wide association study of hypertriglyceridemia. Nat Genet 2010;42(8):684–7.

14. Dallinga-Thie GM, Franssen R, Mooij HL, et al. The metabolism of triglyceride-rich lipoproteins revisited: new players, new insight. Atherosclerosis 2010;211(1):1–8.

15. Surendran RP, Visser ME, Heemelaar S, et al. Mutations in LPL, APOC2, APOA5, GPIHBP1 and LMF1 in patients with severe hypertriglyceridaemia. J Intern Med 2012. http://dx.doi.org/10.1111/j.1365-2796.2012.02516.x. [Epub ahead of print].

16. Young SG, Davies BS, Voss CV, et al. GPIHBP1, an endothelial cell transporter for lipoprotein lipase. J Lipid Res 2011;52(11):1869–84.

17. van de Woestijne AP, Monajemi H, Kalkhoven E, et al. Adipose tissue dysfunction and hypertriglyceridemia: mechanisms and management. Obesity 2011;12(10):829–40.

18. Unger RH. Minireview: weapons of lean body mass destruction: the role of ectopic lipids in the metabolic syndrome. Endocrinology 2003;144(12):5159–65.

19. Hokanson JE, Austin MA. Plasma triglyceride level is a risk factor for cardiovascular disease independent of high-density lipoprotein cholesterol level: a meta-analysis of population-based prospective studies. J Cardiovasc Risk 1996;3(2):213–9.

20. Xiang GD, Xiang LW, He HL, et al. Postprandial lipaemia suppresses endothelium-dependent arterial dilation in patients with hypothyroidism. Endocrine 2012 Feb 22. [Epub ahead of print].

21. Yunoki K, Nakamura K, Miyoshi T, et al. Impact of hypertriglyceridemia on endothelial dysfunction during statin +/- ezetimibe therapy in patients with coronary heart disease. Am J Cardiol 2011; 108(3):333–9.

22. Yunoki K, Nakamura K, Miyoshi T, et al. Ezetimibe improves postprandial hyperlipemia and its induced endothelial dysfunction. Atherosclerosis 2011;217(2):486–91.

23. Kastelein JJ, Akdim F, Stroes ES, et al. Simvastatin with or without ezetimibe in familial hypercholesterolemia. N Engl J Med 2008;358(14):1431–43.

24. Alipour A, van Oostrom AJ, Izraeljan A, et al. Leukocyte activation by triglyceride-rich lipoproteins. Arterioscler Thromb Vasc Biol 2008;28(4): 792–7.

25. Schwartz EA, Reaven PD. Lipolysis of triglyceride-rich lipoproteins, vascular inflammation, and atherosclerosis. Biochim Biophys Acta 2012;1821(5): 858–66 [Epub 2011 Oct 7].

26. van Oostrom AJ, Sijmonsma TP, Verseyden C, et al. Postprandial recruitment of neutrophils may contribute to endothelial dysfunction. J Lipid Res 2003;44(3):576–83.

27. Sinha R, Dufour S, Petersen KF, et al. Assessment of skeletal muscle triglyceride content by (1)H nuclear magnetic resonance spectroscopy in lean and obese adolescents: relationships to insulin sensitivity, total body fat, and central adiposity. Diabetes 2002;51(4):1022–7.

28. Virkamaki A, Korsheninnikova E, Seppala-Lindroos A, et al. Intramyocellular lipid is associated with resistance to in vivo insulin actions on glucose uptake, antilipolysis, and early insulin signaling pathways in human skeletal muscle. Diabetes 2001;50(10):2337–43.

29. Inoue T, Kobayashi K, Inoguchi T, et al. Reduced expression of adipose triglyceride lipase enhances tumor necrosis factor alpha-induced intercellular adhesion molecule-1 expression in human aortic endothelial cells via protein kinase C-dependent activation of nuclear factor-kappaB. J Biol Chem 2011;286(37):32045-53.

30. Sharma S, Adrogue JV, Golfman L, et al. Intramyocardial lipid accumulation in the failing human heart resembles the lipotoxic rat heart. FASEB J 2004;18(14):1692-700.

31. Hirano K. A novel clinical entity: triglyceride deposit cardiomyovasculopathy. J Atheroscler Thromb 2009;16(5):702-5.

32. Bergman RN, Ader M. Free fatty acids and pathogenesis of type 2 diabetes mellitus. Trends Endocrinol Metab 2000;11(9):351-6.

33. Kahn SE, Hull RL, Utzschneider KM. Mechanisms linking obesity to insulin resistance and type 2 diabetes. Nature 2006;444(7121):840-6.

34. Patti ME, Butte AJ, Crunkhorn S, et al. Coordinated reduction of genes of oxidative metabolism in humans with insulin resistance and diabetes: potential role of PGC1 and NRF1. Proc Natl Acad Sci U S A 2003;100(14):8466-71.

35. Boden G, Chen X, Ruiz J, et al. Mechanisms of fatty acid-induced inhibition of glucose uptake. J Clin Invest 1994;93(6):2438-46.

36. Staehr P, Hother-Nielsen O, Landau BR, et al. Effects of free fatty acids per se on glucose production, gluconeogenesis, and glycogenolysis. Diabetes 2003;52(2):260-7.

37. Kruszynska YT, Mulford MI, Yu JG, et al. Effects of nonesterified fatty acids on glucose metabolism after glucose ingestion. Diabetes 1997;46(10):1586-93.

38. Steinberg HO, Paradisi G, Hook G, et al. Free fatty acid elevation impairs insulin-mediated vasodilation and nitric oxide production. Diabetes 2000; 49(7):1231-8.

39. Steinberg HO, Tarshoby M, Monestel R, et al. Elevated circulating free fatty acid levels impair endothelium-dependent vasodilation. J Clin Invest 1997;100(5):1230-9.

40. Kumar S, Durrington PN, Bhatnagar D, et al. Suppression of non-esterified fatty acids to treat type A insulin resistance syndrome. Lancet 1994; 343(8905):1073-4.

41. de Jongh RT, Serne EH, Ijzerman RG, et al. Free fatty acid levels modulate microvascular function: relevance for obesity-associated insulin resistance, hypertension, and microangiopathy. Diabetes 2004;53(11):2873-82.

42. Pilz S, Scharnagl H, Tiran B, et al. Free fatty acids are independently associated with all-cause and cardiovascular mortality in subjects with coronary artery disease. J Clin Endocrinol Metab 2006; 91(7):2542-7.

43. Il'yasova D, Wang F, D'Agostino RB Jr, et al. Prospective association between fasting NEFA and type 2 diabetes: impact of post-load glucose. Diabetologia 2010;53(5):866-74.

44. Byrne CD, Maison P, Halsall D, et al. Cross-sectional but not longitudinal associations between non-esterified fatty acid levels and glucose intolerance and other features of the metabolic syndrome. Diabet Med 1999;16(12):1007-15.

45. Karpe F, Dickmann JR, Frayn KN. Fatty acids, obesity, and insulin resistance: time for a reevaluation. Diabetes 2011;60(10):2441-9.

46. Opie LH, Walfish PG. Plasma free fatty acid concentrations in obesity. N Engl J Med 1963; 268:757-60.

47. Fielding BA, Callow J, Owen RM, et al. Postprandial lipemia: the origin of an early peak studied by specific dietary fatty acid intake during sequential meals. Am J Clin Nutr 1996;63(1):36-41.

48. McQuaid SE, Hodson L, Neville MJ, et al. Downregulation of adipose tissue fatty acid trafficking in obesity: a driver for ectopic fat deposition? Diabetes 2011;60(1):47-55.

49. Halcox JP, Donald AE, Ellins E, et al. Endothelial function predicts progression of carotid intima-media thickness. Circulation 2009;119(7):1005-12.

50. Steinberg HO, Bayazeed B, Hook G, et al. Endothelial dysfunction is associated with cholesterol levels in the high normal range in humans. Circulation 1997;96(10):3287-93.

51. Feron O, Dessy C, Moniotte S, et al. Hypercholesterolemia decreases nitric oxide production by promoting the interaction of caveolin and endothelial nitric oxide synthase. J Clin Invest 1999;103(6): 897-905.

52. Duvillard L, Pont F, Florentin E, et al. Metabolic abnormalities of apolipoprotein B-containing lipoproteins in non-insulin-dependent diabetes: a stable isotope kinetic study. Eur J Clin Invest 2000;30(8):685-94.

53. Verges B, Florentin E, Baillot-Rudoni S, et al. Effects of 20 mg rosuvastatin on VLDL1-, VLDL2-, IDL- and LDL-ApoB kinetics in type 2 diabetes. Diabetologia 2008;51(8):1382-90.

54. Koh KK, Quon MJ, Han SH, et al. Simvastatin improves flow-mediated dilation but reduces adiponectin levels and insulin sensitivity in hypercholesterolemic patients. Diabetes Care 2008;31(4): 776-82.

55. Adnitt PI, Frayn KN. Effects of metformin on glucose uptake by the isolated rat diaphragm. Br J Pharmacol 1972;45(1):152P-3P.

56. Blair A, Shaul PW, Yuhanna IS, et al. Oxidized low density lipoprotein displaces endothelial nitric-oxide synthase (eNOS) from plasmalemmal caveolae and impairs eNOS activation. J Biol Chem 1999;274(45):32512-9.

57. Uittenbogaard A, Shaul PW, Yuhanna IS, et al. High density lipoprotein prevents oxidized low density lipoprotein-induced inhibition of endothelial nitric-oxide synthase localization and activation in caveolae. J Biol Chem 2000;275(15):11278–83.

58. Kita T, Yokode M, Ishii K, et al. The role of oxidized lipoproteins in the pathogenesis of atherosclerosis. Clin Exp Pharmacol Physiol Suppl 1992;20: 37–42.

59. Maor I, Aviram M. Oxidized low density lipoprotein leads to macrophage accumulation of unesterified cholesterol as a result of lysosomal trapping of the lipoprotein hydrolyzed cholesteryl ester. J Lipid Res 1994;35(5):803–19.

60. Verges B, Brun JM, Vaillant G, et al. Influence of obesity and hypertriglyceridaemia on the low HDL2-cholesterol level and on its relationship with prevalence of atherosclerosis in type 2 diabetes. Diabete Metab 1992;18(4):289–97.

61. Golay A, Zech L, Shi MZ, et al. High density lipoprotein (HDL) metabolism in noninsulin-dependent diabetes mellitus: measurement of HDL turnover using tritiated HDL. J Clin Endocrinol Metab 1987;65(3):512–8.

62. Duvillard L, Pont F, Florentin E, et al. Inefficiency of insulin therapy to correct apolipoprotein A-I metabolic abnormalities in non-insulin-dependent diabetes mellitus. Atherosclerosis 2000;152(1):229–37.

63. Besler C, Heinrich K, Rohrer L, et al. Mechanisms underlying adverse effects of HDL on eNOS-activating pathways in patients with coronary artery disease. J Clin Invest 2011;121(7):2693–708.

64. Persegol L, Verges B, Foissac M, et al. Inability of HDL from type 2 diabetic patients to counteract the inhibitory effect of oxidised LDL on endothelium-dependent vasorelaxation. Diabetologia 2006; 49(6):1380–6.

65. Abel ED, Litwin SE, Sweeney G. Cardiac remodeling in obesity. Physiol Rev 2008;88(2):389–419.

66. Lopaschuk GD, Folmes CD, Stanley WC. Cardiac energy metabolism in obesity. Circ Res 2007; 101(4):335–47.

67. Hall JE, da Silva AA, do Carmo JM, et al. Obesity-induced hypertension: role of sympathetic nervous system, leptin, and melanocortins. J Biol Chem 2010;285(23):17271–6.

68. Kenchaiah S, Evans JC, Levy D, et al. Obesity and the risk of heart failure. N Engl J Med 2002;347(5): 305–13.

69. Dyntar D, Eppenberger-Eberhardt M, Maedler K, et al. Glucose and palmitic acid induce degeneration of myofibrils and modulate apoptosis in rat adult cardiomyocytes. Diabetes 2001;50(9): 2105–13.

70. Park TS, Hu Y, Noh HL, et al. Ceramide is a cardiotoxin in lipotoxic cardiomyopathy. J Lipid Res 2008; 49(10):2101–12.

71. Chess DJ, Lei B, Hoit BD, et al. Effects of a high saturated fat diet on cardiac hypertrophy and dysfunction in response to pressure overload. J Diabet Complications 2008;14(1):82–8.

72. Galvao TF, Brown BH, Hecker PA, et al. High intake of saturated fat, but not polyunsaturated fat, improves survival in heart failure despite persistent mitochondrial defects. Cardiovasc Res 2012;93(1): 24–32.

73. Okere IC, Chandler MP, McElfresh TA, et al. Differential effects of saturated and unsaturated fatty acid diets on cardiomyocyte apoptosis, adipose distribution, and serum leptin. Am J Physiol Heart Circ Physiol 2006;291(1):H38–44.

74. Okere IC, Chess DJ, McElfresh TA, et al. High-fat diet prevents cardiac hypertrophy and improves contractile function in the hypertensive dahl salt-sensitive rat. Clin Exp Pharmacol Physiol 2005; 32(10):825–31.

75. Stanley WC, Dabkowski ER, Ribeiro RF Jr, et al. Dietary fat and heart failure: moving from lipotoxicity to lipoprotection. Circ Res 2012;110(5):764–76.

76. Halton TL, Willett WC, Liu S, et al. Low-carbohydrate-diet score and the risk of coronary heart disease in women. N Engl J Med 2006;355(19): 1991–2002.

77. Hu FB, Willett WC. Optimal diets for prevention of coronary heart disease. JAMA 2002;288(20): 2569–78.

78. Lavie CJ, Milani RV, Mehra MR, et al. Omega-3 polyunsaturated fatty acids and cardiovascular diseases. J Am Coll Cardiol 2009;54(7): 585–94.

79. Mozaffarian D, Wu JH. Omega-3 fatty acids and cardiovascular disease: effects on risk factors, molecular pathways, and clinical events. J Am Coll Cardiol 2011;58(20):2047–67.

80. Foley R. Cardiac disease in diabetic patients with renal disease. Acta Diabetol 2002;39(Suppl 1): S9–14.

81. Mogensen CE, Christensen CK, Vittinghus E. The stages in diabetic renal disease. With emphasis on the stage of incipient diabetic nephropathy. Diabetes 1983;32(Suppl 2):64–78.

82. Stam F, van Guldener C, Becker A, et al. Endothelial dysfunction contributes to renal function-associated cardiovascular mortality in a population with mild renal insufficiency: the Hoorn study. J Am Soc Nephrol 2006;17(2):537–45.

83. Stehouwer CD. Endothelial dysfunction in diabetic nephropathy: state of the art and potential significance for non-diabetic renal disease. Nephrol Dial Transplant 2004;19(4):778–81.

84. Attia DM, Ni ZN, Boer P, et al. Proteinuria is preceded by decreased nitric oxide synthesis and prevented by a NO donor in cholesterol-fed rats. Kidney Int 2002;61(5):1776–87.

85. Vaziri ND, Moradi H. Mechanisms of dyslipidemia of chronic renal failure. Hemodial Int 2006;10(1):1–7.

86. Vaziri ND. Dyslipidemia of chronic renal failure: the nature, mechanisms, and potential consequences. Am J Physiol Renal Physiol 2006;290(2):F262–72.

87. Kronenberg F, Kuen E, Ritz E, et al. Lipoprotein(a) serum concentrations and apolipoprotein(a) phenotypes in mild and moderate renal failure. J Am Soc Nephrol 2000;11(1):105–15.

88. Prinsen BH, de Sain-van der Velden MG, de Koning EJ, et al. Hypertriglyceridemia in patients with chronic renal failure: possible mechanisms. Kidney Int Suppl 2003;(84):S121–4.

89. Dalrymple LS, Kaysen GA. The effect of lipoproteins on the development and progression of renal disease. Am J Nephrol 2008;28(5):723–31.

90. Baines RJ, Brunskill NJ. Tubular toxicity of proteinuria. Nat Rev Nephrol 2011;7(3):177–80.

91. Iacobini C, Menini S, Ricci C, et al. Advanced lipoxidation end-products mediate lipid-induced glomerular injury: role of receptor-mediated mechanisms. J Pathol 2009;218(3):360–9.

92. Nosadini R, Tonolo G. Role of oxidized low density lipoproteins and free fatty acids in the pathogenesis of glomerulopathy and tubulointerstitial lesions in type 2 diabetes. Nutr Metab Cardiovasc Dis 2011;21(2):79–85.

93. Obrosova IG. Diabetic painful and insensate neuropathy: pathogenesis and potential treatments. Neurotherapeutics 2009;6(4):638–47.

94. Andersen H. Motor dysfunction in diabetes. Diabetes Metab Res Rev 2012;28(Suppl 1):89–92.

95. Said G, Baudoin D, Toyooka K. Sensory loss, pains, motor deficit and axonal regeneration in length-dependent diabetic polyneuropathy. J Neurol 2008;255(11):1693–702.

96. Cameron NE, Cotter MA. Diabetes causes an early reduction in autonomic ganglion blood flow in rats. J Diabet Complications 2001;15(4):198–202.

97. Zent R, Pozzi A. Angiogenesis in diabetic nephropathy. Semin Nephrol 2007;27(2):161–71.

98. Tesfaye S, Chaturvedi N, Eaton SE, et al. Vascular risk factors and diabetic neuropathy. N Engl J Med 2005;352(4):341–50.

99. Witte DR, Tesfaye S, Chaturvedi N, et al. Risk factors for cardiac autonomic neuropathy in type 1 diabetes mellitus. Diabetologia 2005;48(1):164–71.

100. Lacigova S, Bartunek L, Cechurova D, et al. Influence of cardiovascular autonomic neuropathy on atherogenesis and heart function in patients with type 1 diabetes. Diabetes Res Clin Pract 2009; 83(1):26–31.

101. Obrosova IG, Ilnytska O, Lyzogubov VV, et al. High-fat diet induced neuropathy of pre-diabetes and obesity: effects of "healthy" diet and aldose reductase inhibition. Diabetes 2007;56(10): 2598–608.

102. Padilla A, Descorbeth M, Almeyda AL, et al. Hyperglycemia magnifies Schwann cell dysfunction and cell death triggered by PA-induced lipotoxicity. Brain Res 2011;1370:64–79.

103. Nowicki M, Muller K, Serke H, et al. Oxidized low-density lipoprotein (oxLDL)-induced cell death in dorsal root ganglion cell cultures depends not on the lectin-like oxLDL receptor-1 but on the toll-like receptor-4. J Neurosci Res 2010;88(2):403–12.

104. Yan SS, Chen D, Yan S, et al. RAGE is a key cellular target for Abeta-induced perturbation in Alzheimer's disease. Front Biosci 2012;4:240–50.

105. Johannsen DL, Ravussin E. Can increased muscle ROS scavenging keep older animals young and metabolically fit? Cell Metab 2010;12(6):557–8.

106. Preedy VR, Adachi J, Asano M, et al. Free radicals in alcoholic myopathy: indices of damage and preventive studies. Free Radic Biol Med 2002; 32(8):683–7.

107. Victor VM, Rocha M, Herance R, et al. Oxidative stress and mitochondrial dysfunction in type 2 diabetes. Curr Pharm Des 2011;17(36):3947–58.

108. Hayek T, Kaplan M, Kerry R, et al. Macrophage NADPH oxidase activation, impaired cholesterol fluxes, and increased cholesterol biosynthesis in diabetic mice: a stimulatory role for D-glucose. Atherosclerosis 2007;195(2):277–86.

109. Maloney E, Sweet IR, Hockenbery DM, et al. Activation of NF-kappaB by palmitate in endothelial cells: a key role for NADPH oxidase-derived superoxide in response to TLR4 activation. Arterioscler Thromb Vasc Biol 2009;29(9):1370–5.

110. Steinbeck MJ, Robinson JM, Karnovsky MJ. Activation of the neutrophil NADPH-oxidase by free fatty acids requires the ionized carboxyl group and partitioning into membrane lipid. J Leukoc Biol 1991;49(4):360–8.

111. Chinen I, Shimabukuro M, Yamakawa K, et al. Vascular lipotoxicity: endothelial dysfunction via fatty-acid-induced reactive oxygen species overproduction in obese Zucker diabetic fatty rats. Endocrinology 2007;148(1):160–5.

112. Curnutte JT, Erickson RW, Ding J, et al. Reciprocal interactions between protein kinase C and components of the NADPH oxidase complex may regulate superoxide production by neutrophils stimulated with a phorbol ester. J Biol Chem 1994;269(14): 10813–9.

113. Nauseef WM, Volpp BD, McCormick S, et al. Assembly of the neutrophil respiratory burst oxidase. Protein kinase C promotes cytoskeletal and membrane association of cytosolic oxidase components. J Biol Chem 1991;266(9):5911–7.

114. Hulsmans M, Van Dooren E, Holvoet P. Mitochondrial reactive oxygen species and risk of atherosclerosis. Curr Atheroscler Rep 2012; 14(3):264–76.

115. Schonfeld P, Wojtczak L. Fatty acids as modulators of the cellular production of reactive oxygen species. Free Radic Biol Med 2008;45(3):231–41.

116. Rocha M, Apostolova N, Hernandez-Mijares A, et al. Oxidative stress and endothelial dysfunction in cardiovascular disease: mitochondria-targeted therapeutics. Curr Med Chem 2010;17(32): 3827–41.

117. Kim JA, Wei Y, Sowers JR. Role of mitochondrial dysfunction in insulin resistance. Circ Res 2008; 102(4):401–14.

118. Moukdar F, Robidoux J, Lyght O, et al. Reduced antioxidant capacity and diet-induced atherosclerosis in uncoupling protein-2-deficient mice. J Lipid Res 2009;50(1):59–70.

119. Erdei N, Toth A, Pasztor ET, et al. High-fat diet-induced reduction in nitric oxide-dependent arteriolar dilation in rats: role of xanthine oxidase-derived superoxide anion. Am J Physiol Heart Circ Physiol 2006;291(5):H2107–15.

120. Pannirselvam M, Verma S, Anderson TJ, et al. Cellular basis of endothelial dysfunction in small mesenteric arteries from spontaneously diabetic (db/db -/-) mice: role of decreased tetrahydrobiopterin bioavailability. Br J Pharmacol 2002;136(2): 255–63.

121. Vasquez-Vivar J, Kalyanaraman B, Martasek P. The role of tetrahydrobiopterin in superoxide generation from eNOS: enzymology and physiological implications. Free Radic Res 2003;37(2): 121–7.

122. Wellen KE, Hotamisligil GS. Obesity-induced inflammatory changes in adipose tissue. J Clin Invest 2003;112(12):1785–8.

123. Xu H, Barnes GT, Yang Q, et al. Chronic inflammation in fat plays a crucial role in the development of obesity-related insulin resistance. J Clin Invest 2003;112(12):1821–30.

124. Linton MF, Fazio S. Macrophages, inflammation, and atherosclerosis. Int J Obes Relat Metab Disord 2003;27(Suppl 3):S35–40.

125. Kim F, Pham M, Luttrell I, et al. Toll-like receptor-4 mediates vascular inflammation and insulin resistance in diet-induced obesity. Circ Res 2007; 100(11):1589–96.

126. Shi H, Kokoeva MV, Inouye K, et al. TLR4 links innate immunity and fatty acid-induced insulin resistance. J Clin Invest 2006;116(11):3015–25.

127. Nguyen MT, Favelyukis S, Nguyen AK, et al. A subpopulation of macrophages infiltrates hypertrophic adipose tissue and is activated by free fatty acids via toll-like receptors 2 and 4 and JNK-dependent pathways. J Biol Chem 2007;282(48): 35279–92.

128. Michelsen KS, Doherty TM, Shah PK, et al. Role of Toll-like receptors in atherosclerosis. Circ Res 2004;95(12):e96–7.

129. Son JW, Jang EH, Kim MK, et al. Serum BMP-4 levels in relation to arterial stiffness and carotid atherosclerosis in patients with Type 2 diabetes. Biomark Med 2011;5(6):827–35.

130. Geng H, Wang A, Rong G, et al. The effects of ox-LDL in human atherosclerosis may be mediated in part via the toll-like receptor 4 pathway. Mol Cell Biochem 2010;342(1–2):201–6.

131. Holland WL, Bikman BT, Wang LP, et al. Lipid-induced insulin resistance mediated by the proinflammatory receptor TLR4 requires saturated fatty acid-induced ceramide biosynthesis in mice. J Clin Invest 2011;121(5):1858–70.

132. Montagnani M, Chen H, Barr VA, et al. Insulin-stimulated activation of eNOS is independent of Ca2+ but requires phosphorylation by Akt at Ser(1179). J Biol Chem 2001;276(32):30392–8.

133. Montagnani M, Ravichandran LV, Chen H, et al. Insulin receptor substrate-1 and phosphoinositide-dependent kinase-1 are required for insulin-stimulated production of nitric oxide in endothelial cells. Mol Endocrinol 2002;16(8):1931–42.

134. Gao Z, Hwang D, Bataille F, et al. Serine phosphorylation of insulin receptor substrate 1 by inhibitor kappa B kinase complex. J Biol Chem 2002; 277(50):48115–21.

135. Lee S, Lynn EG, Kim JA, et al. Protein kinase C-zeta phosphorylates insulin receptor substrate-1, -3, and -4 but not -2: isoform specific determinants of specificity in insulin signaling. Endocrinology 2008;149(5):2451–8.

136. Steinberg HO, Brechtel G, Johnson A, et al. Insulin-mediated skeletal muscle vasodilation is nitric oxide dependent. A novel action of insulin to increase nitric oxide release. J Clin Invest 1994; 94(3):1172–9.

137. Bikman BT, Summers SA. Ceramides as modulators of cellular and whole-body metabolism. J Clin Invest 2011;121(11):4222–30.

138. Wilson-Fritch L, Burkart A, Bell G, et al. Mitochondrial biogenesis and remodeling during adipogenesis and in response to the insulin sensitizer rosiglitazone. Mol Cell Biol 2003;23(3):1085–94.

139. Bogacka I, Xie H, Bray GA, et al. Pioglitazone induces mitochondrial biogenesis in human subcutaneous adipose tissue in vivo. Diabetes 2005; 54(5):1392–9.

140. Nisoli E, Clementi E, Carruba MO, et al. Defective mitochondrial biogenesis: a hallmark of the high cardiovascular risk in the metabolic syndrome? Circ Res 2007;100(6):795–806.

141. Le Gouill E, Jimenez M, Binnert C, et al. Endothelial nitric oxide synthase (eNOS) knockout mice have defective mitochondrial beta-oxidation. Diabetes 2007;56(11):2690–6.

142. Petersen KF, Dufour S, Befroy D, et al. Impaired mitochondrial activity in the insulin-resistant

offspring of patients with type 2 diabetes. N Engl J Med 2004;350(7):664–71.

143. Ozcan U, Cao Q, Yilmaz E, et al. Endoplasmic reticulum stress links obesity, insulin action, and type 2 diabetes. Science 2004;306(5695): 457–61.

144. Ozcan U, Yilmaz E, Ozcan L, et al. Chemical chaperones reduce ER stress and restore glucose homeostasis in a mouse model of type 2 diabetes. Science 2006;313(5790):1137–40.

145. Boden G, Duan X, Homko C, et al. Increase in endoplasmic reticulum stress-related proteins and genes in adipose tissue of obese, insulin-resistant individuals. Diabetes 2008;57(9):2438–44.

146. Kars M, Yang L, Gregor MF, et al. Tauroursodeoxycholic acid may improve liver and muscle but not adipose tissue insulin sensitivity in obese men and women. Diabetes 2010;59(8):1899–905.

147. Hotamisligil GS. Inflammation and endoplasmic reticulum stress in obesity and diabetes. Int J Obes (Lond) 2008;32(Suppl 7):S52–4.

148. Vladykovskaya E, Sithu SD, Haberzettl P, et al. The lipid peroxidation product, 4-hydroxy-trans-2-nonenal causes endothelial activation by inducing endoplasmic reticulum stress. J Biol Chem 2012 Jan 6. [Epub ahead of print].

149. Zhang Y, Xue R, Zhang Z, et al. Palmitic and linoleic acids induce ER stress and apoptosis in hepatoma cells. Lipids Health Dis 2012;11:1.

150. Fu S, Yang L, Li P, et al. Aberrant lipid metabolism disrupts calcium homeostasis causing liver endoplasmic reticulum stress in obesity. Nature 2011; 473(7348):528–31.

151. Tabas I. The role of endoplasmic reticulum stress in the progression of atherosclerosis. Circ Res 2010; 107(7):839–50.

152. Ji C, Kaplowitz N. ER stress: can the liver cope? J Hepatol 2006;45(2):321–33.

153. Gregor MF, Yang L, Fabbrini E, et al. Endoplasmic reticulum stress is reduced in tissues of obese subjects after weight loss. Diabetes 2009;58(3): 693–700.

154. Aguirre V, Uchida T, Yenush L, et al. The c-Jun NH(2)-terminal kinase promotes insulin resistance during association with insulin receptor substrate-1 and phosphorylation of Ser(307). J Biol Chem 2000;275(12):9047–54.

155. Carlson CJ, White MF, Rondinone CM. Mammalian target of rapamycin regulates IRS-1 serine 307 phosphorylation. Biochem Biophys Res Commun 2004;316(2):533–9.

156. Hilder TL, Tou JC, Grindeland RE, et al. Phosphorylation of insulin receptor substrate-1 serine 307 correlates with JNK activity in atrophic skeletal muscle. FEBS Lett 2003;553(1–2):63–7.

157. Chun L, Junlin Z, Aimin W, et al. Inhibition of ceramide synthesis reverses endothelial dysfunction and atherosclerosis in streptozotocin-induced diabetic rats. Diabetes Res Clin Pract 2011;93(1): 77–85.

158. Datta SR, Dudek H, Tao X, et al. Akt phosphorylation of BAD couples survival signals to the cell-intrinsic death machinery. Cell 1997;91(2):231–41.

159. Zhou H, Summers SA, Birnbaum MJ, et al. Inhibition of Akt kinase by cell-permeable ceramide and its implications for ceramide-induced apoptosis. J Biol Chem 1998;273(26):16568–75.

160. Katsuyama K, Shichiri M, Marumo F, et al. Role of nuclear factor-kappaB activation in cytokine- and sphingomyelinase-stimulated inducible nitric oxide synthase gene expression in vascular smooth muscle cells. Endocrinology 1998;139(11):4506–12.

161. Pahan K, Sheikh FG, Khan M, et al. Sphingomyelinase and ceramide stimulate the expression of inducible nitric-oxide synthase in rat primary astrocytes. J Biol Chem 1998;273(5):2591–600.

162. Dimmeler S, Haendeler J, Galle J, et al. Oxidized low-density lipoprotein induces apoptosis of human endothelial cells by activation of CPP32-like proteases. A mechanistic clue to the 'response to injury' hypothesis. Circulation 1997;95(7):1760–3.

163. Suc I, Escargueil-Blanc I, Troly M, et al. HDL and ApoA prevent cell death of endothelial cells induced by oxidized LDL. Arterioscler Thromb Vasc Biol 1997;17(10):2158–66.

164. Noor R, Shuaib U, Wang CX, et al. High-density lipoprotein cholesterol regulates endothelial progenitor cells by increasing eNOS and preventing apoptosis. Atherosclerosis 2007;192(1):92–9.

165. Hoffmann J, Haendeler J, Aicher A, et al. Aging enhances the sensitivity of endothelial cells toward apoptotic stimuli: important role of nitric oxide. Circ Res 2001;89(8):709–15.

166. Barlow CE, LaMonte MJ, Fitzgerald SJ, et al. Cardiorespiratory fitness is an independent predictor of hypertension incidence among initially normotensive healthy women. Am J Epidemiol 2006;163(2):142–50.

167. Sui X, LaMonte MJ, Laditka JN, et al. Cardiorespiratory fitness and adiposity as mortality predictors in older adults. JAMA 2007;298(21):2507–16.

168. Carter SL, Rennie C, Tarnopolsky MA. Substrate utilization during endurance exercise in men and women after endurance training. Am J Physiol Endocrinol Metab 2001;280(6):E898–907.

169. Schrauwen P, van Aggel-Leijssen DP, Hul G, et al. The effect of a 3-month low-intensity endurance training program on fat oxidation and acetyl-CoA carboxylase-2 expression. Diabetes 2002;51(7): 2220–6.

170. Liu L, Shi X, Bharadwaj KG, et al. DGAT1 expression increases heart triglyceride content but ameliorates lipotoxicity. J Biol Chem 2009;284(52): 36312–23.

171. Criswell D, Powers S, Dodd S, et al. High intensity training-induced changes in skeletal muscle antioxidant enzyme activity. Med Sci Sports Exerc 1993;25(10):1135–40.

172. Pinto A, Di Raimondo D, Tuttolomondo A, et al. Effects of physical exercise on inflammatory markers of atherosclerosis. Curr Pharm Des 2012; 287(14):11398–409.

173. Menshikova EV, Ritov VB, Ferrell RE, et al. Characteristics of skeletal muscle mitochondrial biogenesis induced by moderate-intensity exercise and weight loss in obesity. J Appl Phys 2007;103(1): 21–7.

174. Richter EA, Ruderman NB. AMPK and the biochemistry of exercise: implications for human health and disease. Biochem J 2009;418(2):261–75.

175. Ropelle ER, Flores MB, Cintra DE, et al. IL-6 and IL-10 anti-inflammatory activity links exercise to hypothalamic insulin and leptin sensitivity through IKKbeta and ER stress inhibition. PLoS Biol 2010; 8(8):e1000465.

176. Christ-Roberts CY, Pratipanawatr T, Pratipanawatr W, et al. Exercise training increases glycogen synthase activity and GLUT4 expression but not insulin signaling in overweight nondiabetic and type 2 diabetic subjects. Metabolism 2004;53(9):1233–42.

177. Maiorana A, O'Driscoll G, Taylor R, et al. Exercise and the nitric oxide vasodilator system. Sports Med 2003;33(14):1013–35.

178. Colberg SR, Albright AL, Blissmer BJ, et al. Exercise and Type 2 Diabetes. Med Sci Sports Exerc 2010 Dec;42(12):2283–303.

179. Lim S, Despres JP, Koh KK. Prevention of atherosclerosis in overweight/obese patients. - In need of novel multi-targeted approaches. Circ J 2011; 75(5):1019–27.

180. Istvan ES, Deisenhofer J. Structural mechanism for statin inhibition of HMG-CoA reductase. Science 2001;292(5519):1160–4.

181. Group HPSC. MRC/BHF Heart Protection Study of cholesterol lowering with simvastatin in 20,536 high-risk individuals: a randomised placebo-controlled trial. Lancet 2002;360(9326):7–22.

182. Ridker PM, Cannon CP, Morrow D, et al. C-reactive protein levels and outcomes after statin therapy. N Engl J Med 2005;352(1):20–8.

183. Ridker PM, Danielson E, Fonseca FA, et al. Reduction in C-reactive protein and LDL cholesterol and cardiovascular event rates after initiation of rosuvastatin: a prospective study of the JUPITER trial. Lancet 2009;373(9670):1175–82.

184. Sorrentino S, Landmesser U. Nonlipid-lowering effects of statins. Curr Treat Options Cardiovasc Med 2005;7(6):459–66.

185. Zhou Q, Liao JK. Pleiotropic effects of statins. - Basic research and clinical perspectives. Circ J 2010;74(5):818–26.

186. Wang CY, Liu PY, Liao JK. Pleiotropic effects of statin therapy: molecular mechanisms and clinical results. Trends Mol Med 2008;14(1):37–44.

187. Colhoun HM, Betteridge DJ, Durrington PN, et al. Primary prevention of cardiovascular disease with atorvastatin in type 2 diabetes in the Collaborative Atorvastatin Diabetes Study (CARDS): multicentre randomised placebo-controlled trial. Lancet 2004; 364(9435):685–96.

188. Koh KK, Quon MJ, Rosenson RS, et al. Vascular and metabolic effects of treatment of combined hyperlipidemia: focus on statins and fibrates. Int J Cardiol 2008;124(2):149–59.

189. Rawlings R, Nohria A, Liu PY, et al. Comparison of effects of rosuvastatin (10 mg) versus atorvastatin (40 mg) on rho kinase activity in caucasian men with a previous atherosclerotic event. Am J Cardiol 2009;103(4):437–41.

190. Liu PY, Liu YW, Lin LJ, et al. Evidence for statin pleiotropy in humans: differential effects of statins and ezetimibe on rho-associated coiled-coil containing protein kinase activity, endothelial function, and inflammation. Circulation 2009;119(1):131–8.

191. Gabay C, Kushner I. Acute-phase proteins and other systemic responses to inflammation. N Engl J Med 1999;340(6):448–54.

192. Wang CH, Li SH, Weisel RD, et al. C-reactive protein upregulates angiotensin type 1 receptors in vascular smooth muscle. Circulation 2003; 107(13):1783–90.

193. Kleemann R, Verschuren L, de Rooij BJ, et al. Evidence for anti-inflammatory activity of statins and PPARalpha activators in human C-reactive protein transgenic mice in vivo and in cultured human hepatocytes in vitro. Blood 2004;103(11): 4188–94.

194. Laufs U, La Fata V, Plutzky J, et al. Upregulation of endothelial nitric oxide synthase by HMG CoA reductase inhibitors. Circulation 1998;97(12):1129–35.

195. Laufs U, Liao JK. Post-transcriptional regulation of endothelial nitric oxide synthase mRNA stability by Rho GTPase. J Biol Chem 1998;273(37): 24266–71.

196. Kosmidou I, Moore JP, Weber M, et al. Statin treatment and 3' polyadenylation of eNOS mRNA. Arterioscler Thromb Vasc Biol 2007;27(12):2642–9.

197. Wenzel P, Daiber A, Oelze M, et al. Mechanisms underlying recoupling of eNOS by HMG-CoA reductase inhibition in a rat model of streptozotocin-induced diabetes mellitus. Atherosclerosis 2008;198(1):65–76.

198. Antoniades C, Bakogiannis C, Leeson P, et al. Rapid, direct effects of statin treatment on arterial redox state and nitric oxide bioavailability in human atherosclerosis via tetrahydrobiopterin-mediated endothelial nitric oxide synthase coupling. Circulation 2011;124(3):335–45.

199. Hattori Y, Nakanishi N, Akimoto K, et al. HMG-CoA reductase inhibitor increases GTP cyclohydrolase I mRNA and tetrahydrobiopterin in vascular endothelial cells. Arterioscler Thromb Vasc Biol 2003; 23(2):176–82.

200. Rueckschloss U, Galle J, Holtz J, et al. Induction of NAD(P)H oxidase by oxidized low-density lipoprotein in human endothelial cells: antioxidative potential of hydroxymethylglutaryl coenzyme A reductase inhibitor therapy. Circulation 2001; 104(15):1767–72.

201. Mason RP, Kubant R, Heeba G, et al. Synergistic effect of amlodipine and atorvastatin in reversing LDL-induced endothelial dysfunction. Pharm Res 2008;25(8):1798–806.

202. Otto A, Fontaine J, Tschirhart E, et al. Rosuvastatin treatment protects against nitrate-induced oxidative stress in eNOS knockout mice: implication of the NAD(P)H oxidase pathway. Br J Pharmacol 2006;148(4):544–52.

203. Cangemi R, Loffredo L, Carnevale R, et al. Early decrease of oxidative stress by atorvastatin in hypercholesterolaemic patients: effect on circulating vitamin E. Eur Heart J 2008;29(1):54–62.

204. Morawietz H, Erbs S, Holtz J, et al. Endothelial protection, AT1 blockade and cholesterol-dependent oxidative stress: the EPAS trial. Circulation 2006;114(Suppl 1):I296–301.

205. Nickenig G, Baumer AT, Temur Y, et al. Statin-sensitive dysregulated AT1 receptor function and density in hypercholesterolemic men. Circulation 1999;100(21):2131–4.

206. Plutzky J. The PPAR-RXR transcriptional complex in the vasculature: energy in the balance. Circ Res 2011;108(8):1002–16.

207. Yki-Jarvinen H. Thiazolidinediones. N Engl J Med 2004;351(11):1106–18.

208. Friedland SN, Leong A, Filion KB, et al. The cardiovascular effects of peroxisome proliferator-activated receptor agonists. Am J Med 2012; 125(2):126–33.

209. Willson TM, Brown PJ, Sternbach DD, et al. The PPARs: from orphan receptors to drug discovery. J Med Chem 2000;43(4):527–50.

210. Marx N, Sukhova GK, Collins T, et al. PPARalpha activators inhibit cytokine-induced vascular cell adhesion molecule-1 expression in human endothelial cells. Circulation 1999;99(24):3125–31.

211. Ziouzenkova O, Perrey S, Asatryan L, et al. Lipolysis of triglyceride-rich lipoproteins generates PPAR ligands: evidence for an antiinflammatory role for lipoprotein lipase. Acad Sci U S A 2003; 100(5):2730–5.

212. Marx N, Mackman N, Schonbeck U, et al. PPARalpha activators inhibit tissue factor expression and activity in human monocytes. Circulation 2001; 103(2):213–9.

213. Muhlestein JB, May HT, Jensen JR, et al. The reduction of inflammatory biomarkers by statin, fibrate, and combination therapy among diabetic patients with mixed dyslipidemia: the DIACOR (Diabetes and Combined Lipid Therapy Regimen) study. J Am Coll Cardiol 2006;48(2): 396–401.

214. Rigamonti E, Chinetti-Gbaguidi G, Staels B. Regulation of macrophage functions by PPAR-alpha, PPAR-gamma, and LXRs in mice and men. Arterioscler Thromb Vasc Biol 2008;28(6):1050–9.

215. Babaev VR, Ishiguro H, Ding L, et al. Macrophage expression of peroxisome proliferator-activated receptor-alpha reduces atherosclerosis in low-density lipoprotein receptor-deficient mice. Circulation 2007;116(12):1404–12.

216. Diep QN, Amiri F, Touyz RM, et al. PPARalpha activator effects on Ang II-induced vascular oxidative stress and inflammation. Hypertension 2002; 40(6):866–71.

217. Koh KK, Han SH, Quon MJ, et al. Beneficial effects of fenofibrate to improve endothelial dysfunction and raise adiponectin levels in patients with primary hypertriglyceridemia. Diabetes Care 2005;28(6):1419–24.

218. Rubins HB, Robins SJ, Collins D, et al. Gemfibrozil for the secondary prevention of coronary heart disease in men with low levels of high-density lipoprotein cholesterol. Veterans Affairs High-Density Lipoprotein Cholesterol Intervention Trial Study Group. N Engl J Med 1999;341(6):410–8.

219. Rubins HB, Robins SJ, Collins D, et al. Diabetes, plasma insulin, and cardiovascular disease: subgroup analysis from the Department of Veterans Affairs high-density lipoprotein intervention trial (VA-HIT). Arch Intern Med 2002;162(22): 2597–604.

220. Keech A, Simes RJ, Barter P, et al. Effects of long-term fenofibrate therapy on cardiovascular events in 9795 people with type 2 diabetes mellitus (the FIELD study): randomised controlled trial. Lancet 2005;366(9500):1849–61.

221. Ginsberg HN, Elam MB, Lovato LC, et al. Effects of combination lipid therapy in type 2 diabetes mellitus. N Engl J Med 2010;362(17):1563–74.

222. Elam M, Lovato LC, Ginsberg H. Role of fibrates in cardiovascular disease prevention, the ACCORD-Lipid perspective. Curr Opin Lipidol 2010;22(1): 55–61.

223. Miyazaki Y, Glass L, Triplitt C, et al. Effect of rosiglitazone on glucose and non-esterified fatty acid metabolism in Type II diabetic patients. Diabetologia 2001;44(12):2210–9.

224. Miyazaki Y, Mahankali A, Matsuda M, et al. Effect of pioglitazone on abdominal fat distribution and insulin sensitivity in type 2 diabetic patients. J Clin Endocrinol Metab 2002;87(6):2784–91.

225. Miyazaki Y, He H, Mandarino LJ, et al. Rosiglitazone improves downstream insulin receptor signaling in type 2 diabetic patients. Diabetes 2003;52(8):1943–50.

226. Bajaj M, Baig R, Suraamornkul S, et al. Effects of pioglitazone on intramyocellular fat metabolism in patients with type 2 diabetes mellitus. J Clin Endocrinol Metab 2010;95(4):1916–23.

227. Bays H, Mandarino L, DeFronzo RA. Role of the adipocyte, free fatty acids, and ectopic fat in pathogenesis of type 2 diabetes mellitus: peroxisomal proliferator-activated receptor agonists provide a rational therapeutic approach. J Clin Endocrinol Metab 2004;89(2):463–78.

228. Kubota N, Terauchi Y, Yamauchi T, et al. Disruption of adiponectin causes insulin resistance and neointimal formation. J Biol Chem 2002;277(29):25863–6.

229. Yamauchi T, Kadowaki T. Physiological and pathophysiological roles of adiponectin and adiponectin receptors in the integrated regulation of metabolic and cardiovascular diseases. Int J Obes(Lond) 2008;32(Suppl 7):S13–8.

230. Puigserver P, Spiegelman BM. Peroxisome proliferator-activated receptor-gamma coactivator 1 alpha (PGC-1 alpha): transcriptional coactivator and metabolic regulator. Endocr Rev 2003;24(1):78–90.

231. Coletta DK, Sriwijitkamol A, Wajcberg E, et al. Pioglitazone stimulates AMP-activated protein kinase signalling and increases the expression of genes involved in adiponectin signalling, mitochondrial function and fat oxidation in human skeletal muscle in vivo: a randomised trial. Diabetologia 2009;52(4):723–32.

232. Brown JD, Plutzky J. Peroxisome proliferator-activated receptors as transcriptional nodal points and therapeutic targets. Circulation 2007;115(4):518–33.

233. Calnek DS, Mazzella L, Roser S, et al. Peroxisome proliferator-activated receptor gamma ligands increase release of nitric oxide from endothelial cells. Arterioscler Thromb Vasc Biol 2003;23(1):52–7.

234. Chen NG, Sarabia SF, Malloy PJ, et al. PPARgamma agonists enhance human vascular endothelial adhesiveness by increasing ICAM-1 expression. Biochem Biophys Res Commun 1999;263(3):718–22.

235. Marx N, Mach F, Sauty A, et al. Peroxisome proliferator-activated receptor-gamma activators inhibit IFN-gamma-induced expression of the T cell-active CXC chemokines IP-10, Mig, and I-TAC in human endothelial cells. J Immunol 2000;164(12):6503–8.

236. Inoue I, Goto S, Matsunaga T, et al. The ligands/activators for peroxisome proliferator-activated receptor alpha (PPARalpha) and PPARgamma increase Cu2+, Zn2+-superoxide dismutase and decrease p22phox message expressions in primary endothelial cells. Metabolism 2001;50(1):3–11.

237. Delerive P, Martin-Nizard F, Chinetti G, et al. Peroxisome proliferator-activated receptor activators inhibit thrombin-induced endothelin-1 production in human vascular endothelial cells by inhibiting the activator protein-1 signaling pathway. Circ Res 1999;85(5):394–402.

238. Satoh H, Tsukamoto K, Hashimoto Y, et al. Thiazolidinediones suppress endothelin-1 secretion from bovine vascular endothelial cells: a new possible role of PPARgamma on vascular endothelial function. Biochem Biophys Res Commun 1999;254(3):757–63.

239. Sugawara A, Takeuchi K, Uruno A, et al. Transcriptional suppression of type 1 angiotensin II receptor gene expression by peroxisome proliferator-activated receptor-gamma in vascular smooth muscle cells. Endocrinology 2001;142(7):3125–34.

240. Dormandy JA, Charbonnel B, Eckland DJ, et al. Secondary prevention of macrovascular events in patients with type 2 diabetes in the PROactive Study (PROspective pioglitAzone Clinical Trial In macroVascular Events): a randomised controlled trial. Lancet 2005;366(9493):1279–89.

241. Nissen SE, Nicholls SJ, Wolski K, et al. Comparison of pioglitazone vs glimepiride on progression of coronary atherosclerosis in patients with type 2 diabetes: the PERISCOPE randomized controlled trial. JAMA 2008;299(13):1561–73.

242. Mazzone T, Meyer PM, Feinstein SB, et al. Effect of pioglitazone compared with glimepiride on carotid intima-media thickness in type 2 diabetes: a randomized trial. JAMA 2006;296(21):2572–81.

243. Davidson M, Meyer PM, Haffner S, et al. Increased high-density lipoprotein cholesterol predicts the pioglitazone-mediated reduction of carotid intima-media thickness progression in patients with type 2 diabetes mellitus. Circulation 2008;117(16):2123–30.

244. Nicholls SJ, Tuzcu EM, Wolski K, et al. Lowering the triglyceride/high-density lipoprotein cholesterol ratio is associated with the beneficial impact of pioglitazone on progression of coronary atherosclerosis in diabetic patients: insights from the PERISCOPE (Pioglitazone Effect on Regression of Intravascular Sonographic Coronary Obstruction Prospective Evaluation) study. J Am Coll Cardiol 2011;57(2):153–9.

245. Nissen SE, Wolski K. Effect of rosiglitazone on the risk of myocardial infarction and death from cardiovascular causes. N Engl J Med 2007;356(24):2457–71.

246. Simo R, Rodriguez A, Caveda E. Different effects of thiazolidinediones on cardiovascular risk in

patients with type 2 diabetes mellitus: pioglitazone versus rosiglitazone. Curr Drug Saf 2010;5(3): 234–44.

247. Sgarra L, Addabbo F, Potenza MA, et al. Determinants of evolving cardiovascular benefit/risk profile of rosiglitazone during the natural history of diabetes. Am J Physiol Endocrinol Metab 2012; 302(10):E1171–82 [Epub 2012 Feb 28].

248. Goldberg RB, Kendall DM, Deeg MA, et al. A comparison of lipid and glycemic effects of pioglitazone and rosiglitazone in patients with type 2 diabetes and dyslipidemia. Diabetes Care 2005; 28(7):1547–54.

249. Balakumar P, Rose M, Ganti SS, et al. PPAR dual agonists: are they opening Pandora's Box? Pharm Res 2007;56(2):91–8.

250. Tozzo E, Ponticiello R, Swartz J, et al. The dual peroxisome proliferator-activated receptor alpha/ gamma activator muraglitazar prevents the natural progression of diabetes in db/db mice. J Pharmacol Exp Ther 2007;321(1):107–15.

251. Kendall DM, Rubin CJ, Mohideen P, et al. Improvement of glycemic control, triglycerides, and HDL cholesterol levels with muraglitazar, a dual (alpha/ gamma) peroxisome proliferator-activated receptor activator, in patients with type 2 diabetes inadequately controlled with metformin monotherapy: A double-blind, randomized, pioglitazone-comparative study. Diabetes Care 2006;29(5):1016–23.

252. Chira EC, McMillen TS, Wang S, et al. Tesaglitazar, a dual peroxisome proliferator-activated receptor alpha/gamma agonist, reduces atherosclerosis in female low density lipoprotein receptor deficient mice. Atherosclerosis 2007;195(1):100–9.

253. Liao J, Soltani Z, Ebenezer P, et al. Tesaglitazar, a dual peroxisome proliferator-activated receptor agonist (PPAR alpha/gamma), improves metabolic abnormalities and reduces renal injury in obese Zucker rats. Nephron Exp Nephrol 2009;114(2): e61–8.

254. Cha DR, Zhang X, Zhang Y, et al. Peroxisome proliferator activated receptor alpha/gamma dual agonist tesaglitazar attenuates diabetic nephropathy in db/db mice. Diabetes 2007;56(8):2036–45.

255. Cox SL. Tesaglitazar: a promising approach in type 2 diabetes. Drugs Today (Barc) 2006;42(3): 139–46.

256. Li PP, Shan S, Chen YT, et al. The PPARalpha/ gamma dual agonist chiglitazar improves insulin resistance and dyslipidemia in MSG obese rats. Br J Pharmacol 2006;148(5):610–8.

257. Henry RR, Lincoff AM, Mudaliar S, et al. Effect of the dual peroxisome proliferator-activated receptor-alpha/gamma agonist aleglitazar on risk of cardiovascular disease in patients with type 2 diabetes (SYNCHRONY): a phase II, randomised, dose-ranging study. Lancet 2009;374(9684):126–35.

258. Ferrario CM, Richmond RS, Smith R, et al. Renin-angiotensin system as a therapeutic target in managing atherosclerosis. Am J Ther 2004;11(1): 44–53.

259. Yusuf S, Gerstein H, Hoogwerf B, et al. Ramipril and the development of diabetes. JAMA 2001; 286(15):1882–5.

260. Barzilay JI, Davis BR, Cutler JA, et al. Fasting glucose levels and incident diabetes mellitus in older nondiabetic adults randomized to receive 3 different classes of antihypertensive treatment: a report from the Antihypertensive and Lipid-Lowering Treatment to Prevent Heart Attack Trial (ALLHAT). Arch Intern Med 2006;166(20): 2191–201.

261. Bosch J, Yusuf S, Gerstein HC, et al. Effect of ramipril on the incidence of diabetes. N Engl J Med 2006;355(15):1551–62.

262. McMurray JJ, Holman RR, Haffner SM, et al. Effect of valsartan on the incidence of diabetes and cardiovascular events. N Engl J Med 2010; 362(16):1477–90.

263. Van Linthout S, Spillmann F, Lorenz M, et al. Vascular-protective effects of high-density lipoprotein include the downregulation of the angiotensin II type 1 receptor. Hypertension 2009;53(4):682–7.

264. Olsen MH, Wachtell K, Beevers G, et al. Effects of losartan compared with atenolol on lipids in patients with hypertension and left ventricular hypertrophy: the Losartan Intervention For Endpoint reduction in hypertension study. J Hypertens 2009;27(3): 567–74.

265. Nishida Y, Takahashi Y, Nakayama T, et al. Effect of candesartan monotherapy on lipid metabolism in patients with hypertension: a retrospective longitudinal survey using data from electronic medical records. Cardiovasc Diabetol 2010;9:38.

Insulin Resistance and Heart Failure: Molecular Mechanisms

Annayya R. Aroor, MD, PhD[a,b], Chirag H. Mandavia, MD[a,b],
James R. Sowers, MD[a,b,c,d],*

KEYWORDS

- Cardiac insulin resistance • Cardiorenal metabolic syndrome • Heart failure
- Molecular mechanisms

KEY POINTS

- Heart failure is increasing in parallel with aging and diabetes in westernized industrialized countries.
- Insulin resistance is associated with diastolic dysfunction in the cardiorenal metabolic syndrome and type 2 diabetes.
- Insulin metabolic signaling is important in cardiac metabolic flexibility and postischemic reconditioning, and impairment in signaling compromises both processes.

Heart failure (HF) is a major cause of morbidity and mortality in the Western world. HF is present in more than 5 million people in the United States, accounting for nearly US$40 billion in annual health care costs.[1] Coronary heart disease (CHD), diabetes, hypertension, and cardiorenal syndrome (CRS) are the major factors causing HF.[1,2] CRS is a constellation of metabolic disorders including obesity, hypertension, insulin resistance, and myocardial and renal abnormalities. CRS increases the risk for the development of T2DM mellitus (T2DM) and renal and cardiovascular disease (CVD)-related CHD and HF.[3] At least 25% of adults in the United States have been diagnosed with CRS. The incidence of CRS is increasing at an alarming rate, owing to an increase in the aging population and an epidemic increase in overnutrition and sedentary lifestyle. Epidemiologic studies indicate that more than 60% of American adults are overweight and more than 40% of Americans older than 60 years have CRS. In addition, childhood and adult obesity is also emerging as a global health problem that predisposes to CRS and T2DM.[1–4]

THE CHICKEN AND THE EGG: INSULIN RESISTANCE AND HEART FAILURE
Insulin Resistance Contributing to Cardiomyopathy

A strong association exists between insulin resistance and HF. Insulin resistance predicted the development of HF in several clinical studies.[5] Although association of insulin resistance to HF may be attributed to associated conditions such as CRS, hypertension, and CHD, the recognition

This research was supported by NIH (R01 HL73101-01A and R01 HL107910-01) and the Veterans Affairs Merit System (0018) for JRS.
The authors have nothing to disclose.
a Department of Internal Medicine, University of Missouri School of Medicine, One Hospital Drive, Columbia, MO 65212, USA; b Diabetes and Cardiovascular Research Center, University of Missouri School of Medicine, One Hospital Drive, Columbia, MO 65212, USA; c Department of Medical Pharmacology and Physiology, University of Missouri School of Medicine, One Hospital Drive, Columbia, MO 65212, USA; d Harry S. Truman Memorial Veterans' Hospital, 800 Hospital Drive, Columbia, MO 65201, USA
* Corresponding author. University of Missouri–Columbia School of Medicine, Columbia, MO 65212.
E-mail address: sowersj@health.missouri.edu

of HF in association with diabetes in the absence of CHD and hypertension (diabetic cardiomyopathy), and obesity in the absence of diabetes, hypertension, and CHD (obesity cardiomyopathy) raises the intriguing hypothesis that insulin resistance alone has profound adverse effects on cardiac function.[6,7] Although moderate alcohol consumption is considered beneficial for cardiovascular risk, heavy alcohol consumption is associated with the development of insulin resistance and cardiac dysfunction (alcoholic cardiomyopathy).[8] The causal association between insulin resistance and cardiac dysfunction is seen in the development of insulin resistance by both genetic and environmental factors.[9] Transgenic mice with cardiomyocyte-specific deletion of insulin receptor (CIRKO) or insulin receptor substrate (CIRSKO) have reduced insulin-stimulated glucose uptake and also have impairment in cardiac function. Moreover, glucose transporter 4 (GLUT4) knockout mice also develop cardiac dysfunction, thereby implicating insulin resistance as a contributing factor in the development of contractile dysfunction in CRS.[10–12]

Heart Failure Contributing to Insulin Resistance

The presence of HF may predict the development of insulin resistance, and the risk of T2DM in HF is 18% to 22% higher per 10 years than in treated hypertension. Twenty-eight percent of elderly HF patients developed diabetes mellitus over a period of 3 years and in multivariate analysis, congestive HF predicted development of T2DM. HF patients may have both systemic and cardiac insulin resistance. Insulin resistance is also seen after myocardial infarction.[13–15]

INSULIN SIGNALING AND ITS REGULATION IN THE HEART AND VASCULATURE
Insulin Signaling in the Heart and Vasculature

Insulin signaling occurs through 2 different pathways: the phosphatidylinositol-3 kinase (PI3-kinase)/protein kinase B (Akt) signaling pathway, eliciting mainly metabolic responses, and the mitogen-activated protein kinase (MAPK) signaling pathway, eliciting growth factor–like responses.[16,17] In this path-selective signaling (**Fig. 1**), activation of ligand-activated insulin receptor phosphorylates insulin receptor substrate 1 (IRS-1). Phosphorylation of tyrosine residues on IRS-1 results in the engagement of Src homology 2 (SH2) domain-binding motifs for SH2 domain signaling molecules, including PI3-kinase and growth factor receptor bound protein 2 (GRB2). When SH2 domains of the

p85 regulatory subunit of PI3-kinase bind to the tyrosine-phosphorylated motifs on IRS-1, this activates the preassociated p110 catalytic subunit to generate phosphatidylinositol-3,4,5-triphosphate. This molecule then binds to the pleckstrin homology domain in 3-phosphoinositide–dependent protein kinase 1 (PDK-1), resulting in its phosphorylation and the activation of other downstream kinases including Akt and atypical protein kinase C (PKC) isoforms, which mediate several actions including GLUT-4 translocation to the membrane, leading to glucose uptake in myocardial tissue and skeletal muscle, nitric oxide (NO)-mediated coronary vasodilation, metabolic flexibility, and energy homeostasis.[16,17] The MAPK signaling pathway involves tyrosine-phosphorylated IRS-1 or SH2 and collagen homologous region–containing protein (Shc) binding to the SH2 domain of GRB2, which results in the activation of the preassociated guanosine triphosphate (GTP) exchange factor son-of-sevenless (SOS) and GTP-binding protein rat sarcoma (RAS), which phosphorylates/activates extracellular signal–regulated kinase (ERK) 1/2. These signaling pathways contribute to growth and remodeling responses and the resultant myocardial hypertrophy, cardiac fibrosis, impaired myocardial-endothelial signaling, and death of myocardial and endothelial cells. The regulation of phosphorylation by protein tyrosine phosphatases or lipid phosphatases provides a negative regulation loop.[16–18]

Regulation of Insulin Signaling

The major converging point in the insulin signaling pathway contributing to insulin resistance is the docking protein IRS-1. The phosphorylation of serine residues of IRS-1 by several kinases, including PKC, C-Jun N-terminal kinase (JNK), mammalian target of rapamycin (mTOR), and ribosomal p70 S6 kinase 1 (S6K1), is the major mechanism for regulation of IRS-1 function.[16–18] Phosphorylation of serine residues of IRS-1 attenuates IRS-1 tyrosine phosphorylation and its association with the p85 subunit of PI3-kinase, and triggers its proteasome-dependent degradation. Proteasome degradation can occur by a suppressor of cytokine signaling (SOCS)-3–mediated, but phosphorylation-independent, mechanism. Inappropriate activation of tyrosine or lipid phosphatases, Akt, FOXO transcription factors, adenosine monophosphate–activated protein kinase (AMPK) signaling inhibiting mTOR/S6K, regulation of IRS-1 expression and IRS-1 signaling components by micro-RNA, and increased expression of tribbles homolog protein 3 (TRIB3) modulating IRS-1 tyrosine phosphorylation and Akt activation, also

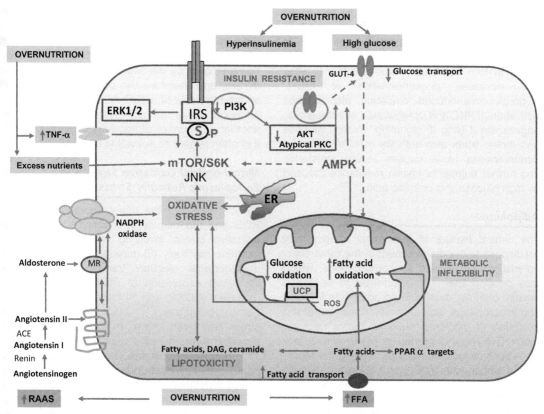

Fig. 1. Overnutrition and impaired insulin metabolic signaling leading to cardiomyopathy. The major signaling pathway causing insulin resistance is the convergence of multiple stimuli leading to the activation of S6 kinase. Overnutrition results in increased levels of circulating fatty acids, amino acids, and excess glucose that cause activation of mTOR/S6 kinase. Activation of RAAS results in oxidative stress caused by activation of NADPH oxidase by Ang II and aldosterone. Oxidative stress–induced activation of kinases, including JNK and S6 kinase, results in serine phosphorylation of IRS-1 and inhibition of insulin metabolic signaling. Cytokine-induced insulin resistance also involves activation of S6 kinase. Oxidative stress and insulin resistance is also accompanied by impaired AMPK signaling, which is a negative regulator of mTOR/S6 kinase. Persistent hyperactivation of mTOR/S6 kinase also leads to ER stress, oxidative stress, and activation of JNK. Excess accumulation and enhanced oxidation of fatty acids concomitant with increased accumulation of lipid intermediates result in lipotoxicity and metabolic inflexibility. These 4 overnutrition-induced cellular events are further amplified by their feed-forward interactions. ACE, angiotensin-converting enzyme; AKT, protein kinase B; AMPK, adenosine monophosphate–activated protein kinase; DAG, diacylglycerol; ER, endoplasmic reticulum; ERK, extracellular signal–regulated kinase; FFA, free fatty acid; GLUT, glucose transporter; IRS, insulin receptor substrate; JNK, C-Jun N-terminal kinase; MR, mineralocorticoid receptor; mTOR, mammalian target of rapamycin; NADPH, nicotinamide adenine dinucleotide phosphate; PKC, protein kinase C; PPAR, peroxisome-proliferator activator receptor; RAAS, renin–angiotensin II–aldosterone system; ROS, reactive oxygen species; S6K, ribosomal p70 S6 kinase 1; TNF, tumor necrosis factor; UCP, uncoupling protein.

contribute to impaired insulin signaling and insulin resistance.[16,18–21]

MOLECULAR MECHANISMS OF CARDIAC INSULIN RESISTANCE

The development of cardiac insulin resistance may occur independently of systemic insulin resistance, but systemic insulin resistance significantly contributes to cardiac insulin resistance secondary to increased circulating levels of nutrients, oxidative stress, and alterations in neurohumoral and cytokine balance (see **Fig. 1**).

Overnutrition

Increased levels of circulating free fatty acids (FFAs) and triglycerides caused by peripheral insulin resistance or overnutrition accumulate in the myocardial cells by increased uptake. The consequences are increased accumulation of lipid molecules such as diacylglycerol (DAG), fatty acids, and ceramide that contribute to insulin resistance through activation of kinases resulting in increased serine phosphorylation of IRS-1. In addition, hyperglycemia induces oxidative stress, which in turn activates redox-sensitive kinases and increases phosphorylation of IRS-1. Hyperglycemia-induced oxidation also causes activation of PKC and upregulation of intracardiac angiotensin II (Ang II) signaling. Excess glucose and amino acids also activate mTOR/S6K1. Hyperinsulinemia alone causes insulin resistance and further augments insulin resistance induced by high glucose and palmitic acid.[16–22]

Adipokines

The central feature of abdominal obesity may predispose to the development of the other characteristics of CRS and its complications, which may develop later.[16–18] In addition to increased release of FFAs, dysregulated adipocyte function and macrophage activation results in increased secretion of cytokines such as tumor necrosis factor (TNF)-α and interleukin (IL)-6, and adipokines such as resistin, while decreasing the secretion of adiponectin. TNF-α and IL-6 cause insulin resistance through activation of MAPK, PKC, mTOR/S6K1, and SOCS-3 mediated proteasomal degradation of IRS-1. Resistin induces insulin resistance and inflammation, whereas adiponectin improves insulin resistance.[3,12,16,17,23–25]

Activation of Renin–Angiotensin II– Aldosterone and Sympathetic Nervous Systems

Activation of the renin–angiotensin II–aldosterone system (RAAS) and the sympathetic nervous system (SNS) is seen not only in early stages of HF associated with insulin resistance but also in chronic HF or myocardial infraction.[24–27] In addition to the synthesis of aldosterone by Ang II, the mechanisms contributing to the link between aldosterone and insulin resistance include triggering of aldosterone release from adrenals by cytokines including TNF α and IL-6, and release of a lipid factor from adipose tissue. Both aldosterone and Ang II can activate the membrane-bound nicotinamide adenine dinucleotide phosphate (NADPH)-oxidase enzyme complex in vascular smooth muscle cells, and heart and skeletal muscle tissue, which results in the generation of reactive oxygen species (ROS). Positive cross-talk between Ang II and aldosterone for the nongenomic effects results in potentiating effects on ROS production. ROS production leads, in turn, to activation of redox-sensitive kinases such as protein S6K, PKC isoenzymes, and MAPKs, thereby causing

serine phosphorylation of IRS-1 leading to insulin resistance. Recent studies are suggestive of cross-talk between RAAS and mammalian target of rapamycin complex I (mTORC1)/S6K1 activation mediated by the angiotensin type-2 receptor (AT2R), and therefore the possible existence of an adaptive role of mTOR-AT2R signaling loop.[28] Although abnormal activation of the SNS is another component of insulin resistance and HF, it is often related to activation of RAAS.[26,27]

Mitochondrial Oxidative Stress and Endoplasmic Reticular Stress

Mitochondria are the major sources of cellular ROS, and this occurs (1) secondary to cytosolic oxidative stress involving NADPH oxidase or xanthine oxidase, (2) through dysregulation of mitochondrial electron transport, (3) through increased expression of mitochondrial NADPH oxidase 4 (NOX4), and (4) through altered protein lysine acetylation.[27,28] Mitochondrial oxidative stress has been shown to compromise insulin signaling through serine phosphorylation of IRS-1.[27,28] The endoplasmic reticulum (ER) stress contributes to mitochondrial oxidative stress and insulin resistance. Although the mechanism of ER stress–induced insulin resistance is not yet clearly known, activation of stress-activated MAPK JNK has been proposed as one of the signaling pathways linking ER stress and insulin resistance.[28,29]

MOLECULAR MECHANISMS OF HEART FAILURE IN THE CONTEXT OF INSULIN RESISTANCE

HF is associated with left ventricular (LV) hypertrophy, with increases in wall thickness and LV mass index, myocardial cell death, dilated cardiomyopathy, extracellular fibrosis, and functional abnormalities affecting diastolic and systolic function. The development of cardiac dysfunction results from cardiovascular insulin resistance as well as peripheral and hepatic insulin resistance.[5,9,14,18,22] The factors contributing to cardiac injury are impaired calcium signaling, changes in substrate metabolism, mitochondrial dysfunction and oxidative stress, ER stress, and dysregulated myocardial-endothelial interactions. The consequences are impaired calcium handling and contractility, decreased cardiac energy efficiency, myocardial cell death, and cardiac fibrosis (Fig. 2).

Impaired Calcium Handling

Intracellular calcium plays a critical role in modulating cardiac function. Calcium-induced calcium

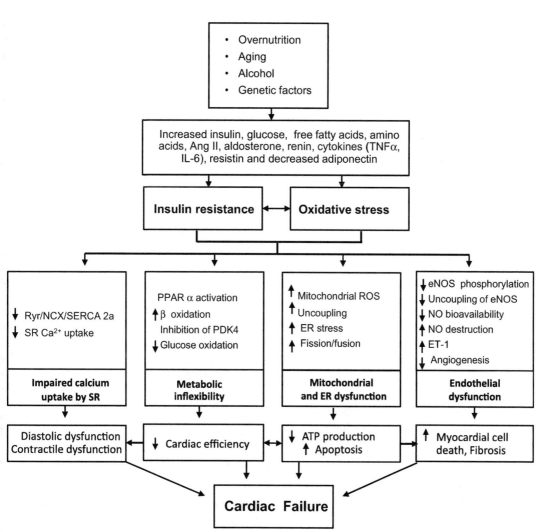

Fig. 2. Molecular mechanisms of cardiac insulin resistance and consequences of impaired insulin signaling and overnutrition, leading to cardiac dysfunction. The major consequences of insulin resistance and oxidative stress causing cardiac dysfunction are impaired calcium handling, metabolic inflexibility, mitochondrial and ER dysfunction, and endothelial dysfunction. These events contribute to cardiac inefficiency, myocardial cell death, and cardiac fibrosis and diastolic dysfunction. The progression of cardiac injury leads to contractile dysfunction and cardiac failure. Ang, angiotensin; ATP, adenosine triphosphate; eNOS, endothelial nitric oxide synthase; ER, endoplasmic reticulum; ET, endothelin; IL, interleukin; NCX, sodium/calcium exchanger; NO, nitric oxide; PDK, 3-phosphoinositide–dependent protein kinase; PPAR, peroxisome-proliferator activator receptor; ROS, reactive oxygen species; Ryr, ryanodine receptor; SERCA, sarcoplasmic endoplasmic reticulum Ca^{2+}-ATPase; SR, sarcoplasmic reticulum; TNF, tumor necrosis factor.

release regulates myocardial contractility through activation of ion channels, activation of ryanodine receptor (Ryr), and activity of sodium/calcium exchanger (NCX). Myocardial relaxation mainly occurs though resequestration of Ca^{2+} in the sarcoplasmic reticulum by the activity of sarcoplasmic ER Ca^{2+}–adenosine triphosphatase 2a (SERCA2a). Impaired diastolic function is the earliest cardiac dysfunction observed in CRS and T2DM. Abnormalities in the expression or activity of Ryr receptor, SERCA2a, and NCX, and impaired uptake of calcium by the sarcoplasmic reticulum have been reported in CRS and diabetic cardiomyopathy. PI3-kinase/Akt signaling has been shown to regulate intracellular calcium thorough potentiation of function of L-type calcium channel and up-regulation of SERCA2a expression and activity, while cardiac insulin resistance blunts PI3-kinase/Akt signaling thereby contributing to impaired calcium handling.[3,6,30–35]

Alterations in Substrate Metabolism and Impaired Cardiac Efficiency

Early metabolic abnormalities in substrate metabolism

Decreased glucose oxidation mainly occurs as a result of decreased entry of glucose though GLUT-4 and increased accumulation of fatty acid through inhibition of glucokinase and pyruvate dehydrogenase.[3] Increased flux of fatty acids into myocardial cells caused by systemic/adipose tissue insulin resistance and insulin resistance–associated redistribution of cluster differentiation protein 36 (CD36) to plasma membrane results in increased fatty acid oxidation. Under these conditions, the expression of cardiac peroxisome-proliferator activator receptor α (PPAR-α) is increased. Moreover, the PPARs are activated by ligands including fatty acids. Once activated, PPAR-α enhances the transcription of proteins controlling fatty acid uptake (lipoprotein lipase, CD36, and fatty acid–binding protein) and oxidation (medium- and long-chain acyl coenzyme A [CoA] dehydrogenase and hydroxyl acyl CoA dehydrogenase). Because glucose is a more efficient substrate, the cardiac metabolic switch from glucose metabolism to fatty acid oxidation decreases cardiac efficiency. This process results in further metabolic stress to the failing heart. Prevention of altered substrate metabolism in db/db mice by perinatal expression of the GLUT-4 glucose transporter prevented cardiac dysfunction in db/db mice, which further favors the existence of a metabolic switch in insulin resistance associated with T2DM.[34,35]

Late metabolic alterations in substrate metabolism and decompensated heart failure

As the disease progresses and myocardium assumes the phenotype of the fetal gene program, the expression of genes regulating β-oxidation of fatty acids is downregulated, thereby further dampening the metabolic efficiency of the myocardium. Under these conditions AMPK signaling is impaired, peroxisome-proliferator activator receptor γ coactivator (PGC)-1α is downregulated, and PPAR-α expression is decreased.[33–35]

Myocardial injury and superimposed insulin resistance

Another situation that has been increasingly recognized and that makes clinical management challenging is the development of insulin resistance accompanied by activation of RAAS, SNS, and oxidative stress after myocardial infarction or long-standing HF and ischemic heart disease. Under these conditions, the presence of insulin resistance abolishes the adaptation of myocardial switching to glucose oxidation necessary for the survival of the myocardium, resulting in increased myocardial cell death and poor outcome.[9,14,15,33–35]

Mitochondrial Dysfunction, Oxidative Stress, and Endoplasmic Reticular Stress

Both reduced and increased myocardial mitochondrial biogenesis associated with altered mitochondrial dynamics (fission and fusion) have been observed in humans and animals with CRS, coinciding with a reduced level of adenosine triphosphate and dysfunctional mitochondrial electron transport. The distinct findings are related to either the duration of CRS or associated underlying disorders. Mitochondrial oxidative stress and ER stress also contribute to myocardial apoptosis.[27,28,36,37] The role of myocardial autophagy in cardiac dysfunction is not clear at present.[38,39]

Impaired Cardiomyocyte–Endothelial Nitric Oxide Signaling

Endothelial dysfunction is an important link between insulin resistance and HF. Insulin resistance in endothelial cells results in impaired generation of NO or uncoupling of endothelial nitric oxide synthase. This process results in hypoxia and inhibition of angiogenesis, leading to myocardial cell death. Endothelial insulin resistance also results in increased release of endothelin-1 (ET-1), which causes cardiac hypertrophy and fibrosis.[3,6,7,40]

TARGETING INSULIN RESISTANCE IN HEART FAILURE

Lifestyle Interventions

The clinical significance of insulin resistance in patients with chronic HF often represents potentially reversible metabolic derangements in these individuals, especially at early stages of cardiac dysfunction. Lifestyle interventions, such as reductions in caloric intake and alcohol intake as well as increased exercise, appear to improve systemic and tissue insulin resistance. These measures target several insulin signaling cascades implicated in insulin resistance, including suppression of TRIB3 expression thereby overcoming TRIB3-mediated insulin resistance.[3,5,21,41]

Insulin Resistance

Apart from improving hepatic and peripheral insulin resistance, treatment of impaired glucose tolerance by metformin has been shown to actually reverse ventricular dysfunction in animal models. In insulin-resistant cardiomyocytes, metformin promotes translocation of glucose transporter 1 (GLUT-1) and GLUT-4 to the sarcolemma. It promotes glucose uptake in an AMPK-dependent manner and prevents high-glucose–induced abnormalities in relaxation by reducing intracellular Ca transients. Metformin increases fatty acid oxidation (FAO), but effects on glucose metabolism and AMPK activation appear to maintain metabolic flexibility.[9,13,42,43]

RAAS and SNS Activation

Given the importance of insulin resistance as an independent risk factor for mortality in HF, the use of both angiotensin-converting enzyme inhibitors (ACEIs) and angiotensin receptor blockers (ARBs) has been reported to significantly reduce the incidence of new-onset diabetes in large trials of patients with HF. ACEIs and ARBs are not completely effective in improving insulin resistance or hypertension, and aldosterone escape often impedes their efficacy.[26,44,45] The direct renin inhibitor aliskiren is a potent and selective inhibitor of renin,[26] the enzyme considered to be the rate-limiting step in the RAAS.[26,44] Renin inhibition is associated with attenuation of Ang II levels and reduction in blood pressure.[46,47] Mineralocorticoid receptor (MR) antagonists (MRAs) also improve LV function and clinical outcomes when they are taken in combination with ACEIs, ARBs, and β-blockers. However, some clinical studies linked MRAs to abnormal glucose homeostasis, thereby being suggestive of the complexity of MR receptor signaling.[26,44,45] Nonselective β-blockers that do not worsen insulin sensitivity, such as nebivolol and carvedilol, appear to exert beneficial effects in HF.[48] Nebivolol also inhibits Ang II–induced activation of NADPH oxidase and ROS, thereby providing a rationale for having beneficial effects on insulin sensitivity.[49]

Substrate Metabolism

Drugs modulating glucagon-like peptide 1 (GLP-1) signaling comprising GLP-1 mimetics or dipeptidyl peptidase (DPP)-4 inhibitors have been reported to be useful in controlling hyperglycemia by stimulating insulin secretion from the pancreas as well as enhancing myocardial glucose uptake via the translocation of GLUT-1 and GLUT-4 to the sarcolemma.[9,50] Chronic infusion of GLP-1 also improves LV dysfunction, exercise tolerance, and quality of life, in addition to improving cardiac insulin sensitivity. The DPP-4 inhibitor sitagliptin improved LV performance in response to stress and reduced postischemic stunning in patients with CHD, and preserved LV ejection fraction. Linagliptin has also been shown to have cardiovascular benefits in patients with T2DM.[9,50,51]

Trimetazidine affects use of myocardial substrates by inhibiting oxidative phosphorylation and by shifting the metabolism from FFAs to glucose oxidation though inhibition of long-chain 3-ketoacyl CoA, the last enzyme in β-oxidation. In small clinical studies, the drug showed small but statistically significant improvement in decreasing FAO, improvement in ventricular function, and decrease in insulin resistance in HF patients.[13,33,52,53]

Mitochondrial Oxidative Stress and Endoplasmic Reticular Stress

New compounds targeting mitochondrial oxidative stress and ER stress are being developed. In this regard, targeting mitochondrial production by synthetic Szezo-Schiller peptide S-31 prevented cardiac hypertrophy and fibrosis and improved LV diastolic function in a model of cardiomyopathy induced by Ang II and hypertension.[54] Drugs approved by the Food and Drug Administration that have been shown to decrease ER stress also improve cardiac function in animal studies, suggesting their potential use in suppression of insulin resistance in humans.[55]

SUMMARY

Insulin resistance is closely linked to HF and is associated with major factors contributing to HF. In clinical situations both conditions most often coexist, but the presence of insulin resistance contributes adversely to the progression of HF. The cardiovascular insulin resistance is also modulated by systemic insulin resistance. The signaling pathways contributing to insulin resistance converge mainly at IRS-1. In addition to glucotoxicity and lipotoxicity, dysregulation of neurohumoral and cytokine imbalance and oxidative stress are mainly responsible for cardiac insulin resistance and impaired cardiac function. Although targeting the RAAS and SNS has markedly improved clinical outcomes, drugs targeting metabolic pathways, GLP-1 signaling, mitochondrial dysfunction, and ER stress may show additional benefits based on underlying metabolic abnormality. Therefore, identifying mechanism-based new therapeutic targets to improve insulin resistance holds promise for better management of insulin resistance and HF.

ACKNOWLEDGMENTS

The authors would like to thank Brenda Hunter for her editing assistance.

REFERENCES

1. Norton C, Georgiopoulou VV, Kalogeropoulos AP, et al. Epidemiology and cost of advanced heart failure. Prog Cardiovasc Dis 2011;54:78–85.
2. Sowers JR, Whaley-Connell A, Hayden MR. The role of overweight and obesity in the cardiorenal syndrome. Cardiorenal Med 2011;1:5–12.
3. Falcão-Pires I, Leite-Moreira AF. Diabetic cardiomyopathy: understanding the molecular and cellular basis to progress in diagnosis and treatment. Heart Fail Rev 2012;17(3):325–44.
4. Reaven GM. Insulin resistance: the link between obesity and cardiovascular disease. Med Clin North Am 2011;95:875–92.
5. Horwich TB, Fonarow GC. Glucose, obesity, metabolic syndrome, and diabetes relevance to incidence of heart failure. J Am Coll Cardiol 2010;55:283–93.
6. Wong C, Marwick TH. Obesity cardiomyopathy: pathogenesis and pathophysiology. Nat Clin Pract Cardiovasc Med 2007;4:436–43.
7. Witteles RM, Fowler MB. Insulin-resistant cardiomyopathy clinical evidence, mechanisms, and treatment options. J Am Coll Cardiol 2008;51:93–102.
8. Zhang Y, Ren J. ALDH2 in alcoholic heart diseases: molecular mechanism and clinical implications. Pharmacol Ther 2011;132:86–95.
9. Ashrafian H, Frenneaux MP, Opie LH. Metabolic mechanisms in heart failure. Circulation 2007;116:434–48.
10. McQueen AP, Zhang D, Hu P, et al. Contractile dysfunction in hypertrophied hearts with deficient insulin receptor signaling: possible role of reduced capillary density. J Mol Cell Cardiol 2005;39:882–92.
11. Sena S, Hu P, Zhang D, et al. Impaired insulin signaling accelerates cardiac mitochondrial dysfunction after myocardial infarction. J Mol Cell Cardiol 2009;46:910–8.
12. Domenighetti AA, Danes VR, Curl CL, et al. Targeted GLUT-4 deficiency in the heart induces cardiomyocyte hypertrophy and impaired contractility linked with Ca (2+) and proton flux dysregulation. J Mol Cell Cardiol 2010;48:663–72.
13. Mamas MA, Deaton C, Rutter MK, et al. Impaired glucose tolerance and insulin resistance in heart failure: underrecognized and undertreated? J Card Fail 2010;16:761–8.
14. Heck PM, Dutka DP. Insulin resistance and heart failure. Curr Heart Fail Rep 2009;6:89–94.
15. Coats AJ, Anker SD. Insulin resistance in chronic heart failure. J Cardiovasc Pharmacol 2000;35(7 Suppl 4):S9–14.
16. Bertrand L, Horman S, Beauloye C, et al. Insulin signaling in the heart. Cardiovasc Res 2008;79(2):238–48.

17. Saha AK, Xu XJ, Balon TW, et al. Insulin resistance due to nutrient excess: is it a consequence of AMPK downregulation? Cell Cycle 2011;10:3447–51.
18. Kim JA, Jang HJ, Martinez-Lemus LA, et al. Activation of mTOR/p70S6 kinase by ANG II inhibits insulin-stimulated endothelial nitric oxide synthase and vasodilation. Am J Physiol Endocrinol Metab 2012;302:E201–8.
19. Zhang J, Gao Z, Yin J, et al. S6K directly phosphorylates IRS-1 on Ser-270 to promote insulin resistance in response to TNF-(alpha) signaling through IKK2 J Biol Chem 2008;283:35375–82.
20. Pulakat L, Aroor AR, Gul R, et al. Cardiac insulin resistance and microRNA modulators. Exp Diabetes Res 2012;2012:654904 [Epub 2011 Jul 31].
21. Sowers JR. Role of TRIB3 in diabetic and overnutrition-induced atherosclerosis. Diabetes 2012;61:265–6.
22. Gray S, Kim JK. New insights into insulin resistance in the diabetic heart. Trends Endocrinol Metab 2011;22:394–403.
23. Rocha VZ, Folco EJ. Inflammatory concepts of obesity. Int J Inflamm 2011;2011:529061 [Epub 2011 Aug 3].
24. Putnam K, Shoemaker R, Yiannikouris F, et al. The renin angiotensin system: a target of and contributor to dyslipidemias, altered glucose homeostasis and hypertension of the metabolic syndrome. Am J Physiol Heart Circ Physiol 2012;302(6):H1219–30 [Epub 2012 Jan 6].
25. Whaley-Connell A, McCullough PA, Sowers JR. The role of oxidative stress in the metabolic syndrome. Rev Cardiovasc Med 2011;12:21–9.
26. Lastra G, Dhuper S, Johnson MS, et al. Salt, aldosterone, and insulin resistance: impact on the cardiovascular system. Nat Rev Cardiol 2010;7:577–84.
27. Kim J, Wei Y, Sowers JR. Role of mitochondrial dysfunction in insulin resistance. Circ Res 2008;102:401–14.
28. Aroor AR, Mandavia C, Ren J, et al. Mitochondria and oxidative stress in cardiorenal metabolic syndrome. Cardiorenal Med 2012;2:87–109.
29. Cnop M, Foufelle F, Velloso LA. Endoplasmic reticulum stress, obesity and diabetes. Trends Mol Med 2012;18:59–68.
30. Lebeche D, Davidoff AJ, Hajjar RJ. Interplay between impaired calcium regulation and insulin signaling abnormalities in diabetic cardiomyopathy. Nat Clin Pract Cardiovasc Med 2008;5:715–24.
31. Ren J, Pulakat L, Whaley-Connell A, et al. Mitochondrial biogenesis in the metabolic syndrome and cardiovascular disease. J Mol Med (Berl) 2010;88:993–1001.
32. Mandavia CH, Pulakat L, DeMarco V, et al. Overnutrition, obesity and metabolic Cardiomyopathy. Metabolism 2012, Mar 30. [Epub ahead of print].

33. Tuunanen H, Knuuti J. Metabolic remodelling in human heart failure. Cardiovasc Res 2011;90:251–7.

34. Nagoshi T, Yoshimura M, Rosano GM, et al. Optimization of cardiac metabolism in heart failure. Curr Pharm Des 2011;17:3846–53.

35. van de Weijer T, Schrauwen-Hinderling VB, Schrauwen P. Lipotoxicity in type 2 diabetic cardiomyopathy. Cardiovasc Res 2011;92:10–8.

36. Boudina S, Bugger H, Sena S, et al. Contribution of impaired myocardial insulin signaling to mitochondrial dysfunction and oxidative stress in the heart. Circulation 2009;119:1272–83.

37. Santos CX, Tanaka LY, Wosniak J, et al. Mechanisms and implications of reactive oxygen species generation during the unfolded protein response: roles of endoplasmic reticulum oxidoreductases, mitochondrial electron transport, and NADPH oxidase. Antioxid Redox Signal 2009;11:2409–27.

38. Mellor KM, Bell JR, Young MJ, et al. Myocardial autophagy activation and suppressed survival signaling is associated with insulin resistance in fructose-fed mice. J Mol Cell Cardiol 2011;50: 1035–43 [Epub 2011 Mar 6].

39. Xu X, Ren J. Unmasking the Janus faces of autophagy in obesity-associated insulin resistance and cardiac dysfunction. Clin Exp Pharmacol Physiol 2012;39:200–8.

40. Takeda N, Manabe I. Cellular interplay between cardiac myocytes and nonmyocytes in cardiac remodeling. Int J Inflamm 2011;13. Article ID 535241.

41. Sullivan SD, Ratner RE. Should the metabolic syndrome patient with prediabetes be offered pharmacotherapy? Curr Diab Rep 2011;11:91–8.

42. Wong AK, Al Zadjali MA, Choy AM, et al. Insulin resistance: a potential new target for therapy in patients with heart failure. Cardiovasc Ther 2008;26:203–13.

43. Cittadini A, Napoli R, Monti MG, et al. Metformin prevents the development of chronic heart failure in the SHHF rat model. Diabetes 2012;61(4): 944–53 [Epub 2012 Feb 16].

44. Tamargo J, López-Sendón J. Novel therapeutic targets for the treatment of heart failure. Nat Rev Drug Discov 2011;10:536–55.

45. Messaoudi S, Azibani F, Delcayre C, et al. Aldosterone, mineralocorticoid receptor, and heart failure. Mol Cell Endocrinol 2012;350:266–72.

46. Marchionne EM, Diamond-Stanic MK, Prasonnarong M, et al. Chronic renin inhibition with aliskiren improves glucose tolerance, insulin sensitivity, and skeletal muscle glucose transport activity in obese Zucker rats. Am J Physiol Regul Integr Comp Physiol 2012; 302:R137–42.

47. Lastra G, Habibi J, Whaley-Connell AT, et al. Direct renin inhibition improves systemic insulin resistance and skeletal muscle glucose transport in a transgenic rodent model of tissue renin overexpression. Endocrinology 2009;150:2561–8.

48. Ladage D, Schwinger RH, Brixius K. Cardio-selective beta-blocker: pharmacological evidence and their influence on exercise capacity. Cardiovasc Ther 2012 Jan 26. http://dx.doi.org/10.1111/j.1755-5922.2011.00306.x. [Epub ahead of print].

49. Manrique C, Lastra G, Habibi J, et al. Nebivolol improves insulin sensitivity in the TGR(Ren2)27 rat. Metabolism 2011;60:1757–66.

50. Sivertsen J, Rosenmeier J, Holst JJ, et al. The effect of glucagon-like peptide 1 on cardiovascular risk. Nat Rev Cardiol 2012;9(4):209–22.

51. Barnett AH. Linagliptin: a novel dipeptidyl peptidase 4 inhibitor with a unique place in therapy. Adv Ther 2011;28:447–59.

52. Horowitz JD, Chirkov YY, Kennedy JA, et al. Modulation of myocardial metabolism: an emerging therapeutic principle. Curr Opin Cardiol 2010;25:329–34.

53. Ardehali H, Sabbah HN, Burke MA, et al. Targeting myocardial substrate metabolism in heart failure: potential for new therapies. Eur J Heart Fail 2012; 14:120–9.

54. Maack C, Böhm M. Targeting mitochondrial oxidative stress in heart failure throttling the afterburner. J Am Coll Cardiol 2011;58:83–6.

55. Minamino T, Komuro I, Kitakaze M. Endoplasmic reticulum stress as a therapeutic target in cardiovascular disease. Circ Res 2010;107: 1071–82.

Diabetic Cardiomyopathy
Bench to Bedside

Joel D. Schilling, MD, PhD[a],*, Douglas L. Mann, MD[b]

KEYWORDS

- Diabetic cardiomyopathy • Mitochondria • Heart failure • Metabolism

KEY POINTS

- Diabetes is associated with an increased risk of developing heart failure and portends a worse prognosis in patients with heart failure.
- The pathophysiology of diabetic cardiomyopathy is multifactorial, but mitochondrial dysfunction may represent a final common pathway leading to heart failure.
- The diabetic myocardium is more susceptible to injury induced by myocardial ischemia or pressure overload, leading to a further increase in heart failure among people with diabetes with other cardiac risk factors.
- Current pharmacologic therapies for diabetes improve hyperglycemia, but the benefit in heart failure is unknown. Metformin and incretin-modulating drugs show promise as cardioprotective antidiabetic agents.

CASE VIGNETTE

A 58-year-old man with no past medical history presents with 3 months of progressive dyspnea on exertion and mild lower-extremity edema. On initial evaluation his hemoglobin A_{1c} is elevated at 7.8%, fasting triglycerides are increased at 220 mg/dL, and his high-density lipoprotein is low at 30 mg/dL. He undergoes an echocardiogram, which reveals moderate left ventricular hypertrophy, low normal ejection fraction (45%), pseudonormal diastolic filling, and a dilated inferior vena cava. He has mild, diffuse coronary artery disease on cardiac catheterization and his blood pressure is 135/80.

  What is the most likely cause of his heart
  failure?
  How does diabetes influence cardiac metabolism and function?
  How should his diabetes be treated given his cardiomyopathy?

INTRODUCTION

The prevalence of obesity in the United States has reached epidemic proportions. As a consequence, obesity-related diseases, such as diabetes, also continue to increase at a staggering rate. Cardiovascular complications are common in people with diabetes and account for most of the morbidity and mortality in this population. In particular, the link between diabetes and heart failure (HF) has gained increased attention over the past several decades. The term "diabetic cardiomyopathy" (diabetic CM) was first coined in the early 1970s by Rubler, who identified four patients at autopsy with diabetic nephrosclerosis and a nonischemic cardiomyopathy.[1] Since that time epidemiologic studies have confirmed that people with diabetes are more than twice as likely to develop HF compared with people without diabetes.[2] Moreover, the survival of patients with diabetes and HF is also reduced relative to those without diabetes.[3] For these reasons, understanding the pathogenic

[a] Diabetic Cardiovascular Disease Center, Division of Cardiology, Department of Medicine, Washington University School of Medicine, St Louis, MO 63110, USA; [b] Center for Cardiovascular Research, Division of Cardiology, Department of Medicine, Washington University School of Medicine, St Louis, MO 63110, USA
* Corresponding author.
E-mail address: jschilli@dom.wustl.edu

Heart Failure Clin 8 (2012) 619–631
http://dx.doi.org/10.1016/j.hfc.2012.06.007
1551-7136/12/$ – see front matter © 2012 Elsevier Inc. All rights reserved.

mechanisms responsible for diabetic myocardial disease is of significant interest.

The accepted clinical definition of diabetic CM is the presence of diastolic or systolic cardiac dysfunction in a patient with diabetes without other obvious causes for cardiomyopathy, such as coronary artery disease (CAD), hypertension (HTN), or valvular heart disease. Given the vague nature of this definition and lack of true diagnostic criteria, diabetic CM remains a somewhat elusive entity. However, extensive clinical and animal model research has identified certain structural and pathologic findings that characterize this metabolic cardiomyopathy. Typically, left ventricular hypertrophy (LVH) and diastolic dysfunction are the earliest manifestations of diabetic CM, with systolic dysfunction occurring later in the course of disease. However, given the loose clinical criterion for diagnosing diabetic CM, there is some uncertainty as to its natural history.

The strong association between diabetes and HF has fueled intense human and animal research aimed at identifying the mechanisms underlying diabetic myocardial disease. Several pathologic abnormalities have been identified in the diabetic heart including myocardial lipid overload, altered substrate use, oxidative stress, fibrosis, inflammation, and mitochondrial dysfunction. Although significant progress has been made, the precise underpinnings of diabetic CM remain controversial. Many still question whether diabetes in and of itself is capable of producing overt HF. This article discusses the current thinking with regards to the pathogenesis and management of diabetic CM, with an emphasis on areas of uncertainty. In addition, the interplay between diabetes and other HF risk factors is discussed.

PATHOGENESIS

The pathogenesis of diabetic CM is complex and multifactorial (**Fig. 1**). However, several common themes have emerged. This section focuses first on the structural and functional abnormalities that occur in the diabetic heart, and then reviews the potential molecular mechanisms contributing to myocyte dysfunction.

Structural and Functional Characterization of Diabetic CM

LVH
LVH is a significant predictor for the development of HF, and is associated with increased mortality.[4,5] Although HTN is the leading risk factor for the development of LVH, substantial evidence indicates that diabetes can also trigger this pathologic remodeling response. Echocardiographic studies performed in patients with diabetes have consistently shown

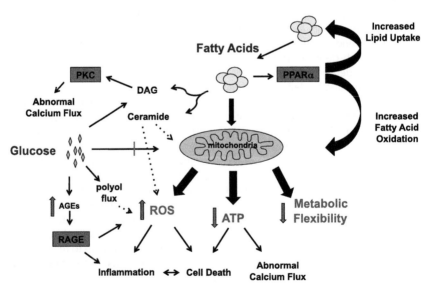

Fig. 1. The multifaceted effects of diabetes on cardiomyocyte biology. In the diabetic state, excess fatty acids are present inside the cell leading to excessive mitochondrial FAO; PPARα activation; and the generation of lipid-signaling molecules, such as ceramide and DAG. This metabolic reprogramming leads to mitochondrial dysfunction manifested by excess ROS production, less efficient ATP generation, and metabolic inflexibility. Stressed mitochondria also amplify inflammatory and cell death responses. Hyperglycemia can further augment cardiac myocyte toxicity by the formation of AGEs and promoting excess ROS and DAG generation. AGE, advanced glycation end products; DAG, diacylglycerol; FAP, fatty acid oxidation; PKC, protein kinase C; ROS, reactive oxygen species.

a strong association between diabetes, increased LV mass, and LVH even in the absence of coexistent HTN.[6,7] Moreover, obesity itself also portends an increased risk of concentric LVH independent of elevated blood pressures.[8] Consistent with this observation, there is evidence to suggest that adipose tissue–derived cytokines may contribute to cardiac hypertrophy in situations of nutrient excess.[9] Moreover, hyperinsulinemia may also contribute to cardiac myocyte hypertrophy.[10] Although the precise mechanisms of the hypertrophic response to metabolic stress remain to be fully elucidated, LVH has become a defining structural characteristic of diabetic CM.

Diastolic dysfunction

LVH and hypertrophic remodeling are associated with abnormal myocardial relaxation and diastolic dysfunction. Similar to the data surrounding LVH in metabolic disease, there is a strong link between diabetes and diastolic dysfunction. Diastolic abnormalities are thought to be among the earliest functional manifestations of diabetic CM. The prevalence of diastolic dysfunction in people with diabetes ranges between 40% and 75%.[11,12] Moreover, most type 1 and type 2 diabetic animal models also reveal diastolic function abnormalities by echocardiography and pressure–volume loop analysis.[13] Importantly, diastolic dysfunction is apparent in these models even in the absence of HTN or CAD. The mechanism of diastolic dysfunction in the diabetic heart may be a consequence of abnormal calcium handling, impaired energetics, cardiac lipid accumulation, or myocardial fibrosis. The early stages of diastolic dysfunction are reversible in people with diabetes who lose weight and normalize their metabolism.[14] This finding implies that the pathogenesis of diabetic CM may have a reversible phase and emphasizes the importance of early, aggressive lifestyle modification in diabetics with impaired myocardial relaxation.

Systolic dysfunction

Reduced LV systolic function is generally considered to be a late manifestation of diabetic CM. It is unknown whether systolic HF is the final common pathway of diabetic CM or is an alternate phenotype determined by the interaction between genetics and diabetes in susceptible individuals. It is also important to recognize that many people with diabetes with "normal" ejection fraction may actually have impaired systolic function when more sophisticated measures, such as myocardial strain measurements or tissue Doppler, are used.[15] As such, the early stages of systolic dysfunction are likely to go unrecognized clinically. Similar to the

general population, the presence of systolic HF is associated with worse prognosis in patients with diabetes.

Cellular and Molecular Defects in Diabetic CM

Glucotoxicity

Hyperglycemia has long been considered a central component in the pathogenesis of diabetic CM. In part, this is supported by evidence that poor blood glucose control correlates with increased risk of developing HF in patients with diabetes.[16] In general, hyperglycemia is thought to contribute to cardiac dysfunction through two potential mechanisms: the generation of advanced glycation end products (AGEs), and the induction of oxidative stress.

Elevated blood glucose levels can lead to the nonenzymatic posttranslational modification of proteins, lipids, and nucleic acids. After rearrangement to the more stable Amadori products these modified molecules are referred to as AGEs.[17] Not surprisingly, the level of AGEs in serum and tissue are significantly elevated in patients with diabetes.[18] In addition to impairing the function of modified proteins or nucleic acids, AGEs can trigger biologic responses by the receptor for AGEs (RAGE). RAGE is a member of the immunoglobulin superfamily that is expressed on a wide variety of cells including macrophages, cardiac myoctyes, endothelial cells, and smooth muscle cells.[19] RAGE signaling leads to the activation of MAP kinases, PI-3 Kinase, rho GTPases, nuclear factor-κB, and NADPH oxidase, which triggers inflammatory cytokine production and reactive oxygen species (ROS) generation. Evidence supporting a role for RAGE activation in the pathogenesis of cardiac dysfunction in diabetes was recently published using a streptozotocin (STZ)-induced model of type 1 diabetes in rats. In this study, treatment of diabetic rats with aminoguanidine, a small molecule that prevents AGE formation, reduced ventricular and vascular stiffening.[20] However, aminoguanidine also has RAGE-independent effects that may be relevant to this phenotype. There is still debate about the importance of AGE/RAGE signaling in diabetic CM because most of the data come from animal models of profound and untreated hyperglycemia. Thus, additional research is necessary to address this question.

Hyperglycemia has also been linked to increased oxidative stress independent of RAGE. The mechanism of ROS generation in this instance can occur by increased glucose flux through the polyol pathway, hexosamine pathway, and mitochrondrial oxidative phosphorylation.[21] A more detailed discussion of oxidative stress in the pathogenesis of diabetic CM is presented later.

Given the dogma that hyperglycemia drives diabetic cardiovascular disease, it is surprising that clinical studies have failed to show that aggressive blood glucose control reduces the incidence of cardiovascular complications in people with diabetes.[22,23] Although this may reflect an inadequate understanding of how best to lower blood glucose, an alternative explanation is that other metabolic factors contribute to the pathogenesis of diabetic myocardial disease independent of hyperglycemia. Potential candidates are altered lipid metabolism, inflammation, and mitochondrial dysfunction. These factors and their sequela are discussed in the following sections.

Altered lipid metabolism

The heart is a metabolic omnivore capable of using diverse substrates for ATP generation. Under normal conditions the heart generates approximately 70% of its ATP from fatty acid oxidation (FAO), with glucose oxidation contributing most of the remainder.[24] Substrate flexibility is also a hallmark of cardiac metabolism. To maintain adequate ATP generation in the face of physiologic or metabolic stress the heart must be able to shift substrate use. This metabolic flexibility is thought to play a crucial role in protecting cardiac myocytes from injury when ATP demand increases or substrate availability decreases.

The impact of obesity and diabetes on myocardial metabolism has been well studied for the past two decades. In diabetes, the heart is bathed in elevated concentrations of fatty acids and glucose. Human studies using positron emission tomography tracers have reproducibly demonstrated increased basal FAO and reduced glucose oxidation rates in patients with obesity and diabetes.[25,26] Consistent with these findings, in vivo and ex vivo animal models have also shown that type 1 and type 2 diabetes lead to increased myocardial FAO capacity.[27,28] As observed in human studies, animal models also confirm that glycolysis and glucose oxidation are reduced in the diabetic myocardium.[29] In part, this is a reflection of myocardial insulin resistance.[30] Thus, despite the presence of elevated glucose in the extracellular environment, its uptake and use is impaired in the diabetic heart.

Metabolic reprogramming in the diabetic heart includes transcriptional and posttranscriptional mechanisms. The PPARα gene expression network is induced in hearts from animals and humans with diabetes based on mRNA and protein analysis.[31,32] PPARα is a nuclear receptor transcription factor whose activity is regulated by fatty acid ligands. The gene targets of PPARα are involved in fatty acid import, FAO, and triglyceride synthesis.[33] In addition, PPARα can suppress glucose oxidation by the transcriptional induction of PDK4, which prevents the entry of glucose into the citric acid cycle.[34] PPARα-independent mechanisms also contribute to the metabolic shift in the diabetic myocardium, including reduced expression of the insulin-responsive glucose transporter GLUT4.[35] As a consequence of reduced myocardial glucose uptake, FAO rates increase to maintain constant levels of cellular ATP.

The augmentation of FAO in diabetes is likely an adaptive mechanism in the short term, designed to handle excessive fatty acid delivery and reduced glucose availability. However, over time this response becomes maladaptive and can potentially lead to myocyte dysfunction. The mechanisms by which altered fatty acid metabolism contributes to cardiac dysfunction is an area of active research, but may include excessive mitochondrial ROS production, less efficient energy generation, and the production of incompletely oxidized acyl-carnatine metabolites and toxic lipid species.[36] Metabolic reprogramming of the diabetic heart also reduces its substrate flexibility. This is relevant in times of stress when the inability to use more efficient substrates, such as glucose, could lead to myocyte energy depletion and dysfunction. There are no clinically available therapies for HF targeted toward modulating myocardial metabolism, making this an attractive area for continued research and clinical translation.

Lipotoxicity

The presence of cardiac myocyte steatosis is a well-established pathologic hallmark of diabetic CM. The accumulation of lipid may seem paradoxic in the setting of increased fatty acid use, but this observation reflects the imbalance between fatty acid uptake and oxidation that occurs in the diabetic heart. Autopsy studies of patients with non-ischemic cardiomyopathy have revealed that patients with diabetes have a significantly more neutral lipid within cardiac myocytes compared with people without diabetes.[37] Consistent with these observations, MRI-based quantification of myocardial triglyceride has also demonstrated that insulin resistance and diabetes are associated with a significant increase in cardiac lipid content.[38,39] Cardiac steatosis is also readily observed in animal models of diabetes, arguing that this is a defining characteristic of diabetic CM.[40] Of note, the accumulation of lipid seems to precede the onset of cardiac dysfunction.

There is a growing body of evidence that supports a role for myocardial lipid accumulation in the pathogenesis of diabetic CM. Several transgenic mouse models of cardiac steatosis have demonstrated that lipid overload can promote LVH and cardiomyopathy in the absence of systemic metabolic perturbations, such as insulin resistance and hyperglycemia.[31,41–43] The mechanisms by which lipids promote cardiac toxicity are not clear, but animal model and cell culture data have implicated endoplasmic reticulum (ER) stress, ceramide accumulation, oxidative stress, and mitochondrial dysfunction.[44,45] Moreover, lipid remodeling of ER and mitochondrial membranes may also be important in the pathogenesis of lipotoxicity. Further investigation with nontransgenic animal models are required to determine the importance of lipotoxicity to the phenotype of diabetic CM.

Oxidative stress

Increased oxidative stress is another common theme in models of diabetic CM. Animal and human data demonstrate increased ROS in the diabetic myocardium. Oxidative stress seems to correlate with excess lipid delivery and elevated mitochondrial FAO rates, arguing that mitochondria are an important source of free radicals in the diabetic heart.[40] However, high rates of FAO do not always lead to excessive ROS generation, implying other derangements in mitochondrial structure and function must also be involved.[46] Hyperglycemia can also trigger oxidative stress by mitochondrial and nonmitochondrial glucose metabolic pathways.[47] Enzymatic sources of ROS, such as that generated by the NAPDH oxidase complex, which is induced by RAGE activation, may also be important for the redox environment in diabetic cardiomyoctyes. In support of this notion, it was recently published that the NAPDH oxidase system is activated in the diabetic heart.[48] Dysfunctional ROS scavenging mechanisms have also been proposed to contribute to the severity of oxidative stress in the diabetic heart.[49] More than likely, a combination of these mechanisms is responsible for the ROS observed in diabetic CM.

The functional importance of oxidative stress in diabetic CM has also been investigated. Mechanistically, it has been postulated that ROS can cause contractile dysfunction through damage of intracellular organelles and proteins. In support of this concept, overexpression of antioxidants, such as superoxide dismutase, catalase, metallothionein, and glutathione peroxidase, significantly improved contractile function in ex vivo hearts and cardiac myocytes from diabetic mice.[50–53] Despite these promising results, most of the data to date come from STZ models of diabetic HF. Whether these findings translate to other diabetic animal models and humans remains to be determined. Nonetheless, the consistent finding of increased oxidant stress in diabetic CM warrants additional research to define the pathologic consequences of excess ROS on cardiac function and to explore the optimal means of reducing this oxidative stress.

Abnormal calcium handling

Cardiac myocyte calcium handling is known to play a key role in the regulation of myocardial contraction and relaxation. In systole, L-type calcium channels allow the influx of calcium, which triggers calcium-mediated calcium release from the sarcoplasmic reticulum (SR). The mobilization of SR calcium is mediated by the ryanodine-sensitive (RyR) calcium channel. During diastole, calcium must be resequestered into the SR to allow for cardiac myocyte relaxation. The SERCA2a channel is necessary for this to occur. In diabetes, the RyR and SERCA channels are dysregulated. The RyR channel is downregulated and hyperphosphorylated in models of type 1 and type 2 diabetes.[54–56] Hyperphosphylation leads to increased calcium leak from the RyR receptor, thereby depleting SR calcium and increasing cytoplasmic calcium during diastole. At the same time, SERCA2a activity is reduced in the diabetic state, further exacerbating SR calcium depletion and impairing calcium sequestration during diastole.[57] In combination, these changes in calcium flux impair systolic contractility and diastolic relaxation. Interestingly, oxidative stress and mitochondrial dysfunction have been implicated in impaired calcium flux.[58]

Protein kinase C signaling

Several protein kinase C (PKC) isoforms are hyperactivated in the diabetic myocardium.[59] The regulation of PKC activity occurs by the lipid signaling molecule diacylglyerol (DAG). In the diabetic heart, DAG levels are elevated as a consequence of enhanced angiotensin II and catacholemine-mediated activation of phospholipase C, the enzyme that cleaves phosphatidylinositol 4,5-bisphosphate to form DAG.[60] In addition, de novo synthesis of DAG is augmented in states of glucose and fatty acid excess, such as occurs in diabetic cardiomyocytes.

Hyperactive PKC signaling in the heart can influence calcium handling, ROS generation, and inflammation all of which can affect cardiac performance. In support of this notion, transgenic mice that overexpress PKCβ in cardiac myocytes develop cardiomyopathy.[61] There is also evidence that PKCβ inhibition can improve the cardiac phenotype of STZ-injected rats.[62] Future investigation is needed to determine the utility of PKC modulation in other models of diabetic myocardial disease.

Apoptosis, inflammation, and fibrosis

Inflammation, cell damage or death, and fibrosis are also pathologic hallmarks of diabetic CM. Inflammation is now recognized as a key participant in the pathogenesis of diabetes and its complications.[63] In models of type 1 and type 2 diabetes, the expression of inflammatory cytokines, such as tumor necrosis factor-α and interleukin-6, is increased in the myocardium.[64,65] A modest increase in macrophages and monocytes has been described in the diabetic myocardium, but the role of these cells in diabetic CM has not been well studied. The initial trigger for metabolic inflammation may be ER stress pathways, ROS, or the release of danger-associated molecular patterns released from damaged myocytes. Inhibition of tumor necrosis factor or caspase 1 (responsible for interleukin-1β production) reduced myocardial inflammation and improved cardiac function in a rat model of STZ-induced diabetes.[64,66] Thus, targeting specific inflammatory pathways may be a novel therapeutic approach for treatment. Future research investigating the initiation and consequences of metabolic inflammation in the diabetic heart is needed. In particular, defining the molecular mechanisms of crosstalk between myocytes and cardiac leukocytes is of interest.

Increased myocyte necrosis and apoptosis is seen in animal and human diabetic hearts.[67–69] Although the mechanism of cell death remains unclear, impaired energetics, oxidative stress, inflammatory cytokines, and fatty acid–induced lipotoxicity have all been implicated in this response.[70] The loss of cardiac myocytes in diabetic CM could contribute directly to LV systolic dysfunction, but more likely the dying cells and their intracellular contents serve to amplify proinflammatory and profibrotic pathways.

Cardiac fibrosis is frequently observed in diabetic hearts and this association is independent of CAD or HTN.[71,72] Animal model and human tissue samples provide evidence that progressive myocardial fibrosis may be a component of diastolic and systolic dysfunction in diabetic CM. However, it should be noted that significant fibrosis is not a feature in all models of diabetic CM.[73] Cardiac myocyte cell death and inflammation can activate profibrotic pathways in the heart. Transforming growth factor-β is thought to play an important role in this process.[74] In addition, the expression and activity of matrix metalloproteinase-2 is significantly diminished in STZ-induced diabetic CM, potentially reducing collagen turnover and increasing fibrosis.[75–77] In combination, increased production

and reduced degradation of collagen may contribute to the pathogenesis of the progressive fibrosis observed in diabetic CM.

Mitochondrial dysfunction

Diabetes dramatically alters mitochondrial substrate use and oxidative flux. Early in the course of insulin resistance there is an increase in mitochondrial number and FAO capacity.[78,79] This seems to be an adaptive response designed to handle the increase in lipid delivery and the reduction in glucose import. However, as overt diabetes develops mitochondrial dysfunction becomes apparent. Specifically, there are changes in the morphology, respiratory capacity, and proteome of mitochondria in the diabetic heart.[80]

Mitochondrial respiratory function has been studied in numerous diabetic models. In type 2 diabetes the expression of mitochondrial uncoupling proteins is increased, which enhances oxygen consumption and reduces ATP generation during mitochondrial oxidative phosphorylation.[81,82] This results in reduced cardiac efficiency and increased ROS generation. These observations were recently extended to humans where freshly isolated human atrial myocytes from diabetic and nondiabetic patients undergoing coronary artery bypass graft were investigated. Consistent with the mouse data, mitochondrial preparations from diabetic myocytes had less efficient ATP generation and increased ROS production compared with nondiabetic samples.[83] Together, these data argue that mitochondria in the diabetic heart are less able to generate ATP and more likely to trigger oxidative stress in cardiac myocytes. However, whether the diabetic myocardium is truly "energy deficient" is still an area of debate.

It is attractive to consider that abnormalities in mitochondrial biology may be a unifying feature of the multitude of derangements present in the diabetic myocardium. Mitochondria play a key role in metabolic flux and energy production, ROS generation, and inflammation, all of which are core features of diabetic HF (see **Fig. 1**). Moreover, alterations in cellular energetics and redox environment likely contribute to many of the stress responses observed in the diabetic heart, such as cell death and dysregulated calcium handling. Thus, modulating mitochondrial function in the heart has the potential to improve numerous aspects of the diabetic CM phenotype.

Summary of Pathogenesis

The last 30 years have witnessed an explosion of research focused on the diabetic heart. As illustrated in the previous sections, the impact of diabetes on myocardial biology is complex and multifactorial. Moreover, much of the cardiac functional data in animal models come from ex vivo assessment of cardiac myocyte performance. Reports of in vivo functional abnormalities in mouse models of type 1 and type 2 diabetes, as determined by echocardiography, have been inconsistent and often underwhelming.[73,84–87] This is further confounded by the large amount of data derived from STZ-induced diabetic models where profound hyperglycemia, volume depletion, tissue atrophy, or the direct effects of STZ on the myocardium likely contribute to the observed phenotypes.[88] In the end, it is still legitimate to question the nature of diabetic CM. It is clear that the diabetic milieu influences myocardial biology and when pushed to extremes can produce cardiac dysfunction. However, the more clinically relevant issue may be how diabetes modulates the myocardial response to other stressors. This is particularly true in humans, where diabetes frequently coexists with other HF risk factors. The next section explores this concept further and discusses the interplay between diabetes and other cardiac stress.

DIABETES AND THE VULNERABLE MYOCARDIUM

The preceding section focused on the mechanisms by which diabetes, as a single disease, can impact myocardial biology. However, most people with diabetes also have other comorbidities that can influence cardiac function, such as CAD and HTN.

For this reason understanding how diabetes impacts the response of the myocardium to other injurious stimuli is clinically relevant. Strong evidence supports the concept that the diabetic heart is more susceptible to damage inflicted by other stressors (**Fig. 2**). Thus, diabetes can function as an amplifier of cardiac injury. This point is illustrated by data investigating the interaction between diabetes and cardiac damage induced by acute myocardial infarction (AMI) and aortic stenosis (AS).

Diabetes and Myocardial Ischemia

Diabetes is associated with accelerated CAD and an increased risk of AMI.[89] What is less well appreciated is that diabetes also alters the response of the myocardium to ischemic stress. Clinical data have consistently demonstrated that people with diabetes have an increased risk of death after acute MI.[90–92] This holds true even when the size of the initial infarct is considered. The excess mortality in this patient population is largely caused by an increased incidence of postinfarction HF.[93–95] These observations highlight the importance of understanding the mechanisms by which diabetes influences the myocardial response to ischemic injury.

Animal models of diabetes and AMI outcomes have replicated the findings of clinical studies. Namely, AMI leads to exaggerated adverse LV remodeling and increased mortality after left anterior descending artery occlusion in type 1 and type 2 diabetic models.[96–99] The similarities in cardiac

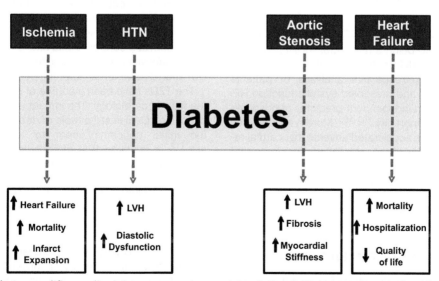

Fig. 2. Diabetes amplifies cardiac injury response to a variety of stimuli. Diabetes augments the risk of adverse cardiovascular outcomes in patients with ischemic heart disease, HTN, aortic stenosis, and heart failure (*blue boxes*). The *dashed arrows* connecting to the text boxes indicate how diabetes influences the outcomes of the previously mentioned cardiovascular diseases.

phenotype between diabetic humans and mice after AMI suggest that animal models may be useful to dissect the mechanisms of this phenomenon. Most data in this area have been descriptive; however, enhanced myocardial injury after ischemia in diabetes has been proposed to involve dysregulated inflammation, increased oxidative stress, or microvascular disease.[100] The molecular basis of these responses and whether they will serve as therapeutic targets in the future remains to be determined.

Diabetes and AS

In addition to acute ischemic stress, the response of the diabetic myocardium to chronic pressure overload, such as seen with AS, is also abnormal. In a recent study of patients with severe AS, diabetes was associated with increased LV mass and reduced systolic function despite similar aortic value gradients.[101] Moreover, this association was independent of coexisting CAD. In a similar study, people with diabetes with AS had increased myocardial fibrosis compared with their nondiabetic counterparts.[102] Interestingly, diabetes was also associated with increased levels of the hypophosphorylated N2B titin isoform. In sum these changes could significantly increase myocardial stiffness, exacerbate diastolic dysfunction, and worsen HF symptoms. There is still much to learn about how diabetes renders the heart more vulnerable to damage from ischemia and pressure overload. Moreover, the impact of diabetes on other myocardial stressors, such as myocarditis and genetic stress, should be explored.

Diabetes and the Progression of HF

In addition to being a risk factor for HF, diabetes can also modulate the natural history of this disease. In retrospective analyses of patients with reduced and preserved systolic function HF, diabetes is an independent predictor of hospitalizations and mortality.[103–105] Moreover, diabetes also promotes accelerated adverse myocardial remodeling in the setting of HTN, another important HF risk factor.[106] Thus, diabetic myocardial remodeling seems to significantly impact the evolution of HF irrespective of the cause. Continued investigation into the mechanism of this phenomenon is warranted.

MANAGEMENT OF DIABETES OF HF

There are no clear guidelines for the management of diabetes in patients with HF. In large part this a consequence of the paucity of clinical trial data in this area. This section briefly discusses issues to consider when managing diabetes in patients with HF.

Insulin-Replacement Strategies

In addition to insulin injections, this group also includes the orally administered sulfonylureas (SU), such as glyburide. In retrospective analyses, the use of insulin for DM was associated with an increased incidence and severity of HF.[107,108] However, given the retrospective, nonrandomized nature of these studies, it is not possible to determine whether insulin treatment truly increases the risk of HF or identifies a higher-risk patient with diabetes. Similar data are present for the SUs. Moreover, the risk of hypoglycemia is increased with the use of insulin or SUs. In general, these agents should not be used as first-line therapy for diabetes in patients with HF.

Insulin-Sensitizing Strategies

The drugs in this class include the biguanides, such as metformin, and the thiozolidendiones (TZDs), such as pioglitazone and rosiglitazone. Metformin was initially contraindicated in patients with HF because of the perceived risk of lactic acidosis. However, more recent observational data argue that the risk of lactic acidosis is very low in this patient population.[109] This has led to renewed interest in metformin as a treatment option for patients with HF and diabetes. In a study by Eurich and colleagues,[110] diabetic patients with HF treated with metformin alone or in combination with an SU had a significant reduction in mortality compared with patients treated with an SU alone. Similar results have also been reported from other retrospective database analyses.[13,111] Although no randomized controlled trial data exist, it seems that metformin treatment is safe in patients with DM and HF, and it may improve outcomes.

The TZDs have been a source of controversy in the field of cardiology. The impact of these medications on CAD is still a topic of debate; however, the initial concerns seem to overstate the risk.[112,113] In 5% to 10% of patients TZDs trigger fluid retention, which leads to an increased risk of HF hospitalization in patients with diastolic or systolic dysfunction.[114] For this reason, many patients with diabetes and HF do not tolerate these medications. Similar to metformin, there are retrospective data that associate TZD-containing regimens with improved mortality in patients with HF.[115] However, given the lack of clinical trials to prove benefit and the potential harm of increasing hospitalization for HF, TZDs should be used with caution in patients with HF. Whether TZDs can reduce the risk of developing

HF in patients with diabetes with normal cardiac function remains an unanswered question. In the future, more selective TZDs may produce the desired metabolic effects without the risk of fluid retention.

Incretin-Based Therapies

Modulation of the incretin system has shown promise as a means to improve blood glucose levels and reduce diabetic complications. Natural incretins, such as glucagon-like peptide-1 (GLP1), are small molecules that are secreted by intestinal epithelial cells in response to food ingestion. GLP-1 mediates its biologic effects by the GLP-1 receptor, which is expressed on a wide variety of cells in the pancreas, heart, lung, kidney, and, hypothalamus. In response to GLP-1, glucose-stimulated insulin release from the pancreas is enhanced. The clearance of GLP-1 is extremely rapid and controlled by the enzyme dipeptidyl peptidase 4 (DPP4). The available agents targeting this pathway function either as the GLP-1 receptor agonists (ie, exentinide/Byetta) or DPP4 inhibitors (sitiglipitin/Januvia).

Evidence supporting the use of incretin-based therapies for reducing cardiovascular complications in diabetes is growing. In an animal model of atherosclerosis, GLP-1 significantly reduced plaque burden.[116] In addition to antiatherogenic effects, the GLP-1 pathway may also have cardioprotective properties. In animal models of AMI and hypertensive CM, GLP-1 infusion reduced adverse LV remodeling, improved cardiac function, and prolonged survival.[117,118] Although the data in humans are less well-established, increased activation of the GLP-1 axis leads to modest weight loss, an improved lipid profile, and lower blood pressures. Moreover, in a small, nonrandomized study GLP-1 infusion was associated with a significant improvement in ejection fraction in patients who presented with AMI and reduced LV function.[119] Currently, there are several ongoing clinical trials designed to address the impact of enhancing GLP-1 signaling on cardiovascular outcomes in diabetes. The results of these studies will provide important information about the use of these agents for the prevention and treatment of diabetic cardiovascular complications.

SUMMARY

Since the term diabetic cardiomyopathy was first coined in 1972 there has been intense interest in this disease entity. With the growing population of patients with diabetes the prevalence of diabetic cardiovascular disease will continue to rise. Although animal model and human studies have elucidated several pathologic features of diabetic CM, understanding of the inciting events that lead to contractile dysfunction or increase myocardial susceptibility to injury remains murky. Moreover, diabetic CM as a cause of clinical HF likely involves the intersection between diabetic-myocardial reprogramming and other cardiac stressors. Given the lack of consensus on how to define or diagnose diabetic CM, there has been limited progress on developing specific treatments for this form of HF. Despite this, mitochondrial dysfunction may explain several of the diabetic CM hallmarks, such as metabolic substrate dysregulation, excess ROS generation, inflammation, and ATP depletion. Thus, targeting mitochondrial biology may lead to important new approaches to improve cardiac function in people with diabetes.

The currently available pharmacologic options for treating diabetes have not been studied rigorously with regards to prevention and treatment of diabetic CM. As a consequence, no specific recommendations can be made for the use of these agents with respect to HF. However, metformin and the incretin-modulator therapies improve metabolic parameters and may be cardioprotective. In contrast, TZDs can exacerbate fluid retention making these drugs problematic in patients with HF. Insulin-replacement therapy should be reserved for those unresponsive to oral therapy because it may be associated with an increased risk of HF incidence and mortality. Further research of these agents in patients with early and late manifestations of diabetic CM is important to define the optimal regimen.

REFERENCES

1. Rubler S, Dlugash J, Yuceoglu YZ, et al. New type of cardiomyopathy associated with diabetic glomerulosclerosis. Am J Cardiol 1972;30:595–602.
2. Kannel WB, McGee DL. Diabetes and cardiovascular disease. The Framingham study. JAMA 1979;241:2035–8.
3. From AM, Leibson CL, Bursi F, et al. Diabetes in heart failure: prevalence and impact on outcome in the population. Am J Med 2006;119:591–9.
4. Artham SM, Lavie CJ, Milani RV, et al. Clinical impact of left ventricular hypertrophy and implications for regression. Prog Cardiovasc Dis 2009; 52:153–67.
5. Devereux RB, Roman MJ. Left ventricular hypertrophy in hypertension: stimuli, patterns, and consequences. Hypertens Res 1999;22:1–9.
6. Devereux RB, Roman MJ, Paranicas M, et al. Impact of diabetes on cardiac structure and function: the strong heart study. Circulation 2000;101: 2271–6.

7. Aneja A, Tang WH, Bansilal S, et al. Diabetic cardiomyopathy: insights into pathogenesis, diagnostic challenges, and therapeutic options. Am J Med 2008;121:748–57.

8. Woodiwiss AJ, Libhaber CD, Majane OH, et al. Obesity promotes left ventricular concentric rather than eccentric geometric remodeling and hypertrophy independent of blood pressure. Am J Hypertens 2008;21:1144–51.

9. Barouch LA, Berkowitz DE, Harrison RW, et al. Disruption of leptin signaling contributes to cardiac hypertrophy independently of body weight in mice. Circulation 2003;108:754–9.

10. Iliadis F, Kadoglou N, Didangelos T. Insulin and the heart. Diabetes Res Clin Pract 2011;93(Suppl 1): S86–91.

11. Brooks BA, Franjic B, Ban CR, et al. Diastolic dysfunction and abnormalities of the microcirculation in type 2 diabetes. Diabetes Obes Metab 2008;10:739–46.

12. Shivalkar B, Dhondt D, Goovaerts I, et al. Flow mediated dilatation and cardiac function in type 1 diabetes mellitus. Am J Cardiol 2006;97:77–82.

13. Aguilar D, Chan W, Bozkurt B, et al. Metformin use and mortality in ambulatory patients with diabetes and heart failure. Circ Heart Fail 2011;4: 53–8.

14. Lin CH, Kurup S, Herrero P, et al. Myocardial oxygen consumption change predicts left ventricular relaxation improvement in obese humans after weight loss. Obesity (Silver Spring) 2011;19:1804–12.

15. Fang ZY, Schull-Meade R, Leano R, et al. Screening for heart disease in diabetic subjects. Am Heart J 2005;149:349–54.

16. Stratton IM, Adler AI, Neil HA, et al. Association of glycaemia with macrovascular and microvascular complications of type 2 diabetes (UKPDS 35): prospective observational study. BMJ 2000;321: 405–12.

17. Barlovic DP, Soro-Paavonen A, Jandeleit-Dahm KA. RAGE biology, atherosclerosis and diabetes. Clin Sci (Lond) 2011;121:43–55.

18. Singh R, Barden A, Mori T, et al. Advanced glycation end-products: a review. Diabetologia 2001;44: 129–46.

19. Ramasamy R, Yan SF, Schmidt AM. Receptor for AGE (RAGE): signaling mechanisms in the pathogenesis of diabetes and its complications. Ann N Y Acad Sci 2011;1243:88–102.

20. Wu MS, Liang JT, Lin YD, et al. Aminoguanidine prevents the impairment of cardiac pumping mechanics in rats with streptozotocin and nicotinamide-induced type 2 diabetes. Br J Pharmacol 2008;154:758–64.

21. Wold LE, Ceylan-Isik AF, Ren J. Oxidative stress and stress signaling: menace of diabetic cardiomyopathy. Acta Pharmacol Sin 2005;26:908–17.

22. Patel A, MacMahon S, Chalmers J, et al. Intensive blood glucose control and vascular outcomes in patients with type 2 diabetes. N Engl J Med 2008;358:2560–72.

23. Gerstein HC, Miller ME, Byington RP, et al. Effects of intensive glucose lowering in type 2 diabetes. N Engl J Med 2008;358:2545–59.

24. Huss JM, Kelly DP. Mitochondrial energy metabolism in heart failure: a question of balance. J Clin Invest 2005;115:547–55.

25. Herrero P, Peterson LR, McGill JB, et al. Increased myocardial fatty acid metabolism in patients with type 1 diabetes mellitus. J Am Coll Cardiol 2006; 47:598–604.

26. Peterson LR, Herrero P, Schechtman KB, et al. Effect of obesity and insulin resistance on myocardial substrate metabolism and efficiency in young women. Circulation 2004;109:2191–6.

27. Hsueh W, Abel ED, Breslow JL, et al. Recipes for creating animal models of diabetic cardiovascular disease. Circ Res 2007;100:1415–27.

28. Lopaschuk GD, Ussher JR, Folmes CD, et al. Myocardial fatty acid metabolism in health and disease. Physiol Rev 2010;90:207–58.

29. Abel ED. Myocardial insulin resistance and cardiac complications of diabetes. Curr Drug Targets Immune Endocr Metabol Disord 2005;5: 219–26.

30. Gray S, Kim JK. New insights into insulin resistance in the diabetic heart. Trends Endocrinol Metab 2011;22:394–403.

31. Finck BN, Han X, Courtois M, et al. A critical role for PPARalpha-mediated lipotoxicity in the pathogenesis of diabetic cardiomyopathy: modulation by dietary fat content. Proc Natl Acad Sci U S A 2003;100:1226–31.

32. Duncan JG. Peroxisome proliferator activated receptor-alpha (PPARalpha) and PPAR gamma coactivator-1alpha (PGC-1alpha) regulation of cardiac metabolism in diabetes. Pediatr Cardiol 2011;32:323–8.

33. Barger PM, Kelly DP. PPAR signaling in the control of cardiac energy metabolism. Trends Cardiovasc Med 2000;10:238–45.

34. Wu P, Peters JM, Harris RA. Adaptive increase in pyruvate dehydrogenase kinase 4 during starvation is mediated by peroxisome proliferator activated receptor alpha. Biochem Biophys Res Commun 2001;287:391–6.

35. Wright JJ, Kim J, Buchanan J, et al. Mechanisms for increased myocardial fatty acid utilization following short-term high-fat feeding. Cardiovasc Res 2009;82:351–60.

36. An D, Rodrigues B. Role of changes in cardiac metabolism in development of diabetic cardiomyopathy. Am J Physiol Heart Circ Physiol 2006;291 H1489–506.

37. Sharma S, Adrogue JV, Golfman L, et al. Intramyocardial lipid accumulation in the failing human heart resembles the lipotoxic rat heart. Faseb J 2004;18:1692–700.

38. McGavock JM, Lingvay I, Zib I, et al. Cardiac steatosis in diabetes mellitus: a 1H-magnetic resonance spectroscopy study. Circulation 2007;116: 1170–5.

39. Rijzewijk LJ, van der Meer RW, Smit JW, et al. Myocardial steatosis is an independent predictor of diastolic dysfunction in type 2 diabetes mellitus. J Am Coll Cardiol 2008;52:1793–9.

40. van de Weijer T, Schrauwen-Hinderling VB, Schrauwen P. Lipotoxicity in type 2 diabetic cardiomyopathy. Cardiovasc Res 2011;92:10–8.

41. Chiu HC, Kovacs A, Ford DA, et al. A novel mouse model of lipotoxic cardiomyopathy. J Clin Invest 2001;107:813–22.

42. Chiu HC, Kovacs A, Blanton RM, et al. Transgenic expression of fatty acid transport protein 1 in the heart causes lipotoxic cardiomyopathy. Circ Res 2005;96:225–33.

43. Yagyu H, Chen G, Yokoyama M, et al. Lipoprotein lipase (LpL) on the surface of cardiomyocytes increases lipid uptake and produces a cardiomyopathy. J Clin Invest 2003;111:419–26.

44. Park TS, Yamashita H, Blaner WS, et al. Lipids in the heart: a source of fuel and a source of toxins. Curr Opin Lipidol 2007;18:277–82.

45. Schaffer JE. Lipotoxicity: when tissues overeat. Curr Opin Lipidol 2003;14:281–7.

46. Chambers KT, Leone TC, Sambandam N, et al. Chronic inhibition of pyruvate dehydrogenase in heart triggers an adaptive metabolic response. J Biol Chem 2011;286:11155–62.

47. Friederich M, Hansell P, Palm F. Diabetes, oxidative stress, nitric oxide and mitochondria function. Curr Diabetes Rev 2009;5:120–44.

48. Serpillon S, Floyd BC, Gupte RS, et al. Superoxide production by NAD(P)H oxidase and mitochondria is increased in genetically obese and hyperglycemic rat heart and aorta before the development of cardiac dysfunction. The role of glucose-6-phosphate dehydrogenase-derived NADPH. Am J Physiol Heart Circ Physiol 2009;297:H153–62.

49. Aliciguzel Y, Ozen I, Aslan M, et al. Activities of xanthine oxidoreductase and antioxidant enzymes in different tissues of diabetic rats. J Lab Clin Med 2003;142:172–7.

50. Shen X, Zheng S, Metreveli NS, et al. Protection of cardiac mitochondria by overexpression of MnSOD reduces diabetic cardiomyopathy. Diabetes 2006; 55:798–805.

51. Ye G, Metreveli NS, Donthi RV, et al. Catalase protects cardiomyocyte function in models of type 1 and type 2 diabetes. Diabetes 2004;53: 1336–43.

52. Ye G, Metreveli NS, Ren J, et al. Metallothionein prevents diabetes-induced deficits in cardiomyocytes by inhibiting reactive oxygen species production. Diabetes 2003;52:777–83.

53. Matsushima S, Kinugawa S, Ide T, et al. Overexpression of glutathione peroxidase attenuates myocardial remodeling and preserves diastolic function in diabetic heart. Am J Physiol Heart Circ Physiol 2006;291:H2237–45.

54. Choi KM, Zhong Y, Hoit BD, et al. Defective intracellular Ca(2+) signaling contributes to cardiomyopathy in type 1 diabetic rats. Am J Physiol Heart Circ Physiol 2002;283:H1398–408.

55. Pereira L, Matthes J, Schuster I, et al. Mechanisms of [Ca2+]i transient decrease in cardiomyopathy of db/db type 2 diabetic mice. Diabetes 2006;55: 608–15.

56. Marx SO, Reiken S, Hisamatsu Y, et al. PKA phosphorylation dissociates FKBP12.6 from the calcium release channel (ryanodine receptor): defective regulation in failing hearts. Cell 2000; 101:365–76.

57. Lebeche D, Davidoff AJ, Hajjar RJ. Interplay between impaired calcium regulation and insulin signaling abnormalities in diabetic cardiomyopathy. Nat Clin Pract Cardiovasc Med 2008;5:715–24.

58. Watanabe K, Thandavarayan RA, Harima M, et al. Role of differential signaling pathways and oxidative stress in diabetic cardiomyopathy. Curr Cardiol Rev 2010;6:280–90.

59. Liu X, Wang J, Takeda N, et al. Changes in cardiac protein kinase C activities and isozymes in streptozotocin-induced diabetes. Am J Physiol 1999;277:E798–804.

60. Wieland T, Lutz S, Chidiac P. Regulators of G protein signalling: a spotlight on emerging functions in the cardiovascular system. Curr Opin Pharmacol 2007;7:201–7.

61. Way KJ, Isshiki K, Suzuma K, et al. Expression of connective tissue growth factor is increased in injured myocardium associated with protein kinase C beta2 activation and diabetes. Diabetes 2002; 51:2709–18.

62. Liu Y, Lei S, Gao X, et al. PKCbeta inhibition with ruboxistaurin reduces oxidative stress and attenuates left ventricular hypertrophy and dysfunction in rats with streptozotocin-induced diabetes. Clin Sci (Lond) 2012;122:161–73.

63. Hotamisligil GS. Inflammation and metabolic disorders. Nature 2006;444:860–7.

64. Westermann D, Van Linthout S, Dhayat S, et al. Tumor necrosis factor-alpha antagonism protects from myocardial inflammation and fibrosis in experimental diabetic cardiomyopathy. Basic Res Cardiol 2007;102:500–7.

65. Ko HJ, Zhang Z, Jung DY, et al. Nutrient stress activates inflammation and reduces glucose metabolism

by suppressing AMP-activated protein kinase in the heart. Diabetes 2009;58:2536–46.

66. Westermann D, Van Linthout S, Dhayat S, et al. Cardioprotective and anti-inflammatory effects of interleukin converting enzyme inhibition in experimental diabetic cardiomyopathy. Diabetes 2007; 56:1834–41.

67. Frustaci A, Kajstura J, Chimenti C, et al. Myocardial cell death in human diabetes. Circ Res 2000;87: 1123–32.

68. Chowdhry MF, Vohra HA, Galinanes M. Diabetes increases apoptosis and necrosis in both ischemic and nonischemic human myocardium: role of caspases and poly-adenosine diphosphate-ribose polymerase. J Thorac Cardiovasc Surg 2007;134: 124–31, 31.e1–3.

69. Barouch LA, Gao D, Chen L, et al. Cardiac myocyte apoptosis is associated with increased DNA damage and decreased survival in murine models of obesity. Circ Res 2006;98:119–24.

70. Cai L, Kang YJ. Cell death and diabetic cardiomyopathy. Cardiovasc Toxicol 2003;3:219–28.

71. Shimizu M, Umeda K, Sugihara N, et al. Collagen remodelling in myocardia of patients with diabetes. J Clin Pathol 1993;46:32–6.

72. Regan TJ, Lyons MM, Ahmed SS, et al. Evidence for cardiomyopathy in familial diabetes mellitus. J Clin Invest 1977;60:884–99.

73. Van den Bergh A, Vanderper A, Vangheluwe P, et al. Dyslipidaemia in type II diabetic mice does not aggravate contractile impairment but increases ventricular stiffness. Cardiovasc Res 2008;77:371–9.

74. Ban CR, Twigg SM. Fibrosis in diabetes complications: pathogenic mechanisms and circulating and urinary markers. Vasc Health Risk Manag 2008;4: 575–96.

75. Van Linthout S, Seeland U, Riad A, et al. Reduced MMP-2 activity contributes to cardiac fibrosis in experimental diabetic cardiomyopathy. Basic Res Cardiol 2008;103:319–27.

76. Li Q, Sun SZ, Wang Y, et al. The roles of MMP-2/TIMP-2 in extracellular matrix remodelling in the hearts of STZ-induced diabetic rats. Acta Cardiol 2007;62:485–91.

77. Bollano E, Omerovic E, Svensson H, et al. Cardiac remodeling rather than disturbed myocardial energy metabolism is associated with cardiac dysfunction in diabetic rats. Int J Cardiol 2007; 114:195–201.

78. Duncan JG, Fong JL, Medeiros DM, et al. Insulin-resistant heart exhibits a mitochondrial biogenic response driven by the peroxisome proliferator-activated receptor-alpha/PGC-1alpha gene regulatory pathway. Circulation 2007;115:909–17.

79. Mitra R, Nogee DP, Zechner JF, et al. The transcriptional coactivators, PGC-1alpha and beta, cooperate to maintain cardiac mitochondrial function during the early stages of insulin resistance. J Mol Cell Cardiol 2012;52(3):701–10 [Epub 2011 Oct 20].

80. Bugger H, Abel ED. Rodent models of diabetic cardiomyopathy. Dis Model Mech 2009;2:454–66.

81. Boudina S, Sena S, O'Neill BT, et al. Reduced mitochondrial oxidative capacity and increased mitochondrial uncoupling impair myocardial energetics in obesity. Circulation 2005;112:2686–95.

82. Boudina S, Sena S, Theobald H, et al. Mitochondrial energetics in the heart in obesity-related diabetes: direct evidence for increased uncoupled respiration and activation of uncoupling proteins. Diabetes 2007;56:2457–66.

83. Anderson EJ, Kypson AP, Rodriguez E, et al. Substrate-specific derangements in mitochondrial metabolism and redox balance in the atrium of the type 2 diabetic human heart. J Am Coll Cardiol 2009;54:1891–8.

84. Daniels A, Linz D, van Bilsen M, et al. Long-term severe diabetes only leads to mild cardiac diastolic dysfunction in Zucker diabetic fatty rats. Eur J Heart Fail 2012;14:193–201.

85. Aasum E, Hafstad AD, Severson DL, et al. Age-dependent changes in metabolism, contractile function, and ischemic sensitivity in hearts from db/db mice. Diabetes 2003;52:434–41.

86. Cosyns B, Droogmans S, Weytjens C, et al. Effect of streptozotocin-induced diabetes on left ventricular function in adult rats: an in vivo pinhole gated SPECT study. Cardiovasc Diabetol 2007;6:30.

87. Basu R, Oudit GY, Wang X, et al. Type 1 diabetic cardiomyopathy in the Akita (Ins2WT/C96Y) mouse model is characterized by lipotoxicity and diastolic dysfunction with preserved systolic function. Am J Physiol Heart Circ Physiol 2009;297:H2096–108.

88. Wold LE, Ren J. Streptozotocin directly impairs cardiac contractile function in isolated ventricular myocytes via a p38 map kinase-dependent oxidative stress mechanism. Biochem Biophys Res Commun 2004;318:1066–71.

89. Nathan DM, Meigs J, Singer DE. The epidemiology of cardiovascular disease in type 2 diabetes mellitus: how sweet it is. or is it? Lancet 1997; 350(Suppl 1):SI4–9.

90. Savage MP, Krolewski AS, Kenien GG, et al. Acute myocardial infarction in diabetes mellitus and significance of congestive heart failure as a prognostic factor. Am J Cardiol 1988;62:665–9.

91. Rytter L, Troelsen S, Beck-Nielsen H. Prevalence and mortality of acute myocardial infarction in patients with diabetes. Diabetes Care 1985;8:230–4.

92. Czyzk A, Krolewski AS, Szablowska S, et al. Clinical course of myocardial infarction among diabetic patients. Diabetes Care 1980;3:526–9.

93. Kouvaras G, Cokkinos D, Spyropoulou M. Increased mortality of diabetics after acute myocardial infarction attributed to diffusely impaired left ventricular

performance as assessed by echocardiography. Jpn Heart J 1988;29:1–9.

94. Yudkin JS, Oswald GA. Determinants of hospital admission and case fatality in diabetic patients with myocardial infarction. Diabetes Care 1988; 11:351–8.

95. Aronson D, Rayfield EJ, Chesebro JH. Mechanisms determining course and outcome of diabetic patients who have had acute myocardial infarction. Ann Intern Med 1997;126:296–306.

96. Greer JJ, Ware DP, Lefer DJ. Myocardial infarction and heart failure in the db/db diabetic mouse. Am J Physiol Heart Circ Physiol 2006;290:H146–53.

97. Thakker GD, Frangogiannis NG, Bujak M, et al. Effects of diet-induced obesity on inflammation and remodeling after myocardial infarction. Am J Physiol Heart Circ Physiol 2006;291:H2504–14.

98. Shiomi T, Tsutsui H, Ikeuchi M, et al. Streptozotocin-induced hyperglycemia exacerbates left ventricular remodeling and failure after experimental myocardial infarction. J Am Coll Cardiol 2003;42:165–72.

99. Cittadini A, Mantzoros CS, Hampton TG, et al. Cardiovascular abnormalities in transgenic mice with reduced brown fat: an animal model of human obesity. Circulation 1999;100:2177–83.

100. Estep JD, Aguilar D. Diabetes and heart failure in the post-myocardial infarction patient. Curr Heart Fail Rep 2006;3:164–9.

101. Lindman BR, Arnold SV, Madrazo JA, et al. The adverse impact of diabetes mellitus on left ventricular remodeling and function in patients with severe aortic stenosis. Circ Heart Fail 2011;4:286–92.

102. Falcao-Pires I, Hamdani N, Borbely A, et al. Diabetes mellitus worsens diastolic left ventricular dysfunction in aortic stenosis through altered myocardial structure and cardiomyocyte stiffness. Circulation 2011;124:1151–9.

103. Aguilar D, Deswal A, Ramasubbu K, et al. Comparison of patients with heart failure and preserved left ventricular ejection fraction among those with versus without diabetes mellitus. Am J Cardiol 2010;105:373–7.

104. Taylor CJ, Roalfe AK, Iles R, et al. Ten-year prognosis of heart failure in the community: follow-up data from the Echocardiographic Heart of England Screening (ECHOES) study. Eur J Heart Fail 2012; 14:176–84.

105. Shi C, Wang LJ, Hu DF, et al. Prevalence, clinical characteristics and outcome in patients with chronic heart failure and diabetes. Chin Med J (Engl) 2010;123:646–50.

106. Eguchi K, Kario K, Hoshide S, et al. Type 2 diabetes is associated with left ventricular concentric remodeling in hypertensive patients. Am J Hypertens 2005;18:23–9.

107. Nichols GA, Koro CE, Gullion CM, et al. The incidence of congestive heart failure associated with

antidiabetic therapies. Diabetes Metab Res Rev 2005;21:51–7.

108. Smooke S, Horwich TB, Fonarow GC. Insulin-treated diabetes is associated with a marked increase in mortality in patients with advanced heart failure. Am Heart J 2005;149:168–74.

109. Tahrani AA, Varughese GI, Scarpello JH, et al. Metformin, heart failure, and lactic acidosis: is metformin absolutely contraindicated? BMJ 2007;335: 508–12.

110. Eurich DT, McAlister FA, Blackburn DF, et al. Benefits and harms of antidiabetic agents in patients with diabetes and heart failure: systematic review. BMJ 2007;335:497.

111. Romero SP, Andrey JL, Garcia-Egido A, et al. Metformin therapy and prognosis of patients with heart failure and new-onset diabetes mellitus. A propensity-matched study in the community. Int J Cardiol 2011. [Epub ahead of print].

112. Pop-Busui R, Lombardero M, Lavis V, et al. Relation of severe coronary artery narrowing to insulin or thiazolidinedione use in patients with type 2 diabetes mellitus (from the Bypass Angioplasty Revascularization Investigation 2 Diabetes Study). Am J Cardiol 2009;104:52–8.

113. Erdmann E, Charbonnel B, Wilcox R. Thiazolidinediones and cardiovascular risk: a question of balance. Curr Cardiol Rev 2009;5:155–65.

114. Erdmann E, Charbonnel B, Wilcox RG, et al. Pioglitazone use and heart failure in patients with type 2 diabetes and preexisting cardiovascular disease: data from the PROactive study (PROactive 08). Diabetes Care 2007;30:2773–8.

115. Masoudi FA, Inzucchi SE, Wang Y, et al. Thiazolidinediones, metformin, and outcomes in older patients with diabetes and heart failure: an observational study. Circulation 2005;111:583–90.

116. Matsubara J, Sugiyama S, Sugamura K, et al. A dipeptidyl peptidase-4 inhibitor, des-fluoro-sitagliptin, improves endothelial function and reduces atherosclerotic lesion formation in apolipoprotein E-deficient mice. J Am Coll Cardiol 2012; 59:265–76.

117. Bose AK, Mocanu MM, Carr RD, et al. Glucagon-like peptide 1 can directly protect the heart against ischemia/reperfusion injury. Diabetes 2005;54:146–51.

118. Poornima I, Brown SB, Bhashyam S, et al. Chronic glucagon-like peptide-1 infusion sustains left ventricular systolic function and prolongs survival in the spontaneously hypertensive, heart failure-prone rat. Circ Heart Fail 2008;1:153–60.

119. Nikolaidis LA, Mankad S, Sokos GG, et al. Effects of glucagon-like peptide-1 in patients with acute myocardial infarction and left ventricular dysfunction after successful reperfusion. Circulation 2004;109: 962–5.

Sphingolipids, Lipotoxic Cardiomyopathy, and Cardiac Failure

Tae-Sik Park, PhD[a], Ira J. Goldberg, MD[b],*

KEYWORDS

- Ceramide - Cardiomyopathy - Diabetes - Ischemia - Sphingosine 1-phosphate

KEY POINTS

- Sphingolipids, elevated in obesity and type 2 diabetes, may cause cardiomyopathy.
- Ceramide alters cardiac energy metabolism and can cause cardiomyocyte apoptosis.
- Sphingosine 1-phosphate protects against ischemia/reperfusion injury.
- Modulation of sphingolipid metabolism in the heart may become a therapy for cardiac disease in patients with obesity and diabetes.

INTRODUCTION

Obesity is associated with an elevated risk of chronic diseases, including diabetes and cardiovascular disease. Accumulation of lipotoxic metabolites in nonadipocyte tissues may be a major cause of dilated cardiomyopathy in patients with obesity or diabetes. Recent studies in humans have related cardiac lipid content with disturbance of cardiac function. Moreover, ectopic disposition of lipids alters substrate metabolism in these tissues and contributes to the development of obesity-mediated diseases.

The heart uses lipids for energy and for cellular structures. Fatty acids supply energy for cardiac muscle contraction and are required substrates for the synthesis of several esters, including phospholipids and sphingolipids. Patients with diabetes and obesity have elevated circulating plasma free fatty acids (FFA) levels. This state might drive greater heart FFA uptake; when uptake exceeds the requirements for energy production, these FFA accumulate as lipid metabolites and

neutral lipids. Lipotoxicity is the term used when lipid overload leads to cellular dysfunction and cell death–mediated organ dysfunction.[1] Because neutral lipids and other lipid metabolites accumulate in the cardiomyocytes of nonischemic failing hearts,[1,2] a hypothesis that lipotoxicity contributes to the development of cardiac dysfunction is gaining credibility.[3] In addition, ischemia has been reported to increase heart levels of some lipids.[4,5]

Of the complex bioactive lipids, ceramide and its metabolites draw particular attention. Studies in animal models of diabetes, obesity, and dilated cardiomyopathy demonstrated that the inhibition of sphingolipid production prevents or delays the onset of the diseases.[6,7] In addition, the activation of ceramidase by adiponectin was associated with reduced cardiac injury after apoptosis.[5] Thus, there is experimental evidence that ceramide is one of the lipotoxic lipids.

Ceramide is a major molecule in sphingolipid metabolism and has been studied extensively. In addition to its structural role in plasma membranes and lipoproteins, ceramide and its metabolites

The authors have nothing to disclose. There is no applicable funding support.

[a] Department of Life Science, Gachon University, Bokjung-dong, Sujung-gu, Seongnam, Gyunggi-do 461-701, South Korea; [b] Division of Preventive Medicine and Nutrition, Columbia University, 630 West 168th Street, PH10-305, New York, NY 10032, USA

* Corresponding author.

E-mail address: ijg3@columbia.edu

Heart Failure Clin 8 (2012) 633–641

http://dx.doi.org/10.1016/j.hfc.2012.06.003

1551-7136/12/$ – see front matter © 2012 Elsevier Inc. All rights reserved.

have profound effects on cellular signaling, such as apoptosis and insulin response.[8] Ceramide is also a precursor for other bioactive sphingolipid metabolites, such as ceramide 1-phosphate, sphingosine, and sphingosine 1-phosphate (S1P) (**Fig. 1**). These sphingolipids regulate cellular processes, including cell proliferation, differentiation, and apoptosis.[9] In this review, the authors intend to describe the role of sphingolipids in cardiovascular pathophysiology as a regulator of cardiac energy metabolism and signaling. Understanding the role of sphingolipids in cardiovascular events may lead to strategies to correct the abnormal signaling pathways in failing hearts.

FAILING HEARTS HAVE ABNORMAL LIPID METABOLISM

The heart requires several forms of lipids, including cholesterol and fatty acids. Most circulating plasma fatty acids are esterified and are incorporated into lipoprotein, phospholipids, and triglycerides. Fatty acids supply energy for heart contraction and are used for structural lipids in cells. Tissue uptake of whole lipoproteins by specific receptors leads to intracellular degradation of phospholipids and triglycerides to varying degrees. FFA uptake caused by either albumin-associated FFA or FFA liberated from lipoproteins supplies cardiac energy substrates. Loss of either lipoprotein lipase (LpL)[10] or the putative FFA transporter CD36[11] in the heart increases cardiac uptake

of glucose, suggesting that the heart is fatty acid deprived and needs an alternative source of energy.

In normal adult hearts, ATP is produced via the oxidation of fatty acids, glucose, lactate, and ketone bodies, with glucose and fatty acids being the principal substrates.[12] Of these substrates, fatty acids are the major fuel supplying 70% of the ATP for normal cardiac function.[13–15] During diabetes, the heart seems to oxidize more fatty acid and less glucose.[16] Heart LpL activity is increased, presumably to allow greater lipoprotein-derived fatty acid uptake.[16,17] One well-studied model is the isolated working heart of obese db/db mice. These hearts have decreased glucose oxidation rates and increased fatty acid oxidation.[18] Although fatty acid oxidation has not been studied in detail, diet-induced obesity rapidly leads to cardiac insulin resistance.[19]

Diabetic cardiomyopathy is a syndrome in which heart failure is not caused by ischemic heart disease or hypertension.[20] The activity of peroxisome proliferator-activated receptor (PPAR) α, a major regulator of fatty acid oxidation in the heart, is increased in diabetic hearts. PPARα overexpression in mice leads to cardiac dysfunction.[21] This cardiomyopathy could result from excess fatty acid oxidation, which is postulated to increase reactive oxygen production, or from accumulation of intracellular lipids, which also occurs in this model. Mice with cardiomyocyte PPARα transgenic expression have enhanced activity of enzymes that catalyze the

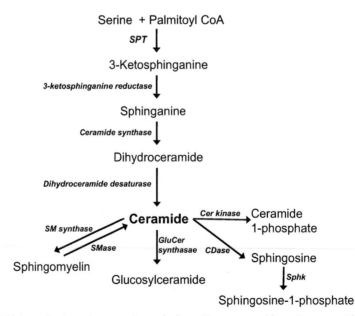

Fig. 1. Sphingolipid biosynthetic pathway and metabolism. CDase, ceramidase; Cer, ceramide; CoA, coenzyme A; GlucCer, glucosylceramide; SM, sphingomyelin; SMase, sphingomyelinase; Sphk, sphingosine kinase; SPT, serine palmitoyltransferase.

synthesis of triglycerides and, like diabetic hearts, have greater intracellular triglyceride stores.[22,23] Hydrolysis of this triglyceride supplies fatty acids to the diabetic hearts.[17] In moderately obese individuals, triglyceride accumulation is detected in the myocardium.[24]

Whether greater reliance on fatty acids is harmful or is an adaptive change is debated. In the setting of ischemia, more specifically hypoxia, the creation of more ATP using less oxygen can occur by the use of glucose and has been proposed as a beneficial therapeutic strategy.[25] Whether this strategy is applicable to nonischemic disease is unclear, and some in vivo studies in animal models fail to support a role for reducing fatty acid oxidation in heart failure. Diets with greater amounts of fat and less carbohydrate lead to better function in some failure models.[26–29]

Another option for the cause of heart failure in diabetic or obese conditions is that toxicity is caused by an alteration of lipid metabolism leading to lipotoxic events. Sphingolipids might be one such lipid.

ELEVATED CERAMIDE CORRELATES WITH LIPOTOXIC CARDIOMYOPATHY

The accumulation of neutral lipids in or around the myocardium is observed in humans or animal models with nonischemic heart failure,[1,2,22,23] and it is hypothesized that excess lipid contributes to the development of cardiac dysfunction.[3,30,31] Several transgenic animal models of lipotoxic cardiomyopathy have been created to support this notion. When hearts internalize excess lipids or have a defect in lipid oxidation, lipid storage is increased. Cardiomyocyte transgenic expression of long-chain acyl coenzyme A synthetase 1 (myosin heavy chain [MHC]-ACS1),[32] fatty acid transport protein 1 (MHC-FATP1),[33] and the cell

membrane anchored form of LpL (LpL^{GPI})[34] are characterized by elevated myocardial fatty acid uptake and lipid deposition and cardiomyopathy.

How does myocardial lipid accumulation lead to cardiomyopathy? Neutral droplets or fatty acids could produce direct toxic effects on myofibrillar function.[35] Fatty acids can induce apoptosis[36] in response to increased levels of reactive oxygen species generated as a toxic by-product of lipid oxidation[35] and activation of protein kinase C signaling pathway.[37] Fatty acids also induce the synthesis of ceramides, which mediate several toxic processes.[6] Although it is still unclear which lipid metabolites directly cause cardiomyopathy, in several models, ceramide accumulation in the heart correlates with these pathophysiological events and heart dysfunction (**Table 1**).[6,32,38] When the balance between fatty acid uptake and oxidation is altered, excess fatty acids are directed toward the synthesis of complex lipids, including triglycerides and phospholipids. An alternative route to use fatty acid surplus is via the ceramide biosynthetic pathway. Increased myocardial ceramide levels are associated with diastolic dysfunction in Akita Ins2 (WT/C96Y) mice and Zucker diabetic fatty (ZDF) rats.[39] To support this notion of ceramide toxicity, improvement in cardiac dysfunction by pharmacologic and genetic intervention in ZDF rats, Akita Ins2 (WT/C96Y), and MHC-ACS1 mice was accompanied by the reduction of cardiac ceramide.[28,36,39] The previously mentioned results suggest that myocardial ceramide levels correlate with the development of cardiac dysfunction found in obese and diabetic hearts.

Methods to reduce ceramide synthesis include the reduction of fatty acid uptake by the heart and conversion of fatty acids to nontoxic triglyceride. Several intervention studies to reduce circulating fatty acids improved cardiac function of

Table 1
Cardiac ceramide, cardiomyocytes apoptosis, and cardiac function in animal models of lipotoxic cardiomyopathy, diabetes, and obesity

Animal Models	References	Cardiac Ceramide Changes	Cardiac Function
MHC-ACS1 mice	Chiu et al[32]	Increased	Decreased
LpL^{GPI} mice	Yagyu et al[34]	Increased	Decreased
MHC-PPARγ mice	Son et al[38]	Increased	Decreased
Akita Ins2 (WT/C96Y) mice	Basu et al[39]	Increased	Decreased
Zucker diabetic fatty rats	Zhou et al[36]	Increased	Decreased
ob/ob mice	Torre-Villalvazo et al[44]	Increased	No change
Rats fed a high-fat diet	Torre-Villalvazo et al[44]	Increased	ND

Abbreviations: LpL^{GPI}, cardiomyocyte-specific overexpression of glycosylphosphatidylinositol-anchored lipoprotein lipase; MHC-ACS1, cardiomyocyte-specific overexpression of long chain acyl coenzyme A synthetase 1; MHC-PPARγ, cardiomyocyte-specific overexpression of peroxisome proliferator-activated receptor γ; ND, not determined.

lipotoxic animals and reduced cardiac ceramide. These interventions include the administration of the PPARγ agonist troglitazone in ZDF rats, insulin treatment of Akita Ins2 (WT/C96Y) mice, and the overexpression of diacylglycerol acyltransferase 1 in MHC-ACS1 mice.[28,36,39]

To find a direct connection between ceramide and lipotoxic cardiomyopathy, the authors studied the involvement of ceramide in the development of lipotoxic cardiomyopathy. LpL[GPI] mice also have increased cardiac ceramide and apoptosis markers, including cytosolic cytochrome c and caspase 3 expression and activity.[40] The authors demonstrated that the inhibition of ceramide biosynthesis by myriocin or heterozygous deletion of Sptlc1, a serine palmitoyltransferase (SPT) subunit, decreased the expression of some apoptotic genes and improved cardiac contraction in LpL[GPI] (**Fig. 2**).[6] In this study, blockage of ceramide biosynthesis seems to modulate mitochondrial substrate oxidation. LpL[GPI] hearts have increased uptake of FFA and rely on fatty acid oxidation for cardiac energy production. A potential mechanism for the improvement with myriocin is that pharmacologic and genetic inhibition of SPT upregulated pyruvate dehydrogenase kinase-4 and decreased the rate of glucose oxidation but led to greater fatty acid (FA) oxidation. However, glucose uptake was increased in LpL[GPI] hearts. This paradoxic fate of glucose is explained by the accumulation of glucose as glycogen with increased phosphorylated glycogen synthase

kinase 3β.[6] In isolated perfused LpL[GPI] hearts, myriocin restored cardiac efficiency, enhancing myocardial energetics by maintaining cardiac performance at a lower oxygen cost. Even with improved cardiac function and balanced substrate use by myriocin treatment, a long-term treatment of LpL[GPI] mice with myriocin only partially rescued the survival rate. A potential reason is the involvement of other lipid metabolites in cardiac dysfunction. Other probable candidates for cardiac failure are diacylglycerol, which alters protein kinase C (PKC) signaling, and FFA. More studies are needed to distinguish the role of ceramide from other lipid metabolites.

CERAMIDE-MEDIATED APOPTOSIS OF CARDIOMYOCYTES

Lipotoxic cardiomyopathy is also associated with the loss of cardiomyocytes via apoptosis.[41,42] Ceramide is a proapoptotic second messenger that activates several signaling pathways, including PKC, protein phosphatase 1 or 2A, and cathepsin D.[43] These signaling pathways are involved in proapoptotic events, including the suppression of Bcl2, the dephosphorylation of protein kinase B (AKT), and the activation of caspases.[43] The accumulation of ceramide was reported to be accompanied by cardiomyocyte apoptosis, and pharmacologic inhibition of ceramide biosynthesis reduced cardiomyocyte apoptosis in ZDF rats and MHC-ACS1 mice.[28,36] However, a recent report

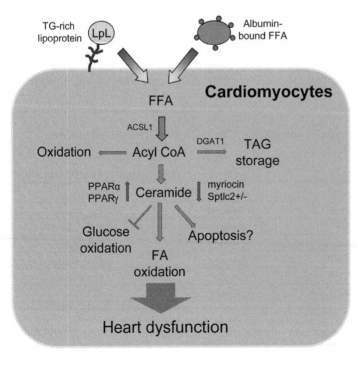

Fig. 2. Lipotoxicity is created by an imbalanced substrate oxidation in heart. Fatty acids are taken up by heart via hydrolysis of triglyceride within lipoproteins by LpL action or transport of albumin-bound free fatty acids. In cardiomyocytes, the free fatty acids are esterified to coenzyme A (CoA) and used for energy or stored as lipid droplets. When lipid uptake exceeds oxidation, more acyl CoAs are shunted to ceramide biosynthesis. Accumulation of ceramide alters the balance of glucose/fatty acid oxidation and leads to cardiac dysfunction. Agonism of PPARα or γ elevates cardiac ceramide levels and leads to cardiac dysfunction. In contrast, myriocin and heterozygous deletion of Sptlc2 prevent cardiac dysfunction. FA, fatty acid; TAG, triacylglycerol; TG, triglyceride.

demonstrated that the myocardium of ob/ob mice and rats fed a high saturated-fat diet did not show increased cardiomyocyte apoptosis even with elevation of ceramide.[44] These conflicting data suggest that the elevation of cardiac ceramide does not always lead to the activation of apoptosis.

The notion that cardiac dysfunction of LpL[GPI] hearts results from its dysregulation of substrate use and not from apoptotic loss of cardiomyocytes suggests that ceramide accumulation does not necessarily accompany apoptosis. The incubation of human cardiomyocyte AC16 cells with C6-ceramide downregulated glucose transporter 4 and upregulated pyruvate dehydrogenase kinase 4 gene expression.[6] These changes in metabolic genes were consistent with what was found in LpL[GPI] mice that has elevated ceramide levels in hearts. These findings also suggest that ceramide modulates cardiac energy metabolism via transcriptional regulation of metabolic genes rather than apoptosis.

PPARs REGULATE CARDIAC SPHINGOLIPID METABOLISM

PPAR transcription factors regulate the oxidation of FA and play an important role in the regulation of substrate metabolism in hearts. There are 3 distinct PPAR isoforms: α, δ, and γ. Of these isoforms, PPARα and δ are highly expressed in hearts and thought to regulate FA metabolism in cardiomyocytes.[45] High fat feeding of cardiac PPARα transgenic mice accelerated the development of cardiomyopathy and was associated with excess FA oxidation and accumulation of ceramide in hearts.[46,47] These effects were not observed in wild-type mice and suggest that PPARα is involved in the regulation of ceramide metabolism in hearts. Baranowski and colleagues[48,49] demonstrated that activation of PPARα by WY-14643, a PPARα agonist, causes ceramide and sphingomyelin accumulation in the myocardium of high fat–fed rats. This result was caused by the activation of de novo sphingolipid synthesis via elevated SPT activity and increased availability of intracellular palmitate, a substrate of SPT. However, it is unclear whether PPARα regulates SPT expression directly or indirectly by elevating FFA pools. Because PPARα agonist activity did not increase myocardial ceramide levels or SPT activity in regular chow-fed rats, both changes in enzymes and substrates (ie, the high-fat diet) are needed to alter de novo ceramide biosynthesis.[48] Alternative pathways for ceramide generation, such as sphingomyelinase

and ceramidase, were not affected by PPARα activation.

The treatment of patients with diabetes with thiazolidinediones, selective PPARγ activators, increases heart failure risk.[50] These clinical observations could have resulted from either greater salt or water retention, despite reduced blood pressure and vasodilation, or direct effects of PPARγ agonists on heart metabolism. In support of this latter hypothesis, Son and colleagues[38] reported that cardiac transgenic expression of PPARγ led to cardiac dysfunction associated with the induction of FA oxidation genes, the accumulation of glycogen and lipids in mouse myocardium, and the disruption of mitochondrial structure. Cardiac ceramide levels were also elevated modestly. The effects of pharmacologic PPARγ agonists on heart metabolism and function in animal models are mixed. These drugs induce glucose transporters 1 and 4 and increase glucose uptake in cultured rat cardiomyocytes and in the heart of diabetic animal models.[51–54] In ZDF rats, the administration of thiazolidinedione reduced cardiac accumulation of ceramide.[36] Similarly, PPARγ agonist treatment of LpL[GPI] mice reduced heart dysfunction and, in this model, was shown to divert circulating lipids to greater adipose and reduced heart uptake.[55] So the use of agonists in vivo is likely to reflect the level of cardiac PPARγ expression and the importance of the induction of PPARγ in adipose.

Another possible action of PPARγ agonists is the induction of ceramide synthesis. In one study, the administration of PPARγ agonists elevated SPT activity and intracellular levels of palmitate, whereas the activation of PPARγ did not change the activities of sphingomyelinase and ceramidase.[56] Thus, the accumulation of cardiac ceramide is via the activation of de novo ceramide biosynthesis. A modest increase in the expression of SPT protein or mRNA did not match the elevated activity, suggesting SPT activity is regulated by posttranscriptional modification. It has been widely accepted that the increased availability of palmitate, a substrate of SPT reaction, increases SPT activity and expression.[57,58] Holland and colleagues[59] found that palmitate activates a toll-like receptor pathway and increases intracellular levels of ceramide by activating de novo ceramide synthesis. These findings indicate that palmitate is not only acting as a substrate for SPT-mediated de novo ceramide synthesis but acting as an activator of the rate-limiting enzyme in this biosynthetic pathway. Collectively, PPARs regulate myocardial sphingolipid metabolism mainly via de novo synthesis (see **Fig. 2**).

CARDIOPROTECTIVE EFFECTS OF S1P

S1P might protect the heart from ischemia-reperfusion injury. S1P is synthesized intracellularly and exerts its function by binding to specific plasma membrane G-protein coupled receptors (S1P$_{1\sim5}$). Intracellular S1P has a proliferative role in cells and is also secreted to the extracellular space (inside-out hypothesis). Secreted S1P binds to the S1P receptors on plasma membrane and elicits its regulatory function. When S1P binds to the S1P receptors, phosphatidylinositol 4-kinase is activated and its downstream targets, AKT and glycogen synthase kinase 3β, are phosphorylated and activate these signaling pathways. Of the 5 subtypes of the S1P receptors, cardiomyocytes express S1P$_1$, S1P$_2$, and S1P$_3$.[60] The incubation of rat neonatal cardiomyocytes with S1P or GM1, a ganglioside that induces sphingosine kinase 1 and elevates endogenous S1P production, prevents hypoxia-induced cell death.[61] Cardioprotection by S1P and GM1 during ischemia/reperfusion injury was confirmed in vivo.[62] The infusion of GM1 reduces cardiac injury through PKCε but S1P exerts cardioprotective effects through the PKCε-independent pathway. Later, it was found that the inactivation of the interaction of G protein and G protein coupled receptor by pertussis toxin or S1P$_{1-3}$ antagonist removed GM-1 mediated cardioprotection.[63] These findings suggest that endogenous S1P is transported from cardiomyocytes and exerts its cardioprotective effects by binding to S1P receptors on the membrane surface. Consistent with these findings, ischemia suppressed sphingosine kinase activity and reduced S1P levels in the heart; these effects were maintained during reperfusion.[64] Sphk1-deficient hearts were susceptible to ischemia/reperfusion injury, and adenoviral Sphk1 gene transfer induced cardioprotection and prevented ischemic heart failure.[65] Although S1P is one of the major lipid components in high-density lipoprotein (HDL), it has been reported that S1P action is independent of HDL.[66]

Of the S1P receptors, S1P$_1$ may be most important for cardioprotection. S1P$_1$-specific agonists protected adult mouse cardiomyocytes from hypoxia.[67] In contrast, VPC23019 and FTY720, the synthetic antagonists of S1P$_1$, prevented cardioprotection elicited by S1P. However, other groups suggested that S1P$_2$ and S1P$_3$ also exert S1P-mediated cardioprotective action. S1P$_{2/3}$ double knockout mice have increased myocardial infarct size during ischemia/reperfusion injury,[68] suggesting the overlapping role of S1P receptor isoforms. In addition, S1P$_3$ deficiency abolished S1P-mediated cardioprotection, and the pharmacologic inhibition of nitric oxide synthase also caused the disappearance of cardioprotective effects, suggesting an important role of this pathway.[69] Recently, it was reported that cardiac-specific S1P$_1$-deficient mice are vulnerable to ischemia/reperfusion injury to the same degree as the wild-type mice.[70] These conflicting data may result from the experimental model systems: S1P$_1$ in cardiomyocytes and S1P$_{2/3}$ in animal hearts. Therefore, the roles of S1P in cardioprotection of nonischemic heart failure deserve further study.

CLINICAL IMPLICATION OF SPHINGOLIPID METABOLISM IN HEART FAILURE

Animal experiments suggest that ceramide is implicated in pathogenesis of cardiac dysfunction associated with obesity and diabetes. However, whether ceramide is relevant to cardiac failure in humans is unclear. Barranowski and colleagues[71] found that the enzymes in sphingolipid biosynthesis were upregulated in the right atrial appendage of overweight patients; the tissue was obtained during coronary bypass graft surgery. These genes include Sptlc1/2, Sphk1, alkaline/acid/neutral ceramidases, and neutral ceramidases. When diabetes was present in the obese patients, the expression of some genes was reduced but higher than lean subjects. They also found increased DNA fragmentation in the hearts of obese nondiabetic patients and it was increased further in obese diabetic hearts. Surprisingly, the elevation of cardiac ceramide was not found. The reason for these conflicting data is likely to be coordinated regulation of ceramide synthesis and degradation. These findings suggested that obesity and type 2 diabetes do not induce ceramide accumulation in the human heart or at least in the atrium.

SUMMARY

All tissues, including the heart, need essential lipids. With obesity and diabetes, hearts are likely to have metabolic imbalance and lipid accumulation. A flurry of recent investigations using animal models suggests that ceramide plays important roles in the pathogenesis of heart failure. In contrast, S1P is implicated in cardioprotection during ischemia/reperfusion injury. Further studies will need to first define the lipid abnormalities that occur in human hearts at various stages of failure, and the associated gene/enzyme alterations associated with heart failure from a variety of causes must be determined. Only then can a reasonable plan be devised to alter sphingolipid metabolism as a method to prevent or treat patients.

REFERENCES

1. Borradaile NM, Schaffer JE. Lipotoxicity in the heart. Curr Hypertens Rep 2005;7:412–7.
2. Harmancey R, Wilson CR, Taegtmeyer H. Adaptation and maladaptation of the heart in obesity. Hypertension 2008;52:181–7.
3. Summers SA. Ceramides in insulin resistance and lipotoxicity. Prog Lipid Res 2006;45:42–72.
4. Perman JC, Bostrom P, Lindbom M, et al. The VLDL receptor promotes lipotoxicity and increases mortality in mice following an acute myocardial infarction. J Clin Invest 2011;121:2625–40.
5. Holland WL, Miller RA, Wang ZV, et al. Receptor-mediated activation of ceramidase activity initiates the pleiotropic actions of adiponectin. Nat Med 2011;17:55–63.
6. Park TS, Hu Y, Noh HL, et al. Ceramide is a cardiotoxin in lipotoxic cardiomyopathy. Journal of lipid research 2008;49:2101–12.
7. Holland WL, Brozinick JT, Wang LP, et al. Inhibition of ceramide synthesis ameliorates glucocorticoid-, saturated-fat-, and obesity-induced insulin resistance. Cell Metab 2007;5:167–79.
8. Guenther GG, Edinger AL. A new take on ceramide: starving cells by cutting off the nutrient supply. Cell Cycle 2009;8:1122–6.
9. Yang J, Yu Y, Sun S, et al. Ceramide and other sphingolipids in cellular responses. Cell Biochem Biophys 2004;40:323–50.
10. Augustus AS, Buchanan J, Park TS, et al. Loss of lipoprotein lipase-derived fatty acids leads to increased cardiac glucose metabolism and heart dysfunction. J Biol Chem 2006;281:8716–23.
11. Hajri T, Ibrahimi A, Coburn CT, et al. Defective fatty acid uptake in the spontaneously hypertensive rat is a primary determinant of altered glucose metabolism, hyperinsulinemia, and myocardial hypertrophy. J Biol Chem 2001;276:23661–6.
12. Stowe KA, Burgess SC, Merritt M, et al. Storage and oxidation of long-chain fatty acids in the C57/BL6 mouse heart as measured by NMR spectroscopy. FEBS Lett 2006;580:4282–7.
13. Opie LH. Cardiac metabolism–emergence, decline, and resurgence. Part II. Cardiovasc Res 1992;26:817–30.
14. Opie LH. Cardiac metabolism–emergence, decline, and resurgence. Part I. Cardiovasc Res 1992;26:721–33.
15. Randle PJ, Garland PB, Hales CN, et al. The glucose fatty-acid cycle. Its role in insulin sensitivity and the metabolic disturbances of diabetes mellitus. Lancet 1963;1:785–9.
16. Rodrigues B, Cam MC, Jian K, et al. Differential effects of streptozotocin-induced diabetes on cardiac lipoprotein lipase activity. Diabetes 1997;46:1346–53.

17. Pulinilkunnil T, Rodrigues B. Cardiac lipoprotein lipase: metabolic basis for diabetic heart disease. Cardiovasc Res 2006;69:329–40.
18. Buchanan J, Mazumder PK, Hu P, et al. Reduced cardiac efficiency and altered substrate metabolism precedes the onset of hyperglycemia and contractile dysfunction in two mouse models of insulin resistance and obesity. Endocrinology 2005;146:5341–9.
19. Ko HJ, Zhang Z, Jung DY, et al. Nutrient stress activates inflammation and reduces glucose metabolism by suppressing AMP-activated protein kinase in the heart. Diabetes 2009;58:2536–46.
20. Gil-Ortega I, Carlos Kaski J. Diabetic miocardiopathy. Med Clin (Barc) 2006;127:584–94.
21. Park SY, Cho YR, Finck BN, et al. Cardiac-specific overexpression of peroxisome proliferator-activated receptor-alpha causes insulin resistance in heart and liver. Diabetes 2005;54:2514–24.
22. Lewis GF, Carpentier A, Adeli K, et al. Disordered fat storage and mobilization in the pathogenesis of insulin resistance and type 2 diabetes. Endocr Rev 2002;23:201–29.
23. Boden G, Lebed B, Schatz M, et al. Effects of acute changes of plasma free fatty acids on intramyocellular fat content and insulin resistance in healthy subjects. Diabetes 2001;50:1612–7.
24. Kankaanpaa M, Lehto HR, Parkka JP, et al. Myocardial triglyceride content and epicardial fat mass in human obesity: relationship to left ventricular function and serum free fatty acid levels. J Clin Endocrinol Metab 2006;91:4689–95.
25. Jaswal JS, Keung W, Wang W, et al. Targeting fatty acid and carbohydrate oxidation–a novel therapeutic intervention in the ischemic and failing heart. Biochim Biophys Acta 2011;1813:1333–50.
26. Okere IC, Young ME, McElfresh TA, et al. Low carbohydrate/high-fat diet attenuates cardiac hypertrophy, remodeling, and altered gene expression in hypertension. Hypertension 2006;48:1116–23.
27. Son NH, Yu S, Tuinei J, et al. PPARgamma-induced cardiolipotoxicity in mice is ameliorated by PPARalpha deficiency despite increases in fatty acid oxidation. J Clin Invest 2010;120:3443–54.
28. Liu L, Shi X, Bharadwaj KG, et al. DGAT1 expression increases heart triglyceride content but ameliorates lipotoxicity. J Biol Chem 2009;284:36312–23.
29. Haemmerle G, Moustafa T, Woelkart G, et al. ATGL-mediated fat catabolism regulates cardiac mitochondrial function via PPAR-alpha and PGC-1. Nat Med 2011;17:1076–85.
30. Young ME, McNulty P, Taegtmeyer H. Adaptation and maladaptation of the heart in diabetes: part II: potential mechanisms. Circulation 2002;105:1861–70.
31. Park TS, Yamashita H, Blaner WS, et al. Lipids in the heart: a source of fuel and a source of toxins. Curr Opin Lipidol 2007;18:277–82.

32. Chiu HC, Kovacs A, Ford DA, et al. A novel mouse model of lipotoxic cardiomyopathy. J Clin Invest 2001;107:813–22.

33. Chiu HC, Kovacs A, Blanton RM, et al. Transgenic expression of fatty acid transport protein 1 in the heart causes lipotoxic cardiomyopathy. Circ Res 2005;96:225–33.

34. Yagyu H, Chen G, Yokoyama M, et al. Lipoprotein lipase (LpL) on the surface of cardiomyocytes increases lipid uptake and produces a cardiomyopathy. J Clin Invest 2003;111:419–26.

35. Dyntar D, Eppenberger-Eberhardt M, Maedler K, et al. Glucose and palmitic acid induce degeneration of myofibrils and modulate apoptosis in rat adult cardiomyocytes. Diabetes 2001;50:2105–13.

36. Zhou YT, Grayburn P, Karim A, et al. Lipotoxic heart disease in obese rats: implications for human obesity. Proc Natl Acad Sci U S A 2000;97:1784–9.

37. Drosatos K, Bharadwaj KG, Lymperopoulos A, et al. Cardiomyocyte lipids impair beta-adrenergic receptor function via PKC activation. Am J Physiol Endocrinol Metab 2011;300:E489–99.

38. Son NH, Park TS, Yamashita H, et al. Cardiomyocyte expression of PPARgamma leads to cardiac dysfunction in mice. J Clin Invest 2007;117:2791–801.

39. Basu R, Oudit GY, Wang X, et al. Type 1 diabetic cardiomyopathy in the Akita (Ins2WT/C96Y) mouse model is characterized by lipotoxicity and diastolic dysfunction with preserved systolic function. Am J Physiol Heart Circ Physiol 2009;297:H2096–108.

40. Yokoyama M, Yagyu H, Hu Y, et al. Apolipoprotein B production reduces lipotoxic cardiomyopathy: studies in heart-specific lipoprotein lipase transgenic mouse. J Biol Chem 2004;279:4204–11.

41. Foo RS, Mani K, Kitsis RN. Death begets failure in the heart. J Clin Invest 2005;115:565–71.

42. Boudina S, Abel ED. Diabetic cardiomyopathy revisited. Circulation 2007;115:3213–23.

43. Pettus BJ, Chalfant CE, Hannun YA. Ceramide in apoptosis: an overview and current perspectives. Biochim Biophys Acta 2002;1585:114–25.

44. Torre-Villalvazo I, Gonzalez F, Aguilar-Salinas CA, et al. Dietary soy protein reduces cardiac lipid accumulation and the ceramide concentration in high-fat diet-fed rats and ob/ob mice. J Nutr 2009;139:2237–43.

45. Yang Q, Li Y. Roles of PPARs on regulating myocardial energy and lipid homeostasis. J Mol Med (Berl) 2007;85:697–706.

46. Finck BN, Lehman JJ, Leone TC, et al. The cardiac phenotype induced by PPARalpha overexpression mimics that caused by diabetes mellitus. J Clin Invest 2002;109:121–30.

47. Finck BN, Han X, Courtois M, et al. A critical role for PPARalpha-mediated lipotoxicity in the pathogenesis of diabetic cardiomyopathy: modulation by dietary fat content. Proc Natl Acad Sci U S A 2003;100: 1226–31.

48. Baranowski M, Blachnio A, Zabielski P, et al. PPAR-alpha agonist induces the accumulation of ceramide in the heart of rats fed high-fat diet. J Physiol Pharmacol 2007;58:57–72.

49. Burkart EM, Sambandam N, Han X, et al. Nuclear receptors PPARbeta/delta and PPARalpha direct distinct metabolic regulatory programs in the mouse heart. J Clin Invest 2007;117:3930–9.

50. Nissen SE, Wolski K. Effect of rosiglitazone on the risk of myocardial infarction and death from cardiovascular causes. N Engl J Med 2007;356: 2457–71.

51. Bahr M, Spelleken M, Bock M, et al. Acute and chronic effects of troglitazone (CS-045) on isolated rat ventricular cardiomyocytes. Diabetologia 1996; 39:766–74.

52. Sidell RJ, Cole MA, Draper NJ, et al. Thiazolidinedione treatment normalizes insulin resistance and ischemic injury in the Zucker fatty rat heart. Diabetes 2002;51:1110–7.

53. Carley AN, Semeniuk LM, Shimoni Y, et al. Treatment of type 2 diabetic db/db mice with a novel PPAR-gamma agonist improves cardiac metabolism but not contractile function. Am J Physiol Endocrinol Metab 2004;286:E449–55.

54. Liu LS, Tanaka H, Ishii S, et al. The new antidiabetic drug MCC-555 acutely sensitizes insulin signaling in isolated cardiomyocytes. Endocrinology 1998;139: 4531–9.

55. Vikramadithyan RK, Hirata K, Yagyu H, et al. Peroxisome proliferator-activated receptor agonists modulate heart function in transgenic mice with lipotoxic cardiomyopathy. J Pharmacol Exp Ther 2005;313:586–93.

56. Baranowski M, Blachnio A, Zabielski P, et al. Pioglitazone induces de novo ceramide synthesis in the rat heart. Prostaglandins Other Lipid Mediat 2007; 83:99–111.

57. Shimabukuro M, Higa M, Zhou YT, et al. Lipoapoptosis in beta-cells of obese prediabetic fa/fa rats. Role of serine palmitoyltransferase overexpression. J Biol Chem 1998;273:32487–90.

58. Blazquez C, Geelen MJ, Velasco G, et al. The AMP-activated protein kinase prevents ceramide synthesis de novo and apoptosis in astrocytes. FEBS Lett 2001;489:149–53.

59. Holland WL, Bikman BT, Wang LP, et al. Lipid-induced insulin resistance mediated by the proinflammatory receptor TLR4 requires saturated fatty acid-induced ceramide biosynthesis in mice. J Clin Invest 2011;121:1858–70.

60. Karliner JS. Sphingosine kinase and sphingosine 1-phosphate in cardioprotection. J Cardiovasc Pharmacol 2009;53:189–97.

61. Karliner JS, Honbo N, Summers K, et al. The lysophospholipids sphingosine-1-phosphate and lysophosphatidic acid enhance survival during hypoxia

in neonatal rat cardiac myocytes. J Mol Cell Cardiol 2001;33:1713–7.

62. Jin ZQ, Zhou HZ, Zhu P, et al. Cardioprotection mediated by sphingosine-1-phosphate and ganglioside GM-1 in wild-type and PKC epsilon knockout mouse hearts. Am J Physiol Heart Circ Physiol 2002;282:H1970–7.

63. Tao R, Zhang J, Vessey DA, et al. Deletion of the sphingosine kinase-1 gene influences cell fate during hypoxia and glucose deprivation in adult mouse cardiomyocytes. Cardiovasc Res 2007;74: 56–63.

64. Vessey DA, Kelley M, Li L, et al. Role of sphingosine kinase activity in protection of heart against ischemia reperfusion injury. Med Sci Monit 2006; 12:BR318–24.

65. Duan HF, Wang H, Yi J, et al. Adenoviral gene transfer of sphingosine kinase 1 protects heart against ischemia/reperfusion-induced injury and attenuates its postischemic failure. Hum Gene Ther 2007;18: 1119–28.

66. Kennedy S, Kane KA, Pyne NJ, et al. Targeting sphingosine-1-phosphate signalling for cardioprotection. Curr Opin Pharmacol 2009;9:194–201.

67. Zhang J, Honbo N, Goetzl EJ, et al. Signals from type 1 sphingosine 1-phosphate receptors enhance adult mouse cardiac myocyte survival during hypoxia. Am J Physiol Heart Circ Physiol 2007;293: H3150–8.

68. Means CK, Xiao CY, Li Z, et al. Sphingosine 1-phosphate S1P2 and S1P3 receptor-mediated Akt activation protects against in vivo myocardial ischemia-reperfusion injury. Am J Physiol Heart Circ Physiol 2007;292:H2944–51.

69. Theilmeier G, Schmidt C, Herrmann J, et al. High-density lipoproteins and their constituent, sphingosine-1-phosphate, directly protect the heart against ischemia/reperfusion injury in vivo via the S1P3 lysophospholipid receptor. Circulation 2006; 114:1403–9.

70. Means CK, Brown JH. Sphingosine-1-phosphate receptor signalling in the heart. Cardiovasc Res 2009;82:193–200.

71. Baranowski M, Blachnio-Zabielska A, Hirnle T, et al. Myocardium of type 2 diabetic and obese patients is characterized by alterations in sphingolipid metabolic enzymes but not by accumulation of ceramide. J Lipid Res 2010;51:74–80.

Myocardial Fatty Acid Metabolism and Lipotoxicity in the Setting of Insulin Resistance

Bernard P.C. Kok, PhD, David N. Brindley, PhD, DSc, FRSC*

KEYWORDS

- Fatty acid oxidation • Lipid accumulation • Metabolic inflexibility • Cardiomyopathy • Diabetes
- Cardiovascular disease

KEY POINTS

- Cardiovascular disease caused by obesity and type 2 diabetes is a major health issue.
- Flexible and dynamic regulation of cardiac metabolism is essential for proper heart function.
- The use of fatty acids in the heart is a major determinant of cardiac adenosine triphosphate production.
- The rates of uptake, storage, and oxidation of fatty acids are increased in diabetes.
- Modulating the plasma lipoprotein profile or cardiac fuel use could alleviate cardiovascular disease phenotypes.

DISEASE DESCRIPTION

The term metabolic syndrome has become all too familiar in a modern society faced with an increase in the rates of obesity and food consumption coupled to a decline in physical activity and an increasingly aging population. The metabolic syndrome is used to describe a set of comorbidities including upper body obesity, insulin resistance, dyslipidemia, and hypertension that increase the risk for developing type 2 diabetes, coronary artery disease, and stroke.[1,2] Increased awareness and treatment of the factors leading to the occurrence of cardiovascular disease has resulted in a decrease in rates of heart disease in both Canada and the United States (**Table 1**).[3,4] However, cardiovascular disease still remains the number 1 cause of death in both countries. Furthermore, the incidence of non–insulin-dependent diabetes mellitus (NIDDM; type 2 diabetes) in the North American (**Tables 2 and 3**) and world populations[5] has not slowed even with the increase in public awareness.

RISK FACTORS ASSOCIATED WITH DIABETES AND CARDIOVASCULAR DISEASE

The risk factors in the development of cardiovascular disease have been studied and reviewed extensively, most notably in the Framingham Heart Study, and they include the following:

- Smoking[6]
- Hypertension[7]
- Age[8]
- Dyslipidemia (eg, low high-density lipoprotein [HDL] to low-density lipoprotein [LDL] ratio and hypertriglyceridemia)[9–11]
- Abdominal obesity (increased waist circumference to height ratio)[12–14]
- Weight gain[15]
- Physical inactivity[16,17]

Financial disclosure and conflict of interest: None.
Signal Transduction Research Group, Department of Biochemistry, School of Translational Medicine, University of Alberta, 357, Heritage Medical Research Centre, 11207 87th Avenue, Edmonton, Alberta T6G 2S2, Canada
* Corresponding author.
E-mail address: david.brindley@ualberta.ca

Heart Failure Clin 8 (2012) 643–661
http://dx.doi.org/10.1016/j.hfc.2012.06.008
1551-7136/12/$ – see front matter © 2012 Elsevier Inc. All rights reserved.

Table 1
Age-adjusted mortality rates due to cardiovascular disease (I00–I78) in Canada and the United States as calculated by population estimates as of July 1 each year, with the exception of the data for the United States population in 2000, which was approximated on April 1

Prevalence/Incidence and Mortality Rates		
Year	Deaths Due to Cardiovascular Disease (Canada)	Deaths Due to Cardiovascular Disease (USA)
2007	151.9	249.9
2006	155.6	261.2
2005	167.4	277.3
2004	175.6	286.5
2003	185.0	306.1
2002	192.1	317.4
2001	197.5	326.5
2000	209.1	339.7

The numbers represent the number of persons afflicted per 100,000 of the population.
Data from Statistics Canada, CANSIM (Table 102-0552) and the Centers for Disease Control and Prevention (GMWK293R).

Of these risk factors, dyslipidemia, physical inactivity, abdominal obesity, and weight gain are also significantly associated with the occurrence of type 2 diabetes.[2,14,18–21] Strikingly, a large

Table 2
Incidence of diagnosed diabetes in the population of Canada

Age Group (Years)	2005	2007	2008	2009	2010
0–44					
Males	83	111	71	59	75
Females	82	57	62	56	58
45–64					
Males	327	401	442	407	502
Females	249	314	335	326	312
65 and over					
Males	299	361	343	436	434
Females	276	320	337	355	369
Total					
Males	715	882	881	937	1058
Females	610	733	775	769	783

The numbers represent the number of persons of the population in thousands.
Data from Statistics Canada, CANSIM (Table 105-0501).

Table 3
Incidence of diagnosed diabetes in the population of the United States

Age Group (Years)	2004	2005	2006	2007	2008
0–44					
Males	1129	1283	1327	1348	1473
Females	1289	1450	1495	1453	1458
45–64					
Males	3605	3834	3999	4219	4606
Females	3327	3603	3814	4137	4734
65 and over					
Males	2803	2843	2905	3022	3256
Females	3068	3283	3472	3667	3767
Total					
Males	7537	7959	8232	8585	9334
Females	7684	8336	8782	9257	9960

The numbers represent the number of persons of the population in thousands.
Data from Centers for Disease Control and Prevention—Diabetes Data and Trends (National Surveillance Data).

proportion of diabetic patients develop cardiovascular disease.[22,23] Moreover, patients diagnosed with diabetes are 2 to 4 times more likely to develop coronary artery disease, heart failure, or diabetic cardiomyopathy.[23–25] Fortunately, the cessation of smoking, the development of antihypertensive drugs, and the availability of drugs used to treat dyslipidemia and insulin resistance (eg, statins, fibrates, and thiazolidinediones) have significantly reduced the incidence of cardiovascular disease in the current population.[3,4] However, the inability to significantly change both diet and lifestyle makes it imperative that we understand and develop novel treatments of the disease phenotypes in patients with type 2 diabetes such that the risk of developing cardiovascular disease is also lessened. One important parameter of healthy cardiac function is the dynamic and tightly regulated process of fuel metabolism in the heart, especially that of fatty acid (FA) metabolism. The regulation of cardiac FA oxidation and storage as well as the consequences of chronic metabolic imbalances on the heart are discussed in the next few sections.

FATTY ACID METABOLISM IN THE HEART
Introduction

On average, the human heart beats 60 to 80 cardiac cycles per minute. With a life expectancy of 78 years, the heart will potentially beat 2.9 billion times in an average lifetime. The continuous pumping of blood driven by the heart throughout the circulatory system is required to sustain a delivery system whereby energy substrates and oxygen can reach other organs in the body. Carbon dioxide is then eliminated through the lungs, and other metabolites are channeled for disposal through the liver and kidneys. It is clear that the proper functioning of the heart is essential, and this is highlighted by the morbidities and mortalities caused by heart failure and cardiovascular disease. The continual work performed by the heart can only be sustained by a constant, uninterrupted stream of energy substrates.

The heart is an "omnivorous" organ that can use various fuels to meet its energy demand:

- Fatty acids
- Glucose
- Ketone bodies
- Amino acids
- Lactate

Out of these substrates, cardiac adenosine triphosphate (ATP) production is obtained from a balance of FA and carbohydrate oxidation, with 50% to 75% of ATP produced from FAs depending on diurnal variations.[26] In fact, the regulation of cardiac fuel use is reliant on plasma FAs and the hydrolysis of triacylglycerol (TG) derived from lipoprotein particles as well as the rate of substrate entry.[27–29]

Regulation of Fatty Acid Supply and Entry

To fully appreciate the mechanisms underlying the metabolism of FAs in the heart and the consequences thereof, one must first comprehend the means by which the heart is supplied by FAs. The hydrolysis of TG stores from the adipose tissue provides a large proportion of circulatory FAs, which are transported, bound to albumin in the plasma. FA supply to the heart is also derived from the hydrolysis of TG in lipoprotein particles such as chylomicrons and very low-density lipoprotein (VLDL) particles (**Fig. 1**). Chylomicron formation in enterocytes mainly in the jejunum occurs postprandially whereby exogenously derived TG (80%–90%) and a small proportion of free and esterified cholesterol (5%–10%) are packaged with apolipoproteins including B48.[30–33] Chylomicrons are then secreted into the mesenteric lymph and enter the vasculature through the thoracic duct.[30–32] VLDLs are mainly secreted from hepatocytes, and each VLDL particle contains one apolipoprotein B100 while consisting of approximately 40% to 50% TG and 20% to 30% cholesterol (free and esterified).[31,33] TG in VLDL particles mainly consist of endogenously derived FAs, for example, from adipose tissue lipolysis,[31]

with some contribution from dietary FAs postprandially.[34] The cardiac uptake and use of TG-derived FAs from VLDLs and chylomicrons depends on lipoprotein lipase (LPL) action (see **Fig. 1**).[29,35,36] LPL is synthesized in the cardiomyocytes[37] and is secreted as an active dimer to the luminal side of the endothelial vessel wall through the action of glycosylphosphatidylinositol-anchored high-density lipoprotein–binding protein 1 (GPIHBP1) (see **Fig. 1**).[38–40] Glycosylphosphatidylinositol-anchored LPL (GPI-LPL) directly expressed on the surface of cardiomyocytes can also facilitate lipid uptake.[41] These investigators proposed that increased FA entry is mediated by GPI-LPL action on partially hydrolyzed lipoprotein particles that exited the vasculature and entered the subendothelial space. It should also be noted that the hydrolysis of lipoprotein TG by LPL as well as the transport of LPL to the capillary lumen appears to be partly dependent on the VLDL receptor.[42–44]

Besides the use of FA hydrolyzed from TG in lipoprotein particles, cardiac FA supply also depends on the uptake of plasma albumin-bound FA by membrane-localized FA transporters including CD36,[45,46] plasma membrane FA binding protein (FABP$_{pm}$),[47] and FA transport proteins, FATP1 and 6 (see **Fig. 1**).[48] The major transporter of FA across the cardiomyocyte plasma membrane appears to be CD36, because inhibition of CD36 decreases cardiac FA uptake by more than 50%.[45,49] Furthermore, CD36 can be dynamically cycled between the plasma membrane and intracellular compartments of cardiomyocytes depending on signals such as insulin and/or contraction, unlike the other FA transporters.[50] CD36 also facilitates the uptake of FAs derived from VLDLs, but it does not appear to be involved in FA uptake from chylomicrons.[29] Although CD36 is thought to be the major mode of cardiac FA uptake, forced overexpression of FATP1 in the heart led to increased FA uptake and metabolism,[51] showing that the other FA transporters could play significant roles in regulating cardiac FA supply. The rate of FA uptake is also dictated by the intracellular flux of FA into oxidative or biosynthetic pathways. Cytoplasmic FA binding protein (FABP$_c$) and long-chain fatty acyl–coenzyme A (CoA) synthases (ACS1-6) can promote FA uptake by binding and directing FAs to the mitochondria for oxidation or to the endoplasmic reticulum for glycerolipid synthesis, thus reducing the intracellular FA concentration and establishing an inward FA gradient (see **Fig. 1**).[52]

Cardiac Fatty Acid Supply in the Diabetic State

Fuel use in the heart is tightly regulated such that any sustained disruption in substrate supply

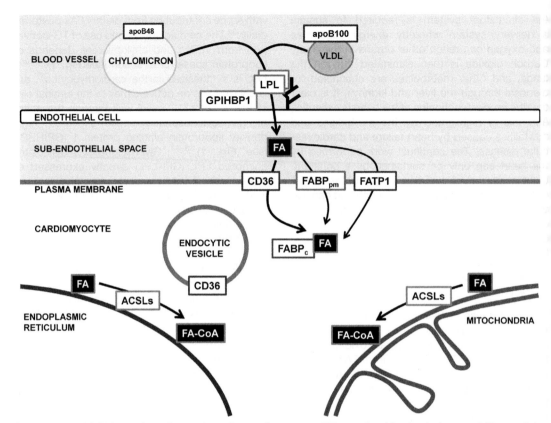

Fig. 1. Fatty acid (FA) supply and entry into the cardiomyocyte. TG contained in circulating apoB48-containing (chylomicrons) and apoB100-containing (very low-density lipoprotein [VLDL]) particles are hydrolyzed by an active dimer of lipoprotein lipase (LPL) anchored to the luminal side of endothelial cells lining the blood vessel by heparan sulfate proteoglycans and glycosylphosphatidylinositol-anchored high-density lipoprotein–binding protein 1 (GPIHBP1). The FAs cross the subendothelial space and enter the cardiomyocyte through facilitated transport by CD36 as well as plasma membrane-localized fatty acid binding protein (FABP$_{pm}$) and fatty acid transport protein 1 (FATP1). CD36 is not permanently localized to the plasma membrane and can cycle into endocytic vesicles. FAs are bound to cytosolic fatty acid binding protein (FABP$_c$) and are activated to acyl-coenzyme A (CoA) esters by different isoforms of long-chain acyl-CoA synthetases (ACSLs) at the mitochondrial or endoplasmic reticulum membranes, before entry into the oxidative or biosynthetic pathways.

and/or oxidation promotes various deleterious phenotypes such as cardiac dysfunction, cardiomyopathies, reduced recovery from ischemia, and heart failure.[53–57] In obese, type 2 diabetic patients, there is increased lipolysis from adipose tissue stores, leading to increased FA delivery and storage in nonadipose tissues such as the liver and heart.[21,58–63] The lack of insulin action coupled to increased glucocorticoid secretion and signaling can also stimulate apolipoprotein B production, VLDL secretion, and gluconeogenesis in the liver.[58,64,65] Furthermore, large quantities of TG and FAs are secreted in chylomicrons owing excessive caloric intake and the lack of dietary control. Therefore, the heart has a considerable source of FAs from the plasma in the diabetic state, available either in VLDL-derived and chylomicron-derived TG or as nonesterified FAs bound to albumin.

The rate of cardiac FA uptake is also increased, because both LPL activity and CD36 expression are increased in diabetes and insulin resistance.[66–71] Besides increased expression in diabetes, CD36 localization to the sarcolemmal membrane is also increased.[72] Furthermore, the supply of FAs is essential in dictating the rate of FA oxidation.[28,73] Finally, cardiac glucose oxidation is downregulated because of the lack of insulin signaling, and FA oxidation (FAO) is heavily favored instead.[74] The effects of increased FAO on the heart is discussed later.

Fate of Fatty Acids on Cardiomyocyte Entry

On entry into the cardiomyocyte, FAs are immediately esterified to acyl-CoA by acyl-CoA synthases (ACSLs), of which there are currently 5 known isoforms (reviewed in Ref.[75]) (see **Fig. 1**). In the heart

ACSL1 appears to be the major isoform, because increases in ACSL activity during development in newborn mice are linked to increases in *Acsl1* transcript levels, whereas *Acsl3* expression is decreased.[76] Furthermore, the use of isoform-dependent inhibitors demonstrated the minor contribution of the remaining isoforms (ACSL4, ACSL5, and ACSL6,) to cardiac ACSL activity as measured by an enzymatic assay using [³H]palmitate as the substrate.[76]

Once formed, acyl-CoA esters are channeled toward oxidation or glycerolipid synthesis. Approximately 75% of FAs entering the heart are oxidized immediately in the mitochondrial matrix under normal conditions.[73] The entry of FAs into the mitochondria is controlled by carnitine palmitoyl transferase (CPT) I, which converts acyl-CoA to acylcarnitine (**Fig. 2**).[74,77] CPT I is inhibited by increased levels of malonyl-CoA,[78,79] which is formed through the action of acetyl-CoA carboxylase (ACC) (see **Fig. 2**).[80] This activity and malonyl-CoA levels are increased when the heart is in the fed state and glycolysis is stimulated.[80–82] Conversely, ACC is inhibited by adenosine monophosphate (AMP)-dependent protein kinase (AMPK) when cellular ATP levels are low, for example, in the fasted state.[26] Furthermore, malonyl-CoA decarboxylase (MCD) can also convert malonyl-CoA to acetyl-CoA, thus relieving the inhibition of CPT I (see **Fig. 2**).[74,83] These differential modes of regulation illustrate the tight and dynamic balance between FA and glucose oxidation in the heart, depending on energy status and substrate availability.

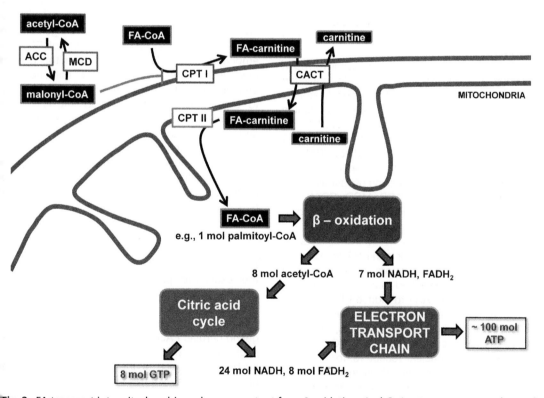

Fig. 2. FA transport into mitochondria and energy output from β-oxidation. Acyl-CoA esters are converted to acyl-carnitines by carnitine palmitoyl transferase I (CPT I) at the outer mitochondrial membrane. CPT I is inhibited by malonyl-CoA synthesized from acetyl-CoA through acetyl-CoA carboxylase (ACC) when the heart is in the fed state and glycolysis is stimulated. Malonyl-CoA de carboxylase (MCD) catalyzes the conversion of malonyl-CoA to acetyl-CoA and can relieve CPT I inhibition. Acylcarnitines are transported across the intermembrane space by carnitine acylcarnitine translocase (CACT), where they are converted back to acyl-CoA esters by CPT II. The acyl-CoA ester can then undergo β-oxidation with the end products of 8 mol acetyl-CoA, 7 mol nicotinamide adenine dinucleotide (NADH), and 7 mol flavin adenine dinucleotide (FADH₂) obtained from 1 mol palmitoyl-CoA. The entry of the 8 mol acetyl-CoA moieties into the citric acid cycle produces 24 mol NADH, 8 mol FADH₂, and 8 mol guanosine triphosphate (GTP). Finally, the reducing equivalents provided by NADH and FADH₂ can produce approximately 100 mol adenosine triphosphate (ATP) through the electron transport chain from the initial 1 mol palmitoyl-CoA based on a calculated theoretical yield of 2.5 mol ATP from 1 mol NADH and 1.5 mol ATP from 1 mol FADH₂.

The acylcarnitine produced by CPT I is transported across the inner mitochondrial membrane by carnitine:acylcarnitine translocase (CACT), followed by its conversion back to acyl-CoA by CPT II (see **Fig. 2**).[74,77] In the mitochondrial matrix, acyl-CoA is metabolized through the β-oxidation cycle, which consists of the sequential actions of acyl-CoA dehydrogenase, enoyl-CoA hydratase, L-3-hydroxylacyl-CoA dehydrogenase, and 3-ketoacyl-CoA thiolase.[74,84] Each cycle results in the hydrolysis of 2 carbons from the acyl-CoA chain and the production of acetyl-CoA, flavin adenine dinucleotide ($FADH_2$), and nicotinamide adenine dinucleotide (NADH). The enzymes 2,4-dienoyl-CoA reductase and enoyl-CoA isomerase are also important for the conversion of *cis* double bonds in unsaturated FAs to *trans* double bonds, which can then be acted on by enoyl-CoA hydratase in the β-oxidation cycle. Acetyl-CoA is then oxidized further in the citric acid cycle to yield more $FADH_2$ and NADH, which are then used to produce ATP through oxidative phosphorylation (see **Fig. 2**).

The coordinated regulation of genes involved in FAO by the peroxisome proliferator-activated receptors (PPARs), and PPARγ coactivator-1α (PGC-1α) has also been shown to be important in controlling cardiac FAO (reviewed in Refs.[57,85–88]). Of the 3 PPAR isoforms, the role of PPARα in FAO has been the most extensively studied. PPARα is a nuclear receptor that acts in conjunction with PGC-1α to induce the expression of various genes including CD36, FATP1, FABP, MCD, CPT1, and medium-chain and long-chain acyl-CoA dehydrogenase, with the net outcome of increasing the cellular capacity for FAO.[57,89] PGC-1α acts as a transcriptional coactivator with PPARα, as previously mentioned. Furthermore, another protein known as lipin-1 is required to act in combination with PGC-1α and PPARα to induce PPARα target genes, at least in the liver.[90] Lipin-1 also acts as an enzyme in glycerolipid synthesis, and this function is discussed in detail later. PGC-1α can also bind to other nuclear receptors, for example, estrogen-related receptors and nuclear respiratory factors, to induce mitochondrial biogenesis and increase oxidative phosphorylation.[85,87] The importance of PPARα and PGC-1α in cardiac metabolism and function is highlighted by studies in knockout mouse models. Fasting-induced expression of PPARα target genes and rates of FAO were blunted in PPARα knockout mice.[91–93] Furthermore, abnormal changes in mitochondrial architecture and the development of myocardial fibrosis were observed in the PPARα null mice as they aged.[91] Mitochondrial gene expression, oxidative metabolism, response to stimulation, and exercise capacity predictably were found to be decreased in PGC-1α knockout mice.[94–96]

Fatty acid oxidation in the diabetic heart

As mentioned previously, diabetic hearts rely predominantly on FAO for ATP production.[27,55,97] Increased consumption of oxygen is required to drive β-oxidation, resulting in augmented levels of reactive oxygen species, which eventually cause mitochondrial damage.[56,74,98–102] Thus, this inflexible dependence on one major substrate leads to decreases in cardiac mechanical efficiency and power as well as reduced recovery from ischemia.[54,55,103,104] The detrimental effects of increased rates of FAO on cardiac function are also demonstrated by studies on transgenic mice, which overexpress PPARα specifically in the heart. Similar to the phenotype of diabetic hearts, these mice have an increased reliance on FAO concurrent with a decrease in glucose oxidation, resulting in cardiac dysfunction.[105,106] By contrast, the major phenotype of transgenic mice with cardiac-specific overexpression of PGC-1α emphasizes the role of PGC-1α in mitochondrial biogenesis. There is excessive mitochondrial proliferation in the hearts of these mice, leading to cardiac hypertrophy, dilated left and right ventricular chambers, decreased cardiac function, and premature death.[107]

Increasing the contribution of glucose oxidation to energy production in hearts after ischemia can improve cardiac function and recovery, because of decreased reliance on FAO.[103,108–111] In addition, one study showed the beneficial effect of preventing FA uptake by knocking out CD36 in transgenic mice with cardiac-specific overexpression of PGC-1α, thus demonstrating the possibility of targeting cardiac FAO in diabetes.[112] Preventing the excessive production of reactive oxygen species could also be another option in alleviating the effects of excessive FAO in diabetic hearts.[100,102] However, it should be clear that targeting cardiac FAO as an intervention in diabetes might only be possible with the use of reversible inhibitors, because of the need to maintain the use of flexible substrates in the heart.[104,113,114]

The Glycerolipid Biosynthetic Pathway

Besides the use of acyl-CoAs in mitochondria β-oxidation, acyl-CoAs also serve as substrates for glycerolipid synthesis through the Kennedy pathway, with the end products being TG or phospholipids.[115,116] All of the enzymes involved in TG synthesis except the lipins are integral membrane proteins localized to the endoplasmic reticulum or the mitochondria.[117,118] The first step of the pathway is the acylation of glycerol-3-phosphate

(G3P) at the *sn*-1 position by glycerol-3-phosphate acyltransferases (GPATs) to form lysophosphatidate (LPA) **(Fig. 3)**. The formation of G3P is catalyzed by the action of G3P dehydrogenase on dihydroxyacetone phosphate, which is a reaction intermediate formed during glycolysis.[118,119] Relatively low levels of glycerol kinase in the heart can also phosphorylate glycerol to form G3P.[120,121]

Out of the 4 GPAT isoforms currently known, GPAT1 is the most extensively studied.[122,123] GPAT1 is localized to the outer mitochondrial membrane and accounts for 30% of the total cardiac GPAT enzymatic activity.[124] The importance of GPAT1 to glycerolipid synthesis is highlighted by the observation that hearts from GPAT1-deficient

mice were protected from diet-induced TG accumulation compared with controls, although this phenotype could be partially attributed to lower plasma TG levels and rates of VLDL secretion in the GPAT1-deficient animals.[124] The microsomal GPATs (GPAT3 and GPAT4) appear to provide the majority of GPAT enzymatic activity in most tissues except the liver.[118] Although the contributions of GPAT3 and 4 to glycerolipid synthesis in adipose tissue and liver have been determined,[122,123] their roles in regulating cardiac glycerolipid metabolism and the effects of GPAT3 and/or GPAT4 deficiencies on cardiac function and metabolism have yet to be elucidated.

Acylglycerol 3-phosphate acyltransferases (AGPATs) catalyze the next step in glycerolipid

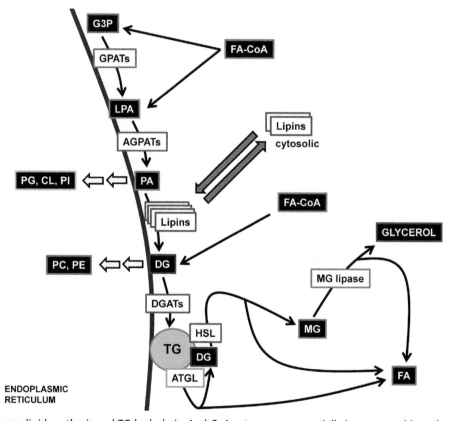

Fig. 3. Glycerolipid synthesis and TG hydrolysis. Acyl-CoA esters are sequentially incorporated into the *sn*-1 and *sn*-2 positions of glycerol-3-phosphate (G3P) by glycerol-3-phosphate acyltransferases (GPATs) and acylglycerol 3-phosphate acyltransferases (AGPATs) to form lysophosphatidate (LPA) and phosphatidate (PA), respectively. These reactions can be catalyzed by endoplasmic reticulum–localized and mitochondrial-localized isoforms of GPATs and AGPATs, as described in the text. PA is dephosphorylated to diacylglycerol (DG) by membrane-associated lipins after they translocate from the cytosol. Alternatively, PA can serve as the substrate for the synthesis of phosphatidylglycerol (PG), cardiolipin (CL), and phosphatidylinositol (PI). Finally, diacylglycerol acyltransferases (DGATs) can incorporate acyl-CoA into DG to form TG. DG is also an essential precursor for phosphatidylcholine (PC) and phosphatidylethanolamine (PC) synthesis. TG stored in lipid droplets can be hydrolyzed by adipose triglyceride lipase (ATGL) to form DG, which is then acted upon by hormone-sensitive lipase (HSL) to form monoacylglycerol (MG). Finally, MG is hydrolyzed by MG lipase to form glycerol. FAs are released from each step of TG hydrolysis and can be used for β-oxidation.

synthesis, which is the formation of phosphatidate (PA) from LPA (see **Fig. 3**). There are at least 4 AGPAT isoforms (AGPAT1, 2, 3, and 5) expressed in the mouse heart,[125] with the caveat that several putative AGPAT isoforms have not been fully characterized.[122] PPARα appears to regulate AGPAT activity and the gene expression of AGPAT3[125]; however, little is known about AGPATs in the heart.

PA can then be hydrolyzed to diacylglycerol (DG) by the phosphatidate phosphatase (PAP) activity of a family of oligomeric, bifunctional proteins called the lipins (lipin-1, -2 and -3) (see **Fig. 3**).[117,126–130] As previously mentioned, the lipins also function as transcriptional coactivators with PGC-1α and PPARα in liver.[90,131] The balance between PA and DG levels represents an important branch-point in phospholipid synthesis. PA is used as the substrate for the synthesis of phosphatidylinositol, phosphatidylglycerol, and cardiolipin whereas DG is the precursor required for the formation of TG, phosphatidylcholine, and phosphatidylethanolamine (see **Fig. 3**).[117,126] The lipins are unique enzymes in this pathway because they are not integral membrane proteins. Instead, lipins are cytosolic proteins that translocate to their sites of action, the endoplasmic reticulum and the nucleus, when stimulated (see **Fig. 3**).[132–134] This translocation is dependent on the presence of a polybasic motif (also called the nuclear localization sequence), which is postulated to bind to negative charges on membrane surfaces.[134,135] These negative charges can be produced by the accumulation of FAs and acyl-CoA esters on the membranes,[135–137] and increased FA supply to the heart, such as in diabetes, acts as a feed-forward signal for TG synthesis.[69,71,138] The SUMOylation of lipin-1 is also required for nuclear localization.[139] Of importance, lipin-1 is phosphorylated on at least 18 serine/threonine residues and hyperphosphorylation promotes its cytosolic localization because of its interaction with 14-3-3 proteins.[132,140] The negatively charged phosphate groups on lipins could also hinder electrostatic interactions with membrane surfaces.

Besides subcellular localization, lipins are also dynamically regulated on the transcriptional level. Lipin-1 gene expression is increased during fasting through glucocorticoid and glucagon signaling and depends on PGC-1α expression; this induction is suppressed by insulin action.[90,141–143] Moreover, lipin-1 gene expression is also modulated by transducer of regulated CREB (cyclic AMP response element binding protein) activity (TORC2),[144] sterol-regulatory binding protein 1 (SREBP1),[145,146] nuclear orphan receptor 1,[147] and estrogen-related receptors α and γ.[143,148] The regulation of cardiac lipin expression is quite dynamic, with decreases in PAP activity and lipin expression demonstrated in rodent models and human patients with heart failure and diabetes.[143,149]

The tissue distribution of the lipins is distinct, with lipin-1 appearing to act as the major lipin isoform in the heart.[127,143,150] However, whole-body deficiency of lipin-1 does not overtly affect cardiac glycerolipid synthesis, and the synthesis of TG and phosphatidylcholine is sustained by the residual activities of lipin-2 and lipin-3.[150] Instead, there were subtle increases reported in phosphatidate accumulation and cellular stress signaling.[143,150]

The final step in the Kennedy pathway for TG synthesis is the conversion of DG to TG by DG acyltransferases (DGAT1 and DGAT2) (see **Fig. 3**).[151,152] Both DGATs are found predominantly at the endoplasmic reticulum,[152,153] and can catalyze the formation of lipid droplets.[154–156] DGAT1 can also function as an acyl-CoA:retinol acyltransferase to esterify retinol,[157,158] whereas DGAT2 activity is more specific for DG.[152] Of note, DGAT2 knockout mice are not viable, owing to impaired TG homeostasis and deficiencies in the permeability barrier of the skin.[159] The overexpression of DGAT1 and DGAT2 in various cell types[152] and mouse models[160–163] leads to increased TG accumulation. It is significant that the consequences of increased TG stores are not detrimental for the most part; instead, DGAT overexpression decreased the levels of potentially toxic lipid metabolites like ceramides and DG.[161,164] Paradoxically, one study showed that TG accumulation caused by overexpressing DGAT2 in glycolytic muscle was accompanied by increased ceramide and DG levels, resulting in insulin resistance.[162] This discrepancy can be explained by the lower contribution of FAs as a fuel in the glycolytic muscle compared with the mitochondrial-rich heart or soleus muscle. However, it is noteworthy that the chronic overexpression of DGAT1 in 52-week-old mice induces cardiomyopathy and cardiac fibrosis, and decreases mitochondrial biogenesis.[165]

Lipid Accumulation in Diabetes

Although the consequences of increased FAO on function and metabolism in the diabetic heart are well characterized, increased cardiac lipid accumulation is an accompanying comorbidity in many of these diabetic models.[166–170] Indeed, FA uptake through CD36 could be an important factor in both increased FAO and lipid accumulation,[69,171] because augmented FAO can still be exceeded by increased uptake of FAs and the excess FAs are channeled into glycerolipid synthesis. Cardiac steatosis has been correlated with cardiac dysfunction in several studies, leading to the term lipotoxic cardiomyopathy.[51,166,167,172] However, studies in the DGAT transgenic mice show that TG accumulation by itself does not cause a detrimental phenotype.[161,163,164] Rather, the deleterious effects of lipid accumulation on the heart appear to be mediated by lipid metabolites such as ceramides, long-chain acyl-CoAs, and DG, which can strongly influence cardiac signaling and viability.[168–170,173–175] Various studies in cellular and mouse models have shown the effects of DG and ceramide accumulation on insulin signaling, β-adrenergic responsiveness, oxidative stress, mitochondrial function, and mechanical efficiency.[41,51,162,172,176–184]

Hydrolysis of Cardiac TG Stores

Cardiac TG stores have been considered as inert lipid droplets; however, it is evident that TG turnover in the heart is rapid and provides a significant source of FAs for ATP production.[185–188] Hydrolysis of TG stores is catalyzed by adipose triglyceride lipase (ATGL),[189,190] hormone-sensitive lipase (HSL),[191] TG hydrolase (TGH),[192] and monoacylglycerol (MG) lipase (see **Fig. 3**).[193] ATGL, in combination with CGI-58 (comparative gene identification 58),[194] catalyzes the first and rate-limiting step in the hydrolysis of TG to DG (see **Fig. 3**).[189,190] Mice deficient in ATGL have decreased TG lipolysis and accumulate high levels of TG in most of the organs, especially the heart.[190,195] In addition, ATGL-mediated lipolysis in the heart releases FAs that act as essential ligands for PPARα activation, which is needed for promoting FAO and maintaining mitochondrial function and substrate use.[196] LPL is critically important in providing the FAs that act as PPARα ligands in the heart, as shown by studies using PPARα transgenic/LPL-knockout mice.[197] Consequently, the absence of ATGL leads to severe metabolic derangements and cardiomyopathy.[190,196] This finding is recapitulated in human patients with mutations in the human *ATGL* gene.[198,199]

The hydrolysis of DG to MG is catalyzed by HSL (see **Fig. 3**).[189] The specificity of HSL for DG as a substrate was demonstrated by the elevated levels of DG in the organs of HSL-deficient mice.[200] Decreased plasma FA levels and reduced FA flux in the adipose tissue of HSL-knockout mice result in decreased myocardial TG accumulation and improved insulin response after a 3-week high-fat diet.[201,202] The importance of HSL in regulating cardiac TG stores is highlighted by studies using cardiac-specific HSL transgenic mice. Fasting-induced TG accumulation is blunted in HSL transgenic mice.[203] Similarly, TG accumulation is lower in streptozotocin-induced diabetic mice with HSL overexpression compared with diabetic controls.[204] Furthermore, the stimulation of gene expression of PPARα and proteins involved in FA uptake was blunted in the streptozotocin-treated HSL transgenic mice.[204] Consequently, there was less myocardial fibrosis and decreased mortality in these mice. Overall, the overexpression of HSL in the heart appears to protect against diabetic cardiomyopathy by modulating the expression of PPARα and its target genes involved in FA uptake. Cardiac overexpression of ATGL in transgenic mice also produces a similar phenotype whereby TG accumulation was reduced and the expression of proteins involved in FA uptake and oxidation were decreased.[205] In this model cardiac glucose oxidation was augmented, and cardiac function and exercise performance was enhanced.[205] Thus, the forced overexpression of ATGL and HSL appears to induce an inhibitory feedback signal to prevent the uptake of FAs and decrease FAO in favor of glucose use. Alternatively, augmented rates of TG hydrolysis in these transgenic mice chronically depletes the cardiac TG pools to such an extent that the release of FAs from these stores does not reach a threshold concentration high enough to activate PPARα and its target genes, as put forth by Haemmerle and colleagues.[196,205] Future studies will be required to clarify these observations.

Finally, MG lipase can hydrolyze MG to FA and glycerol in the heart (see **Fig. 3**).[193] Although studies in MG lipase–deficient mice show that MG lipase is important in adipose and hepatic lipolysis and can influence insulin sensitivity under high-fat fed conditions,[206] the contribution of MG lipase in the heart is unknown. The contribution of TGH to cardiac lipid homeostasis is also unclear. TG hydrolase functions to provide TG for VLDL assembly in hepatocytes.[207,208] As cardiac lipoprotein secretion has been demonstrated,[209,210] TGH might play a similar role in the heart.

Effects of Enhanced Lipolysis in the Diabetic Heart

Recent studies have demonstrated the importance of cardiac TG lipolysis in providing significant quantities of FAs for energy production.[160,186,187,190,196] Of importance is that PPARα appears to be intimately involved in lipolysis because increasing PPARα expression amplifies ATP production from TG-derived FAs.[187] Moreover, the release of exogenous FAs from TG stores by ATGL governs the level of PPARα activation and its target genes involved in FAO in the heart.[196,197]

Table 4
Potential and current drugs used to alleviate disease phenotypes in diabetes and decrease cardiovascular disease and heart failure

	Target/Mechanism of Action	References
(A) Potential Inhibitors		
Etomoxir, oxfenicine	Carnitine palmitoyl transferase-1 inhibitor	110,111,211
Trimetazidine	3-Ketoacyl-CoA thiolase inhibitor	212–214
Ranolazine	Partial fatty acid oxidation inhibitor	215,216
CBM-301940 (isoxazoline-based inhibitor)	Malonyl-CoA decarboxylase inhibitor	109,217
(B) Current Treatments		
Niacin	Modifies lipoprotein profile (increased HDL/LDL ratio)	218,219
Ezetimibe	Cholesterol absorption	220
Metformin	Glycemic control and decreases LDL cholesterol levels	221,222
Fibrates	Improve plasma lipid and lipoprotein profile	223,224
Statins	Inhibit cholesterol synthesis and lower plasma LDL levels	225,226
Thiazolidinediones	Reduce inflammation and improve glycemic control	227,228

Thus, it could be envisaged that ATGL-mediated lipolysis in the heart could exacerbate the dependence on FAO in diabetes and obesity, especially because ATGL and HSL activity are positively regulated by β-adrenergic signaling.[189] Furthermore, ATGL and HSL expression were shown to be increased in streptozotocin-induced diabetes.[204]

TREATMENT OPTIONS

The possibility of alleviating the cardiac metabolic derangements either directly or indirectly with the use of currently available drugs or potential inhibitors represents an attractive option in attempting to address the issue of cardiovascular disease and myopathy in diabetes and obesity.

Drugs used to inhibit FAO directly (**Table 4**) could possibly be used to address aberrant fuel use in diabetes, as numerous studies have demonstrated the benefits of shifting from FA to glucose use in a variety of pathologic conditions.[74,229,230] However, the maintenance of metabolic flexibility has to be achieved because chronic overuse of one substrate over another often results in oxidative stress and cardiac dysfunction.[113,114,231,232]

Drugs used to treat insulin responsiveness and inhibitors with pleiotropic actions (see **Table 4**) can also positively affect cardiovascular function and reduce atherosclerosis by promoting a positive plasma lipoprotein profile and reducing inflammatory signaling.[2,223,227,228,233] In fact, combination drug therapies are now often used in the management of dyslipidemia to lower the risk of cardiovascular disease.[233,234] However, care must be taken to account for the side effects of some drugs alone (eg, rosiglitazone and ezitimibe) or in combination (eg, statin/fibrate) in increasing the risk of stroke, cardiovascular complications, and rhabdomyolysis.[219,227,228,235]

SUMMARY

Cardiovascular disease remains the major cause of mortality in North America, with the increased incidence of obesity and diabetes in the population as a major factor. The derangement of FA and lipid metabolism in diabetes at every step from plasma availability to FA oxidation and lipid synthesis contributes to the development of cardiac dysfunction and myopathy. The current drugs as described in **Table 4**B provide beneficial therapy. Other therapeutic options described in **Table 4**A are still potential treatments, but these could eventually prove to be efficacious in managing this growing epidemic. Furthermore, future studies will ascertain the feasibility of targeting other enzymes involved in FA and lipid turnover to treat dysregulated metabolism in diabetes and cardiovascular disease.

REFERENCES

1. Cornier MA, Dabelea D, Hernandez TL, et al. The metabolic syndrome. Endocr Rev 2008;29(7): 777–822.

2. Moller DE, Kaufman KD. Metabolic syndrome: a clinical and molecular perspective. Annu Rev Med 2005;56:45–62.

3. Ford ES, Ajani UA, Croft JB, et al. Explaining the decrease in U.S. deaths from coronary disease, 1980-2000. N Engl J Med 2007;356(23):2388–98.

4. Brophy JM. The epidemiology of acute myocardial infarction and ischemic heart disease in Canada: data from 1976 to 1991. Can J Cardiol 1997; 13(5):474–8.

5. Shaw JE, Sicree RA, Zimmet PZ. Global estimates of the prevalence of diabetes for 2010 and 2030. Diabetes Res Clin Pract 2010;87(1):4–14.

6. Freund KM, Belanger AJ, D'Agostino RB, et al. The health risks of smoking. The Framingham Study: 34 years of follow-up. Ann Epidemiol 1993;3(4):417–24.

7. Stokes J 3rd, Kannel WB, Wolf PA, et al. Blood pressure as a risk factor for cardiovascular disease. The Framingham Study—30 years of follow-up. Hypertension 1989;13(Suppl 5):I13–8.

8. Turner RC, Millns H, Neil HA, et al. Risk factors for coronary artery disease in non-insulin dependent diabetes mellitus: United Kingdom Prospective Diabetes Study (UKPDS: 23). BMJ 1998;316(7134): 823–8.

9. Manninen V, Tenkanen L, Koskinen P, et al. Joint effects of serum triglyceride and LDL cholesterol and HDL cholesterol concentrations on coronary heart disease risk in the Helsinki Heart Study. Implications for treatment. Circulation 1992;85(1): 37–45.

10. Manttari M, Huttunen JK, Koskinen P, et al. Lipoproteins and coronary heart disease in the Helsinki Heart Study. Eur Heart J 1990;11(Suppl H):26–31.

11. Tenkanen L, Pietila K, Manninen V, et al. The triglyceride issue revisited. Findings from the Helsinki Heart Study. Arch Intern Med 1994; 154(23):2714–20.

12. Méthot J, Houle J, Poirier P. Obesity: how to define central adiposity? Expert Rev Cardiovasc Ther 2010;8(5):639–44.

13. Gabriely I, Ma XH, Yang XM, et al. Removal of visceral fat prevents insulin resistance and glucose intolerance of aging: an adipokine-mediated process? Diabetes 2002;51(10):2951–8.

14. Cannon CP. Cardiovascular disease and modifiable cardiometabolic risk factors. Clin Cornerstone 2007;8(3):11–28.

15. Willett WC, Manson JE, Stampfer MJ, et al. Weight, weight change, and coronary heart disease in women. Risk within the 'normal' weight range. JAMA 1995;273(6):461–5.

16. Kannel WB. Habitual level of physical activity and risk of coronary heart disease: the Framingham study. Can Med Assoc J 1967;96(12):811–2.

17. Sesso HD, Paffenbarger RS Jr, Lee IM. Physical activity and coronary heart disease in men: The Harvard Alumni Health Study. Circulation 2000; 102(9):975–80.

18. Parikh R, Mohan V, Joshi S. Should waist circumference be replaced by index of central obesity (ICO) in definition of metabolic syndrome? Diabetes Metab Res Rev 2012;28(1):3–5.

19. Oguma Y, Sesso HD, Paffenbarger RS Jr, et al. Weight change and risk of developing type 2 diabetes. Obes Res 2005;13(5):945–51.

20. Colditz GA, Willett WC, Rotnitzky A, et al. Weight gain as a risk factor for clinical diabetes mellitus in women. Ann Intern Med 1995;122(7): 481–6.

21. Lewis GF, Carpentier A, Adeli K, et al. Disordered fat storage and mobilization in the pathogenesis of insulin resistance and type 2 diabetes. Endocr Rev 2002;23(2):201–29.

22. Pieske B, Wachter R. Impact of diabetes and hypertension on the heart. Curr Opin Cardiol 2008;23(4):340–9.

23. Aneja A, Tang WH, Bansilal S, et al. Diabetic cardiomyopathy: insights into pathogenesis, diagnostic challenges, and therapeutic options. Am J Med 2008;121(9):748–57.

24. An D, Rodrigues B. Role of changes in cardiac metabolism in development of diabetic cardiomyopathy. Am J Physiol Heart Circ Physiol 2006; 291(4):H1489–506.

25. Fox CS, Coady S, Sorlie PD, et al. Increasing cardiovascular disease burden due to diabetes mellitus: the Framingham Heart Study. Circulation 2007;115(12):1544–50.

26. Lopaschuk GD, Belke DD, Gamble J, et al. Regulation of fatty acid oxidation in the mammalian heart in health and disease. Biochim Biophys Acta 1994;1213(3):263–76.

27. Carley AN, Severson DL. Fatty acid metabolism is enhanced in type 2 diabetic hearts. Biochim Biophys Acta 2005;1734(2):112–26.

28. Longnus SL, Wambolt RB, Barr RL, et al. Regulation of myocardial fatty acid oxidation by substrate supply. Am J Physiol Heart Circ Physiol 2001; 281(4):H1561–7.

29. Bharadwaj KG, Hiyama Y, Hu Y, et al. Chylomicron- and VLDL-derived lipids enter the heart through different pathways: in vivo evidence for receptor- and non-receptor-mediated fatty acid uptake. J Biol Chem 2010;285(49):37976–86.

30. Hussain MM, Kancha RK, Zhou Z, et al. Chylomicron assembly and catabolism: role of apolipoproteins and receptors. Biochim Biophys Acta 1996; 1300(3):151–70.

31. Nakajima K, Nakano T, Tokita Y, et al. Postprandial lipoprotein metabolism: VLDL vs chylomicrons. Clin Chim Acta 2011;412(15–16):1306–18.

32. Havel RJ. Transport and metabolism of chylomicra. Am J Clin Nutr 1958;6(6):662–8.

33. Skipski VP, Barclay M, Barclay RK, et al. Lipid composition of human serum lipoproteins. Biochem J 1967;104(2):340–52.

34. Heath RB, Karpe F, Milne RW, et al. Selective partitioning of dietary fatty acids into the VLDL TG pool in the early postprandial period. J Lipid Res 2003; 44(11):2065–72.

35. Augustus A, Yagyu H, Haemmerle G, et al. Cardiac-specific knock-out of lipoprotein lipase alters plasma lipoprotein triglyceride metabolism and cardiac gene expression. J Biol Chem 2004; 279(24):25050–7.

36. Pillutla P, Hwang YC, Augustus A, et al. Perfusion of hearts with triglyceride-rich particles reproduces the metabolic abnormalities in lipotoxic cardiomyopathy. Am J Physiol Endocrinol Metab 2005; 288(6):E1229–35.

37. Preiss-Landl K, Zimmermann R, Hammerle G, et al. Lipoprotein lipase: the regulation of tissue specific expression and its role in lipid and energy metabolism. Curr Opin Lipidol 2002;13(5):471–81.

38. Davies BS, Beigneux AP, Barnes RH 2nd, et al. GPIHBP1 is responsible for the entry of lipoprotein lipase into capillaries. Cell Metab 2010; 12(1):42–52.

39. Beigneux AP, Davies BS, Tat S, et al. Assessing the role of the glycosylphosphatidylinositol-anchored high density lipoprotein-binding protein 1 (GPIHBP1) three-finger domain in binding lipoprotein lipase. J Biol Chem 2011;286(22):19735–43.

40. Franssen R, Young SG, Peelman F, et al. Chylomicronemia with low postheparin lipoprotein lipase levels in the setting of GPIHBP1 defects. Circ Cardiovasc Genet 2010;3(2):169–78.

41. Yagyu H, Chen G, Yokoyama M, et al. Lipoprotein lipase (LpL) on the surface of cardiomyocytes increases lipid uptake and produces a cardiomyopathy. J Clin Invest 2003;111(3):419–26.

42. Yagyu H, Lutz EP, Kako Y, et al. Very low density lipoprotein (VLDL) receptor-deficient mice have reduced lipoprotein lipase activity. Possible causes of hypertriglyceridemia and reduced body mass with VLDL receptor deficiency. J Biol Chem 2002; 277(12):10037–43.

43. Obunike JC, Lutz EP, Li Z, et al. Transcytosis of lipoprotein lipase across cultured endothelial cells requires both heparan sulfate proteoglycans and the very low density lipoprotein receptor. J Biol Chem 2001;276(12):8934–41.

44. Goudriaan JR, Espirito Santo SM, Voshol PJ, et al. The VLDL receptor plays a major role in chylomicron metabolism by enhancing LPL-mediated triglyceride hydrolysis. J Lipid Res 2004;45(8): 1475–81.

45. Ibrahimi A, Abumrad NA. Role of CD36 in membrane transport of long-chain fatty acids. Curr Opin Clin Nutr Metab Care 2002;5(2):139–45.

46. Brinkmann JF, Abumrad NA, Ibrahimi A, et al. New insights into long-chain fatty acid uptake by heart muscle: a crucial role for fatty acid translocase/CD36. Biochem J 2002;367(Pt 3):561–70.

47. Luiken JJ, Bonen A, Glatz JF. Cellular fatty acid uptake is acutely regulated by membrane-associated fatty acid-binding proteins. Prostaglandins Leukot Essent Fatty Acids 2002;67(2–3):73–8.

48. Gimeno RE, Ortegon AM, Patel S, et al. Characterization of a heart-specific fatty acid transport protein. J Biol Chem 2003;278(18):16039–44.

49. Glatz JF, Luiken JJ, Bonen A. Involvement of membrane-associated proteins in the acute regulation of cellular fatty acid uptake. J Mol Neurosci 2001;16(2–3):123–32 [discussion: 151–7].

50. Luiken JJ, Koonen DP, Willems J, et al. Insulin stimulates long-chain fatty acid utilization by rat cardiac myocytes through cellular redistribution of FAT/CD36. Diabetes 2002;51(10):3113–9.

51. Chiu HC, Kovacs A, Blanton RM, et al. Transgenic expression of fatty acid transport protein 1 in the heart causes lipotoxic cardiomyopathy. Circ Res 2005;96(2):225–33.

52. Mashek DG, Coleman RA. Cellular fatty acid uptake: the contribution of metabolism. Curr Opin Lipidol 2006;17(3):274–8.

53. Chess DJ, Stanley WC. Role of diet and fuel overabundance in the development and progression of heart failure. Cardiovasc Res 2008;79(2): 269–78.

54. Liu Q, Docherty JC, Rendell JC, et al. High levels of fatty acids delay the recovery of intracellular pH and cardiac efficiency in post-ischemic hearts by inhibiting glucose oxidation. J Am Coll Cardiol 2002;39(4):718–25.

55. Buchanan J, Mazumder PK, Hu P, et al. Reduced cardiac efficiency and altered substrate metabolism precedes the onset of hyperglycemia and contractile dysfunction in two mouse models of insulin resistance and obesity. Endocrinology 2005;146(12):5341–9.

56. Boudina S, Sena S, Theobald H, et al. Mitochondrial energetics in the heart in obesity-related diabetes: direct evidence for increased uncoupled respiration and activation of uncoupling proteins. Diabetes 2007;56(10):2457–66.

57. Huss JM, Kelly DP. Nuclear receptor signaling and cardiac energetics. Circ Res 2004;95(6):568–78.

58. Brindley DN. Neuroendocrine regulation and obesity. Int J Obes Relat Metab Disord 1992; 16(Suppl 3):S73–9.

59. McArthur MD, Graham SE, Russell JC, et al. Exaggerated stress-induced release of nonesterified fatty acids in JCR: LA-corpulent rats. Metabolism 1998;47(11):1383–90.

60. Ginsberg HN. Insulin resistance and cardiovascular disease. J Clin Invest 2000;106(4):453–8.

61. Bays H, Mandarino L, DeFronzo RA. Role of the adipocyte, free fatty acids, and ectopic fat in pathogenesis of type 2 diabetes mellitus: peroxisomal proliferator-activated receptor agonists provide a rational therapeutic approach. J Clin Endocrinol Metab 2004;89(2):463–78.

62. Aguilera CM, Gil-Campos M, Canete R, et al. Alterations in plasma and tissue lipids associated with obesity and metabolic syndrome. Clin Sci (Lond) 2008;114(3):183–93.

63. Boden G. Role of fatty acids in the pathogenesis of insulin resistance and NIDDM. Diabetes 1997; 46(1):3–10.

64. Martin-Sanz P, Vance JE, Brindley DN. Stimulation of apolipoprotein secretion in very-low-density and high-density lipoproteins from cultured rat hepatocytes by dexamethasone. Biochem J 1990; 271(3):575–83.

65. Wang CN, McLeod RS, Yao Z, et al. Effects of dexamethasone on the synthesis, degradation, and secretion of apolipoprotein B in cultured rat hepatocytes. Arterioscler Thromb Vasc Biol 1995; 15(9):1481–91.

66. Park TS, Yamashita H, Blaner WS, et al. Lipids in the heart: a source of fuel and a source of toxins. Curr Opin Lipidol 2007;18(3):277–82.

67. Pulinilkunnil T, Rodrigues B. Cardiac lipoprotein lipase: metabolic basis for diabetic heart disease. Cardiovasc Res 2006;69(2):329–40.

68. Ouwens DM, Diamant M, Fodor M, et al. Cardiac contractile dysfunction in insulin-resistant rats fed a high-fat diet is associated with elevated CD36-mediated fatty acid uptake and esterification. Diabetologia 2007;50(9):1938–48.

69. Coort SL, Hasselbaink DM, Koonen DP, et al. Enhanced sarcolemmal FAT/CD36 content and triacylglycerol storage in cardiac myocytes from obese Zucker rats. Diabetes 2004;53(7):1655–63.

70. Coort SL, Luiken JJ, van der Vusse GJ, et al. Increased FAT (fatty acid translocase)/CD36-mediated long-chain fatty acid uptake in cardiac myocytes from obese Zucker rats. Biochem Soc Trans 2004;32(Pt 1):83–5.

71. Koonen DP, Febbraio M, Bonnet S, et al. CD36 expression contributes to age-induced cardiomyopathy in mice. Circulation 2007;116(19):2139–47.

72. Steinbusch LK, Schwenk RW, Ouwens DM, et al. Subcellular trafficking of the substrate transporters GLUT4 and CD36 in cardiomyocytes. Cell Mol Life Sci 2011;68(15):2525–38.

73. Wisneski JA, Gertz EW, Neese RA, et al. Myocardial metabolism of free fatty acids. Studies with ^{14}C-labeled substrates in humans. J Clin Invest 1987;79(2):359–66.

74. Lopaschuk GD, Ussher JR, Folmes CD, et al. Myocardial fatty acid metabolism in health and disease. Physiol Rev 2010;90(1):207–58.

75. Li LO, Klett EL, Coleman RA. Acyl-CoA synthesis, lipid metabolism and lipotoxicity. Biochim Biophys Acta 2010;1801(3):246–51.

76. de Jong H, Neal AC, Coleman RA, et al. Ontogeny of mRNA expression and activity of long-chain acyl-CoA synthetase (ACSL) isoforms in Mus musculus heart. Biochim Biophys Acta 2007;1771(1): 75–82.

77. McGarry JD, Brown NF. The mitochondrial carnitine palmitoyltransferase system. From concept to molecular analysis. Eur J Biochem 1997; 244(1):1–14.

78. Paulson DJ, Ward KM, Shug AL. Malonyl CoA inhibition of carnitine palmitoyltransferase in rat heart mitochondria. FEBS Lett 1984;176(2):381–4.

79. McGarry JD, Leatherman GF, Foster DW. Carnitine palmitoyltransferase I. The site of inhibition of hepatic fatty acid oxidation by malonyl-CoA. J Biol Chem 1978;253(12):4128–36.

80. Saddik M, Gamble J, Witters LA, et al. Acetyl-CoA carboxylase regulation of fatty acid oxidation in the heart. J Biol Chem 1993;268(34):25836–45.

81. Broderick TL, Panagakis G, DiDomenico D, et al. L-carnitine improvement of cardiac function is associated with a stimulation in glucose but not fatty acid metabolism in carnitine-deficient hearts. Cardiovasc Res 1995;30(5):815–20.

82. Awan MM, Saggerson ED. Malonyl-CoA metabolism in cardiac myocytes and its relevance to the control of fatty acid oxidation. Biochem J 1993; 295(Pt 1):61–6.

83. Cuthbert KD, Dyck JR. Malonyl-CoA decarboxylase is a major regulator of myocardial fatty acid oxidation. Curr Hypertens Rep 2005;7(6):407–11.

84. Schulz H. Chapter 5. Oxidation of fatty acids in eukaryotes. In: Dennis E, Vance JE, editors. New comprehensive biochemistry, vol. 36. Elsevier; 2002. p. 127–50.

85. Finck BN, Kelly DP. PGC-1 coactivators: inducible regulators of energy metabolism in health and disease. J Clin Invest 2006;116(3):615–22.

86. Madrazo JA, Kelly DP. The PPAR trio: regulators of myocardial energy metabolism in health and disease. J Mol Cell Cardiol 2008;44(6):968–75.

87. Lin J, Handschin C, Spiegelman BM. Metabolic control through the PGC-1 family of transcription coactivators. Cell Metab 2005;1(6):361–70.

88. Barger PM, Kelly DP. PPAR signaling in the control of cardiac energy metabolism. Trends Cardiovasc Med 2000;10(6):238–45.

89. Yang Q, Li Y. Roles of PPARs on regulating myocardial energy and lipid homeostasis. J Mol Med (Berl) 2007;85(7):697–706.

90. Finck BN, Gropler MC, Chen Z, et al. Lipin 1 is an inducible amplifier of the hepatic PGC-1alpha/PPARalpha regulatory pathway. Cell Metab 2006; 4(3):199–210.

91. Watanabe K, Fujii H, Takahashi T, et al. Constitutive regulation of cardiac fatty acid metabolism through peroxisome proliferator-activated receptor alpha associated with age-dependent cardiac toxicity. J Biol Chem 2000;275(29):22293–9.

92. Campbell FM, Kozak R, Wagner A, et al. A role for peroxisome proliferator-activated receptor alpha (PPARalpha) in the control of cardiac malonyl-CoA levels: reduced fatty acid oxidation rates and increased glucose oxidation rates in the hearts of mice lacking PPARalpha are associated with higher concentrations of malonyl-CoA and reduced expression of malonyl-CoA decarboxylase. J Biol Chem 2002;277(6):4098–103.

93. Leone TC, Weinheimer CJ, Kelly DP. A critical role for the peroxisome proliferator-activated receptor alpha (PPARalpha) in the cellular fasting response: the PPARalpha-null mouse as a model of fatty acid oxidation disorders. Proc Natl Acad Sci U S A 1999;96(13):7473–8.

94. Leone TC, Lehman JJ, Finck BN, et al. PGC-1alpha deficiency causes multi-system energy metabolic derangements: muscle dysfunction, abnormal weight control and hepatic steatosis. PLoS Biol 2005;3(4):e101.

95. Lehman JJ, Boudina S, Banke NH, et al. The transcriptional coactivator PGC-1alpha is essential for maximal and efficient cardiac mitochondrial fatty acid oxidation and lipid homeostasis. Am J Physiol Heart Circ Physiol 2008;295(1):H185–96.

96. Arany Z, He H, Lin J, et al. Transcriptional coactivator PGC-1 alpha controls the energy state and contractile function of cardiac muscle. Cell Metab 2005;1(4):259–71.

97. Herrero P, Peterson LR, McGill JB, et al. Increased myocardial fatty acid metabolism in patients with type 1 diabetes mellitus. J Am Coll Cardiol 2006; 47(3):598–604.

98. Boudina S, Sena S, O'Neill BT, et al. Reduced mitochondrial oxidative capacity and increased mitochondrial uncoupling impair myocardial energetics in obesity. Circulation 2005;112(17):2686–95.

99. Boudina S, Bugger H, Sena S, et al. Contribution of impaired myocardial insulin signaling to mitochondrial dysfunction and oxidative stress in the heart. Circulation 2009;119(9):1272–83.

100. Shen X, Zheng S, Metreveli NS, et al. Protection of cardiac mitochondria by overexpression of MnSOD reduces diabetic cardiomyopathy. Diabetes 2006; 55(3):798–805.

101. Echtay KS, Roussel D, St-Pierre J, et al. Superoxide activates mitochondrial uncoupling proteins. Nature 2002;415(6867):96–9.

102. Ye G, Metreveli NS, Ren J, et al. Metallothionein prevents diabetes-induced deficits in cardiomyocytes by inhibiting reactive oxygen species production. Diabetes 2003;52(3):777–83.

103. Lopaschuk GD, Barr R, Thomas PD, et al. Beneficial effects of trimetazidine in ex vivo working ischemic hearts are due to a stimulation of glucose oxidation secondary to inhibition of long-chain 3-ketoacyl coenzyme a thiolase. Circ Res 2003; 93(3):e33–7.

104. Burgmaier M, Sen S, Philip F, et al. Metabolic adaptation follows contractile dysfunction in the heart of obese Zucker rats fed a high-fat "Western" diet. Obesity (Silver Spring) 2010;18(10):1895–901.

105. Finck BN, Lehman JJ, Leone TC, et al. The cardiac phenotype induced by PPARalpha overexpression mimics that caused by diabetes mellitus. J Clin Invest 2002;109(1):121–30.

106. Hopkins TA, Sugden MC, Holness MJ, et al. Control of cardiac pyruvate dehydrogenase activity in peroxisome proliferator-activated receptor-alpha transgenic mice. Am J Physiol Heart Circ Physiol 2003;285(1):H270–6.

107. Lehman JJ, Barger PM, Kovacs A, et al. Peroxisome proliferator-activated receptor gamma coactivator-1 promotes cardiac mitochondrial biogenesis. J Clin Invest 2000;106(7):847–56.

108. Dyck JR, Hopkins TA, Bonnet S, et al. Absence of malonyl coenzyme A decarboxylase in mice increases cardiac glucose oxidation and protects the heart from ischemic injury. Circulation 2006; 114(16):1721–8.

109. Dyck JR, Cheng JF, Stanley WC, et al. Malonyl coenzyme A decarboxylase inhibition protects the ischemic heart by inhibiting fatty acid oxidation and stimulating glucose oxidation. Circ Res 2004; 94(9):e78–84.

110. Lopaschuk GD, Wall SR, Olley PM, et al. Etomoxir, a carnitine palmitoyltransferase I inhibitor, protects hearts from fatty acid-induced ischemic injury independent of changes in long chain acylcarnitine. Circ Res 1988;63(6):1036–43.

111. Chandler MP, Chavez PN, McElfresh TA, et al. Partial inhibition of fatty acid oxidation increases regional contractile power and efficiency during demand-induced ischemia. Cardiovasc Res 2003; 59(1):143–51.

112. Yang J, Sambandam N, Han X, et al. CD36 deficiency rescues lipotoxic cardiomyopathy. Circ Res 2007;100(8):1208–17.

113. Foley JE. Rationale and application of fatty acid oxidation inhibitors in treatment of diabetes mellitus. Diabetes Care 1992;15(6):773–84.

114. Larsen TS, Aasum E. Metabolic (in)flexibility of the diabetic heart. Cardiovasc Drugs Ther 2008;22(2): 91–5.

115. Kennedy EP. The biological synthesis of phospholipids. Can J Biochem Physiol 1956;34(2):334–48.

116. Weiss SB, Kennedy EP, Kiyasu JY. The enzymatic synthesis of triglycerides. J Biol Chem 1960;235: 40–4.

117. Brindley DN, Kok BP, Kienesberger PC, et al. Shedding light on the enigma of myocardial lipotoxicity: the involvement of known and putative regulators of fatty acid storage and mobilization. Am J Physiol Endocrinol Metab 2010;298(5):E897–908.

118. Coleman RA, Lee DP. Enzymes of triacylglycerol synthesis and their regulation. Prog Lipid Res 2004;43(2):134–76.

119. Kim JY, Park HS, Kang SI, et al. Redox regulation of cytosolic glycerol-3-phosphate dehydrogenase: Cys(102) is the target of the redox control and essential for the catalytic activity. Biochim Biophys Acta 2002;1569(1–3):67–74.

120. Robinson J, Newsholme EA. Glycerol kinase activities in rat heart and adipose tissue. Biochem J 1967;104(1):2C–4C.

121. Golovko MY, Hovda JT, Cai ZJ, et al. Tissue-dependent alterations in lipid mass in mice lacking glycerol kinase. Lipids 2005;40(3):287–93.

122. Takeuchi K, Reue K. Biochemistry, physiology, and genetics of GPAT, AGPAT, and lipin enzymes in triglyceride synthesis. Am J Physiol Endocrinol Metab 2009;296(6):E1195–209.

123. Wendel AA, Lewin TM, Coleman RA. Glycerol-3-phosphate acyltransferases: rate limiting enzymes of triacylglycerol biosynthesis. Biochim Biophys Acta 2009;1791(6):501–6.

124. Lewin TM, de Jong H, Schwerbrock NJ, et al. Mice deficient in mitochondrial glycerol-3-phosphate acyltransferase-1 have diminished myocardial triacylglycerol accumulation during lipogenic diet and altered phospholipid fatty acid composition. Biochim Biophys Acta 2008;1781(6–7):352–8.

125. Lu B, Jiang YJ, Zhou Y, et al. Cloning and characterization of murine 1-acyl-sn-glycerol 3-phosphate acyltransferases and their regulation by PPARalpha in murine heart. Biochem J 2005;385(Pt 2):469–77.

126. Reue K, Brindley DN. Thematic Review Series: glycerolipids. Multiple roles for lipins/phosphatidate phosphatase enzymes in lipid metabolism. J Lipid Res 2008;49(12):2493–503.

127. Donkor J, Sariahmetoglu M, Dewald J, et al. Three mammalian lipins act as phosphatidate phosphatases with distinct tissue expression patterns. J Biol Chem 2007;282(6):3450–7.

128. Han GS, Wu WI, Carman GM. The Saccharomyces cerevisiae Lipin homolog is a Mg^{2+}-dependent phosphatidate phosphatase enzyme. J Biol Chem 2006;281(14):9210–8.

129. Liu GH, Qu J, Carmack AE, et al. Lipin proteins form homo- and hetero-oligomers. Biochem J 2010;432(1):65–76.

130. Han GS, Carman GM. Characterization of the human LPIN1-encoded phosphatidate phosphatase isoforms. J Biol Chem 2010;285(19):14628–38.

131. Donkor J, Zhang P, Wong S, et al. A conserved serine residue is required for the phosphatidate phosphatase activity but not the transcriptional co-activator functions of lipin-1 and lipin-2. J Biol Chem 2009;284(43):29968–78.

132. Harris TE, Huffman TA, Chi A, et al. Insulin controls subcellular localization and multisite phosphorylation of the phosphatidic acid phosphatase, lipin 1. J Biol Chem 2007;282(1):277–86.

133. Peterson TR, Sengupta SS, Harris TE, et al. mTOR complex 1 regulates lipin 1 localization to control the SREBP pathway. Cell 2011;146(3):408–20.

134. Ren H, Federico L, Huang H, et al. A phosphatidic acid binding/nuclear localization motif determines lipin-1 function in lipid metabolism and adipogenesis. Mol Biol Cell 2010;21(18):3171–81.

135. Hopewell R, Martin-Sanz P, Martin A, et al. Regulation of the translocation of phosphatidate phosphohydrolase between the cytosol and the endoplasmic reticulum of rat liver. Effects of unsaturated fatty acids, spermine, nucleotides, albumin and chlorpromazine. Biochem J 1985;232(2):485–91.

136. Martin-Sanz P, Hopewell R, Brindley DN. Long-chain fatty acids and their acyl-CoA esters cause the translocation of phosphatidate phosphohydrolase from the cytosolic to the microsomal fraction of rat liver. FEBS Lett 1984;175(2):284–8.

137. Cascales C, Mangiapane EH, Brindley DN. Oleic acid promotes the activation and translocation of phosphatidate phosphohydrolase from the cytosol to particulate fractions of isolated rat hepatocytes. Biochem J 1984;219(3):911–6.

138. Luiken JJ, Arumugam Y, Dyck DJ, et al. Increased rates of fatty acid uptake and plasmalemmal fatty acid transporters in obese Zucker rats. J Biol Chem 2001;276(44):40567–73.

139. Liu GH, Gerace L. Sumoylation regulates nuclear localization of lipin-1alpha in neuronal cells. PLoS One 2009;4(9):e7031.

140. Peterfy M, Harris TE, Fujita N, et al. Insulin-stimulated interaction with 14-3-3 promotes cytoplasmic localization of lipin-1 in adipocytes. J Biol Chem 2010;285(6):3857–64.

141. Manmontri B, Sariahmetoglu M, Donkor J, et al. Glucocorticoids and cyclic AMP selectively increase hepatic lipin-1 expression, and insulin acts antagonistically. J Lipid Res 2008;49(5):1056–67.

142. Zhang P, O'Loughlin L, Brindley DN, et al. Regulation of lipin-1 gene expression by glucocorticoids during adipogenesis. J Lipid Res 2008;49(7):1519–28.

143. Mitra MS, Schilling JD, Wang X, et al. Cardiac lipin 1 expression is regulated by the peroxisome proliferator activated receptor gamma coactivator 1alpha/estrogen related receptor axis. J Mol Cell Cardiol 2011;51(1):120–8.

144. Ryu D, Oh KJ, Jo HY, et al. TORC2 regulates hepatic insulin signaling via a mammalian phosphatidic acid phosphatase, LIPIN1. Cell Metab 2009;9(3):240–51.

145. Ishimoto K, Nakamura H, Tachibana K, et al. Sterol-mediated regulation of human lipin 1 gene expression in hepatoblastoma cells. J Biol Chem 2009; 284(33):22195–205.

146. Hu M, Wang F, Li X, et al. Regulation of hepatic lipin-1 by ethanol: role of AMP-activated protein kinase/sterol regulatory element-binding protein 1 signaling in mice. Hepatology 2012;55(2):437–46.

147. Pearen MA, Myers SA, Raichur S, et al. The orphan nuclear receptor, NOR-1, a target of beta-adrenergic signaling, regulates gene expression that controls oxidative metabolism in skeletal muscle. Endocrinology 2008;149(6):2853–65.

148. Kim DK, Kim JR, Koh M, et al. Estrogen-related receptor gamma (ERRgamma) is a novel transcriptional regulator of phosphatidic acid phosphatase, LIPIN1, and inhibits hepatic insulin signaling. J Biol Chem 2011;286(44):38035–42.

149. Burgdorf C, Hansel L, Heidbreder M, et al. Suppression of cardiac phosphatidate phosphohydrolase 1 activity and lipin mRNA expression in Zucker diabetic fatty rats and humans with type 2 diabetes mellitus. Biochem Biophys Res Commun 2009;390(1):165–70.

150. Kok BP, Kienesberger PC, Dyck JR, et al. Relationship of glucose and oleate metabolism to cardiac function in lipin-1 deficient (fld) mice. J Lipid Res 2012;53(1):105–18 [Epub 2011 Nov 5].

151. Zammit VA, Buckett LK, Turnbull AV, et al. Diacylglycerol acyltransferases: potential roles as pharmacological targets. Pharmacol Ther 2008;118(3): 295–302.

152. Yen CL, Stone SJ, Koliwad S, et al. Thematic review series: glycerolipids. DGAT enzymes and triacylglycerol biosynthesis. J Lipid Res 2008;49(11): 2283–301.

153. Stone SJ, Levin MC, Farese RV Jr. Membrane topology and identification of key functional amino acid residues of murine acyl-CoA:diacylglycerol acyltransferase-2. J Biol Chem 2006;281(52): 40273–82.

154. Stone SJ, Levin MC, Zhou P, et al. The endoplasmic reticulum enzyme DGAT2 is found in mitochondria-associated membranes and has a mitochondrial targeting signal that promotes its association with mitochondria. J Biol Chem 2009; 284(8):5352–61.

155. McFie PJ, Banman SL, Kary S, et al. Murine diacylglycerol acyltransferase-2 (DGAT2) can catalyze triacylglycerol synthesis and promote lipid droplet formation independent of its localization to the endoplasmic reticulum. J Biol Chem 2011; 286(32):28235–46.

156. Harris CA, Haas JT, Streeper RS, et al. DGAT enzymes are required for triacylglycerol synthesis and lipid droplets in adipocytes. J Lipid Res 2011;52(4):657–67.

157. Yen CL, Monetti M, Burri BJ, et al. The triacylglycerol synthesis enzyme DGAT1 also catalyzes the synthesis of diacylglycerols, waxes, and retinyl esters. J Lipid Res 2005;46(7):1502–11.

158. Shih MY, Kane MA, Zhou P, et al. Retinol esterification by DGAT1 is essential for retinoid homeostasis in murine skin. J Biol Chem 2009;284(7):4292–9.

159. Stone SJ, Myers HM, Watkins SM, et al. Lipopenia and skin barrier abnormalities in DGAT2-deficient mice. J Biol Chem 2004;279(12):11767–76.

160. Liu L, Shi X, Choi CS, et al. Paradoxical coupling of triglyceride synthesis and fatty acid oxidation in skeletal muscle overexpressing DGAT1. Diabetes 2009;58(11):2516–24.

161. Liu L, Shi X, Bharadwaj KG, et al. DGAT1 expression increases heart triglyceride content but ameliorates lipotoxicity. J Biol Chem 2009; 284(52):36312–23.

162. Levin MC, Monetti M, Watt MJ, et al. Increased lipid accumulation and insulin resistance in transgenic mice expressing DGAT2 in glycolytic (type II) muscle. Am J Physiol Endocrinol Metab 2007; 293(6):E1772–81.

163. Monetti M, Levin MC, Watt MJ, et al. Dissociation of hepatic steatosis and insulin resistance in mice overexpressing DGAT in the liver. Cell Metab 2007;6(1):69–78.

164. Liu L, Zhang Y, Chen N, et al. Upregulation of myocellular DGAT1 augments triglyceride synthesis in skeletal muscle and protects against fat-induced insulin resistance. J Clin Invest 2007; 117(6):1679–89.

165. Glenn DJ, Wang F, Nishimoto M, et al. A murine model of isolated cardiac steatosis leads to cardiomyopathy. Hypertension 2011;57(2):216–22.

166. Boudina S, Abel ED. Mitochondrial uncoupling: a key contributor to reduced cardiac efficiency in diabetes. Physiology (Bethesda) 2006;21:250–8.

167. Aasum E, Cooper M, Severson DL, et al. Effect of BM 17.0744, a PPARalpha ligand, on the metabolism of perfused hearts from control and diabetic mice. Can J Physiol Pharmacol 2005;83(2):183–90.

168. Szczepaniak LS, Victor RG, Orci L, et al. Forgotten but not gone: the rediscovery of fatty heart, the most common unrecognized disease in America. Circ Res 2007;101(8):759–67.

169. Brookheart RT, Michel CI, Schaffer JE. As a matter of fat. Cell Metab 2009;10(1):9–12.

170. Harmancey R, Wilson CR, Taegtmeyer H. Adaptation and maladaptation of the heart in obesity. Hypertension 2008;52(2):181–7.

171. Luiken JJ. Sarcolemmal fatty acid uptake vs. mitochondrial beta-oxidation as target to regress cardiac

insulin resistance. Appl Physiol Nutr Metab 2009; 34(3):473–80.

172. Chiu HC, Kovacs A, Ford DA, et al. A novel mouse model of lipotoxic cardiomyopathy. J Clin Invest 2001;107(7):813–22.

173. Schaffer JE. Lipotoxicity: when tissues overeat. Curr Opin Lipidol 2003;14(3):281–7.

174. Kusminski CM, Shetty S, Orci L, et al. Diabetes and apoptosis: lipotoxicity. Apoptosis 2009;14(12): 1484–95.

175. Wende AR, Abel ED. Lipotoxicity in the heart. Biochim Biophys Acta 2010;1801(3):311–9 [Epub 2009 Oct 8].

176. Sparagna GC, Hickson-Bick DL, Buja LM, et al. A metabolic role for mitochondria in palmitate-induced cardiac myocyte apoptosis. Am J Physiol Heart Circ Physiol 2000;279(5):H2124–32.

177. Coll T, Eyre E, Rodriguez-Calvo R, et al. Oleate reverses palmitate-induced insulin resistance and inflammation in skeletal muscle cells. J Biol Chem 2008;283(17):11107–16.

178. Chavez JA, Summers SA. Characterizing the effects of saturated fatty acids on insulin signaling and ceramide and diacylglycerol accumulation in 3T3-L1 adipocytes and C2C12 myotubes. Arch Biochem Biophys 2003;419(2):101–9.

179. Powell DJ, Turban S, Gray A, et al. Intracellular ceramide synthesis and protein kinase Czeta activation play an essential role in palmitate-induced insulin resistance in rat L6 skeletal muscle cells. Biochem J 2004;382(Pt 2):619–29.

180. Russell LK, Finck BN, Kelly DP. Mouse models of mitochondrial dysfunction and heart failure. J Mol Cell Cardiol 2005;38(1):81–91.

181. Basu R, Oudit GY, Wang X, et al. Type 1 diabetic cardiomyopathy in the Akita (Ins2WT/C96Y) mouse model is characterized by lipotoxicity and diastolic dysfunction with preserved systolic function. Am J Physiol Heart Circ Physiol 2009;297(6):H2096–108.

182. Zhang L, Ussher JR, Oka T, et al. Cardiac diacylglycerol accumulation in high fat-fed mice is associated with impaired insulin-stimulated glucose oxidation. Cardiovasc Res 2011;89(1):148–56.

183. Park TS, Hu Y, Noh HL, et al. Ceramide is a cardiotoxin in lipotoxic cardiomyopathy. J Lipid Res 2008; 49(10):2101–12.

184. Drosatos K, Bharadwaj KG, Lymperopoulos A, et al. Cardiomyocyte lipids impair beta-adrenergic receptor function via PKC activation. Am J Physiol Endocrinol Metab 2011;300(3):E489–99.

185. Stanley WC, Recchia FA, Lopaschuk GD. Myocardial substrate metabolism in the normal and failing heart. Physiol Rev 2005;85(3):1093–129.

186. Saddik M, Lopaschuk GD. Myocardial triglyceride turnover and contribution to energy substrate utilization in isolated working rat hearts. J Biol Chem 1991;266(13):8162–70.

187. Banke NH, Wende AR, Leone TC, et al. Preferential oxidation of triacylglyceride-derived fatty acids in heart is augmented by the nuclear receptor PPAR-alpha. Circ Res 2010;107(2):233–41.

188. Swanton EM, Saggerson ED. Effects of adrenaline on triacylglycerol synthesis and turnover in ventricular myocytes from adult rats. Biochem J 1997; 328(Pt 3):913–22.

189. Zechner R, Zimmermann R, Eichmann TO, et al. FAT SIGNALS—lipases and lipolysis in lipid metabolism and signaling. Cell Metab 2012;15(3):279–91.

190. Haemmerle G, Lass A, Zimmermann R, et al. Defective lipolysis and altered energy metabolism in mice lacking adipose triglyceride lipase. Science 2006;312(5774):734–7.

191. Holm C, Kirchgessner TG, Svenson KL, et al. Hormone-sensitive lipase: sequence, expression, and chromosomal localization to 19 cent-q13.3. Science 1988;241(4872):1503–6.

192. Dolinsky VW, Sipione S, Lehner R, et al. The cloning and expression of a murine triacylglycerol hydrolase cDNA and the structure of its corresponding gene. Biochim Biophys Acta 2001; 1532(3):162–72.

193. Karlsson M, Contreras JA, Hellman U, et al. cDNA cloning, tissue distribution, and identification of the catalytic triad of monoglyceride lipase. Evolutionary relationship to esterases, lysophospholipases, and haloperoxidases. J Biol Chem 1997; 272(43):27218–23.

194. Lass A, Zimmermann R, Haemmerle G, et al. Adipose triglyceride lipase-mediated lipolysis of cellular fat stores is activated by CGI-58 and defective in Chanarin-Dorfman syndrome. Cell Metab 2006;3(5):309–19.

195. Schoiswohl G, Schweiger M, Schreiber R, et al. Adipose triglyceride lipase plays a key role in the supply of the working muscle with fatty acids. J Lipid Res 2010;51(3):490–9.

196. Haemmerle G, Moustafa T, Woelkart G, et al. ATGL-mediated fat catabolism regulates cardiac mitochondrial function via PPAR-alpha and PGC-1. Nat Med 2011;17(9):1076–85.

197. Duncan JG, Bharadwaj KG, Fong JL, et al. Rescue of cardiomyopathy in peroxisome proliferator-activated receptor-alpha transgenic mice by deletion of lipoprotein lipase identifies sources of cardiac lipids and peroxisome proliferator-activated receptor-alpha activators. Circulation 2010;121(3):426–35.

198. Schweiger M, Lass A, Zimmermann R, et al. Neutral lipid storage disease: genetic disorders caused by mutations in adipose triglyceride lipase/PNPLA2 or CGI-58/ABHD5. Am J Physiol Endocrinol Metab 2009;297(2):E289–96.

199. Hirano K, Ikeda Y, Zaima N, et al. Triglyceride deposit cardiomyovasculopathy. N Engl J Med 2008;359(22):2396–8.

200. Haemmerle G, Zimmermann R, Hayn M, et al. Hormone-sensitive lipase deficiency in mice causes diglyceride accumulation in adipose tissue, muscle, and testis. J Biol Chem 2002;277(7):4806–15.

201. Park SY, Kim HJ, Wang S, et al. Hormone-sensitive lipase knockout mice have increased hepatic insulin sensitivity and are protected from short-term diet-induced insulin resistance in skeletal muscle and heart. Am J Physiol Endocrinol Metab 2005;289(1):E30–9.

202. Zimmermann R, Haemmerle G, Wagner EM, et al. Decreased fatty acid esterification compensates for the reduced lipolytic activity in hormone-sensitive lipase-deficient white adipose tissue. J Lipid Res 2003;44(11):2089–99.

203. Suzuki J, Shen WJ, Nelson BD, et al. Absence of cardiac lipid accumulation in transgenic mice with heart-specific HSL overexpression. Am J Physiol Endocrinol Metab 2001;281(4):E857–66.

204. Ueno M, Suzuki J, Zenimaru Y, et al. Cardiac overexpression of hormone-sensitive lipase inhibits myocardial steatosis and fibrosis in streptozotocin diabetic mice. Am J Physiol Endocrinol Metab 2008;294(6):E1109–18.

205. Kienesberger PC, Pulinilkunnil T, Sung MM, et al. Myocardial ATGL overexpression decreases the reliance on fatty acid oxidation and protects against pressure overload-induced cardiac dysfunction. Mol Cell Biol 2012;32(4):740–50.

206. Taschler U, Radner FP, Heier C, et al. Monoglyceride lipase deficiency in mice impairs lipolysis and attenuates diet-induced insulin resistance. J Biol Chem 2011;286(20):17467–77.

207. Gilham D, Ho S, Rasouli M, et al. Inhibitors of hepatic microsomal triacylglycerol hydrolase decrease very low density lipoprotein secretion. FASEB J 2003;17(12):1685–7.

208. Wei E, Alam M, Sun F, et al. Apolipoprotein B and triacylglycerol secretion in human triacylglycerol hydrolase transgenic mice. J Lipid Res 2007; 48(12):2597–606.

209. Bartels ED, Nielsen JM, Hellgren LI, et al. Cardiac expression of microsomal triglyceride transfer protein is increased in obesity and serves to attenuate cardiac triglyceride accumulation. PLoS One 2009;4(4):e5300.

210. Boren J, Veniant MM, Young SG. Apo B100-containing lipoproteins are secreted by the heart. J Clin Invest 1998;101(6):1197–202.

211. Stephens TW, Higgins AJ, Cook GA, et al. Two mechanisms produce tissue-specific inhibition of fatty acid oxidation by oxfenicine. Biochem J 1985;227(2):651–60.

212. Fragasso G, Piatti Md PM, Monti L, et al. Short- and long-term beneficial effects of trimetazidine in patients with diabetes and ischemic cardiomyopathy. Am Heart J 2003;146(5):E18.

213. Vitale C, Wajngaten M, Sposato B, et al. Trimetazidine improves left ventricular function and quality of life in elderly patients with coronary artery disease. Eur Heart J 2004;25(20):1814–21.

214. Kantor PF, Lucien A, Kozak R, et al. The antianginal drug trimetazidine shifts cardiac energy metabolism from fatty acid oxidation to glucose oxidation by inhibiting mitochondrial long-chain 3-ketoacyl coenzyme A thiolase. Circ Res 2000;86(5):580–8.

215. Sabbah HN, Chandler MP, Mishima T, et al. Ranolazine, a partial fatty acid oxidation (pFOX) inhibitor, improves left ventricular function in dogs with chronic heart failure. J Card Fail 2002;8(6):416–22.

216. Chaitman BR. Ranolazine for the treatment of chronic angina and potential use in other cardiovascular conditions. Circulation 2006;113(20): 2462–72.

217. Cheng JF, Huang Y, Penuliar R, et al. Discovery of potent and orally available malonyl-CoA decarboxylase inhibitors as cardioprotective agents. J Med Chem 2006;49(14):4055–8.

218. Elam MB, Hunninghake DB, Davis KB, et al. Effect of niacin on lipid and lipoprotein levels and glycemic control in patients with diabetes and peripheral arterial disease: the ADMIT study: a randomized trial. Arterial Disease Multiple Intervention Trial. JAMA 2000;284(10):1263–70.

219. Taylor AJ, Villines TC, Stanek EJ, et al. Extended-release niacin or ezetimibe and carotid intima-media thickness. N Engl J Med 2009;361(22): 2113–22.

220. Garcia-Calvo M, Lisnock J, Bull HG, et al. The target of ezetimibe is Niemann-Pick C1-Like 1 (NPC1L1). Proc Natl Acad Sci U S A 2005;102(23):8132–7.

221. Dunn CJ, Peters DH. Metformin. A review of its pharmacological properties and therapeutic use in non-insulin-dependent diabetes mellitus. Drugs 1995;49(5):721–49.

222. Bolen S, Feldman L, Vassy J, et al. Systematic review: comparative effectiveness and safety of oral medications for type 2 diabetes mellitus. Ann Intern Med 2007;147(6):386–99.

223. Abourbih S, Filion KB, Joseph L, et al. Effect of fibrates on lipid profiles and cardiovascular outcomes: a systematic review. Am J Med 2009; 122(10):962. e1–8.

224. Barter PJ, Rye KA. Cardioprotective properties of fibrates: which fibrate, which patients, what mechanism? Circulation 2006;113(12):1553–5.

225. Law MR, Wald NJ, Rudnicka AR. Quantifying effect of statins on low density lipoprotein cholesterol, ischaemic heart disease, and stroke: systematic review and meta-analysis. BMJ 2003;326(7404):1423.

226. Hebert PR, Gaziano JM, Chan KS, et al. Cholesterol lowering with statin drugs, risk of stroke, and total mortality. An overview of randomized trials. JAMA 1997;278(4):313–21.

227. Zinn A, Felson S, Fisher E, et al. Reassessing the cardiovascular risks and benefits of thiazolidinediones. Clin Cardiol 2008;31(9):397–403.

228. Khanderia U, Pop-Busui R, Eagle KA. Thiazolidinediones in type 2 diabetes: a cardiology perspective. Ann Pharmacother 2008;42(10):1466–74.

229. O'Meara E, McMurray JJ. Myocardial metabolic manipulation: a new therapeutic approach in heart failure? Heart 2005;91(2):131–2.

230. Taegtmeyer H. Cardiac metabolism as a target for the treatment of heart failure. Circulation 2004; 110(8):894–6.

231. Yan J, Young ME, Cui L, et al. Increased glucose uptake and oxidation in mouse hearts prevent high fatty acid oxidation but cause cardiac dysfunction in diet-induced obesity. Circulation 2009;119(21):2818–28.

232. Augustus AS, Buchanan J, Park TS, et al. Loss of lipoprotein lipase-derived fatty acids leads to increased cardiac glucose metabolism and heart dysfunction. J Biol Chem 2006;281(13): 8716–23.

233. Fazio S. Management of mixed dyslipidemia in patients with or at risk for cardiovascular disease: a role for combination fibrate therapy. Clin Ther 2008;30(2):294–306.

234. Brown BG, Zhao XQ, Chait A, et al. Simvastatin and niacin, antioxidant vitamins, or the combination for the prevention of coronary disease. N Engl J Med 2001;345(22):1583–92.

235. Graham DJ, Staffa JA, Shatin D, et al. Incidence of hospitalized rhabdomyolysis in patients treated with lipid-lowering drugs. JAMA 2004;292(21): 2585–90.

Hepatic and Cardiac Steatosis
Are They Coupled?

Elisabetta Bugianesi, MD, PhD[a],*, Amalia Gastaldelli, PhD[b]

KEYWORDS

- Cardiac steatosis • Hepatic steatosis • Nonalcoholic fatty liver disease • Coronary artery disease

KEY POINTS

- Coronary risk factors tend to cluster in patients with nonalcoholic fatty liver disease (NAFLD), who exhibit more advanced carotid atherosclerosis compared with healthy controls.
- Individuals with NAFLD have an increased amount of fat in the epicardial area, which is correlated with abnormal cardiac metabolism, before overt cardiac dysfunction.
- The accumulation of triglyceride in the myocardium of subjects with NAFLD may result from fatty acid overflow in a generalized condition of ectopic fat excess.
- Collectively these findings suggest the presence of complex and intertwined interrelationships between NAFLD, myocardial steatosis, and diastolic dysfunction.

INTRODUCTION

In the last few years several clinical and epidemiologic studies have convincingly associated hepatic steatosis with an increased risk of developing the metabolic syndrome and its related complications, type 2 diabetes and cardiovascular disease (CVD), beyond established predictors. Hepatic steatosis is currently named nonalcoholic fatty liver disease (NAFLD), a term that encompasses a wide spectrum of histologic features, ranging from simple fatty liver (fat infiltration >5% of hepatocytes with or without inflammation) to nonalcoholic steatohepatitis (NASH), which is characterized by the presence of steatosis, necroinflammation, and/or fibrosis, and can lead to cirrhosis.[1] Liver biopsy is the only reliable tool with which to diagnose NAFLD, but noninvasive proxy markers (raised liver enzymes and/or fatty liver at ultrasonography in the absence of viral and alcohol-related liver disease) are usually used in clinical practice. Excess liver fat is very common; as many as 20% of adults in the United States and other Western countries have NAFLD,[2,3] while NASH may be present in up to 3% of the general population and in up to two-thirds of individuals with morbid obesity or type 2 diabetes.[3] An increased risk for CVD events in patients with NAFLD has been highlighted by several epidemiologic reports, although these were biased by the lack of sensitivity of liver enzyme levels, which are normal in the great majority of NAFLD subjects, and by ultrasonography being unable to detect NAFLD for fat infiltration of less than 30%.[4,5]

Early autoptic studies have recognized the heart as an important site of fat accumulation. Fat accumulates preferentially around the heart, within or deep into the pericardium (ie, epicardial fat), but mainly on the external surface of the parietal pericardium within the mediastinum.[6] Excess adipose tissue in the mediastinum is increased in rough proportion to body mass index, but the strongest association is with visceral adipose tissue (VAT) mass.[7] Recent studies using magnetic resonance imaging (MRI) have recognized that a consistent amount of triglyceride accumulates also inside

[a] Division of Gastro-Hepatology, Department of Internal Medicine, San Giovanni Battista Hospital, University of Turin, Corso Dogliotti 14, I-10126 Turin, Italy; [b] Institute of Clinical Physiology, National Research Council, Via G. Moruzzi,1 Località S. Cataldo, Pisa 56124, Italy
* Corresponding author.
E-mail addresses: ebugianesi@yahoo.it; elisabetta.bugianesi@unito.it

Heart Failure Clin 8 (2012) 663–670
http://dx.doi.org/10.1016/j.hfc.2012.06.010
1551-7136/12/$ – see front matter © 2012 Elsevier Inc. All rights reserved.

myocardial cells.[8] The factors that control the differentiation of preadipocytes and the "homing" of triglycerides in the various adipose tissue compartments are still largely unknown. It is now recognized that ectopic fat is increased with obesity and does not accumulate preferably in one organ, but it is simultaneously present in several organs and is associated with increased cardiometabolic risk.[9]

EPIDEMIOLOGIC EVIDENCE OF A LINK BETWEEN FATTY LIVER AND CARDIOVASCULAR DISEASE

Recent studies have highlighted the link between NAFLD and increased CVD.[10] However, the cause-effect relationship is still considered rather weak.[11,12]

NAFLD and Atherosclerosis

Patients with NAFLD have increased markers of subclinical atherosclerosis (impaired flow-mediated vasodilatation and increased carotid-artery intimal medial thickness) independent of obesity and other established risk factors,[10] although this finding has been not universally confirmed. This finding is not surprising because the liver secretes very low-density lipoprotein (VLDL), C-reactive protein (CRP), and fibrinogen, and fatty liver is associated with increased oxidized low-density lipoprotein (LDL) and reactive oxygen species (ROS) (**Fig. 1**), all factors linked to endothelial dysfunction and early atherosclerosis.

The RISC Study showed that subjects with NAFLD are more prone to early carotid atherosclerosis even in the absence of metabolic syndrome and confounding diseases (hypertension, diabetes, CVDs, and dyslipidemia).[13] The same study also documented the relationship between fatty liver and the presence of early plaques at carotid bifurcation, as well as the associations between presence of carotid plaque and established atherosclerotic risk factors, family history of CVD or diabetes, insulin sensitivity, serum liver enzymes, adipokines, fatty free acids, and high-sensitivity C-reactive protein (hsCRP).[13,14]

Hepatic Enzymes and Cardiovascular Disease

In the Hoorn Study, raised alanine aminotransferase (ALT) at baseline increased the 10-year risk of coronary heart disease (CHD) events, after adjustment for components of the metabolic syndrome and other CVD risk factors.[15] By contrast, data from the Framingham Offspring Study showed that 1 standard deviation higher log ALT at baseline was associated with an increased risk of CVD in age- and sex-adjusted models after 20 years of follow-up (hazard ratio [HR] 1.23, 95% confidence interval [CI] 1.12–1.34), but this was attenuated in multivariable adjusted models (HR 1.05, 95% CI 0.96–1.16).[16] Among liver enzymes, γ-glutamyltransferase (GGT) levels rather than ALT levels are most tightly associated with incidental CVD events, even when within the normal range. In a systematic review and a meta-analysis of 10 studies in different ethnic groups,[17] 1 U/L higher GGT (on a log scale) was

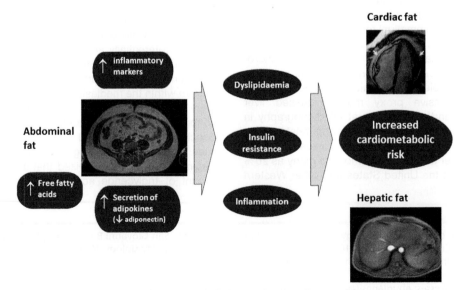

Fig. 1. Relationship between increased abdominal obesity and accumulation of fat around the heart and inside the myocardial and hepatic cells.

associated with a 20% increase in the risk CHD, a 54% increase in the risk of stroke, and a 34% increase in the risk of CHD and stroke combined. The RISC Study demonstrated that the association between GGT and carotid plaques is independent of established atherosclerotic risk factors, insulin sensitivity, adipokines, hsCRP, and physical activity.[14] These results are in line with previous studies that have found a catalytically active GGT within cerebral, carotid, and coronary plaques, co-localized with oxidized LDLs and CD68$^+$ foam cells.[18] It has been hypothesized that GGT binds to LDL lipoproteins and then accumulates in the plaque, where GGT retains its activity and triggers an iron-dependent oxidation of LDL in the extracellular space.[19] Although further studies are needed to explore the mechanisms of GGT action, one can speculate that GGT may add additional information in CVD risk prediction and may be used as a marker of susceptibility to atherogenesis and oxidative stress.

NAFLD and Coronary Heart Disease

Coronary risk factors tend to cluster in patients with NAFLD, who exhibit more advanced carotid atherosclerosis compared with healthy controls.[20] In an Italian study on type 2 diabetic patients, the prevalence of coronary, cerebrovascular, and peripheral vascular disease was remarkably higher among patients with ultrasound-diagnosed fatty liver than in those without, independent of traditional risk factors.[21] In a community-based cohort of 2088 male workers, the presence of ultrasound-diagnosed NAFLD was independently associated with an increased prevalence of ischemic heart disease.[22] In patients consecutively referred for elective coronary angiography, NAFLD was associated with more severe coronary artery disease independently of established risk factors.[23] In a prospective study of 612 patients with clinical indications for coronary angiogram, fatty liver prevalence was 58% and was associated with coronary artery disease (CAD) independently of other metabolic factors.[24] However, presence of fatty liver could not predict cardiovascular mortality and morbidity in patients with established CAD, although the follow-up was relatively short (87 weeks). Cardiac fat, in particular epicardial fat, has been also associated with coronary calcification (CAC score) measured by computed tomography.[25,26]

A small number of prospective studies have been based on gold standard liver biopsy–diagnosed NAFLD. Ekstedt and colleagues[27] found that the 14-year risk of death from CVD was 2-fold higher in patients with NASH but not in patients with simple steatosis. Another study from Sweden recently confirmed that the standardized mortality ratio for all-cause mortality in comparison with the adjusted total Swedish population was 1.55 (95% CI 0.98–2.32) for subjects with simple steatosis and 1.86 (95% CI 1.19–2.76) for nonalcoholic steatohepatitis, during the median period of follow-up of 24 years.[28]

NAFLD and Cardiac Function

In contrast to the data reported above, the information regarding abnormalities in cardiac function among NAFLD patients is limited and controversial. Nondiabetic, normotensive patients with NAFLD have echocardiographic features of early left ventricular (LV) diastolic dysfunction as measured by tissue Doppler echocardiography[29,30] and impaired LV energy metabolism, assessed by cardiac ^{31}P-magnetic resonance spectroscopy (MRS), compared with control subjects without steatosis.[31] In a study involving type 2 diabetic men with known ischemic heart disease, Lautamäki and colleagues[32] found that patients with higher intrahepatic fat content had reduced coronary functional capacity. Rijzewijk and colleagues[31] showed that intramyocardial fat content, as detected by ^{1}H-MRS, was significantly higher in uncomplicated type 2 diabetic men than in nondiabetic control subjects and was associated with impaired LV diastolic function as detected by cardiac MRI. The same investigators also noted a significant, positive association between intramyocardial and intrahepatic fat contents after adjustment for diabetic state.

Direct evidence of the effect of hepatic steatosis on the heart has been provided by Perseghin and colleagues[30] who, using cardiac MRI and ^{31}P-MRS, assessed intrapericardial and extrapericardial fat along with myocardial energy metabolism in young, well-matched nondiabetic men with or without fatty liver, as measured by hepatic ^{1}H-MRS. Individuals with fatty liver had an increased amount of fat in the epicardial area and displayed abnormal cardiac metabolism despite normal LV morphologic features and systolic/diastolic functions. Thus, in subjects with NAFLD cardiac metabolic remodeling appears to be an early event, independent of well-known risk factors for CVD (age, obesity, hypertension, diabetes exercise habits), and may precede the development of functional and structural remodeling of the heart.

PUTATIVE MECHANISMS OF A LINK BETWEEN CARDIAC AND LIVER FAT

In obese or diabetic patients, the metabolic switching of cardiac metabolism from glucose to fat has been attributed to the synergistic action of systemic and myocardial insulin resistance, increased fatty acid availability, and free fatty acid (FFA)-induced changes in transcription of genes involved in cardiac substrate selection, through activation of peroxisome proliferator–activated receptors (PPARs).[33] In NAFLD the pathophysiological mechanisms of defective cardiac efficiency have not been characterized, but the fatty liver constantly clusters with the components of the metabolic syndrome. Conventional wisdom suggests that either hemodynamic or metabolic derangements associated with NAFLD may predispose individuals to CHD and heart failure. However, it is now clear that the relationship between NAFLD and insulin resistance/metabolic syndrome (MetS) is bidirectional: liver fat content is significantly increased in subjects with the MetS and in turn the presence of NAFLD is a strong predictor of MetS and of future risk of CVD.[34]

Fatty Liver as a Major Determinant of Insulin Resistance and the Metabolic Syndrome

The liver is a key site of insulin action: it is the main source of endogenous glucose production (EGP), a major site of lipids disposal and synthesis, and the primary site of insulin degradation. Thus, it is not surprising that excessive liver fat is strongly associated not only with hepatic but also with muscle and adipose tissue insulin resistance and that obese and nonobese subjects who accumulate liver fat are at major risk of developing MetS.[34] There is a strong relation between the amount of hepatic fat and impaired insulin action, which is independent of global or ectopic (visceral, intramyocellular) fat deposition. In fact, once the liver gets fatty, the ability of insulin to inhibit EGP is impaired: hepatic insulin resistance is the major factor responsible for the development of fasting hyperglycemia and of the compensatory hyperinsulinemia. NAFLD is also characterized by a defect in insulin inhibition of VLDL production, leading to hypertriglyceridemia and low concentration of high-density lipoprotein (HDL) cholesterol.[34,35] Liver steatosis was the strongest predictor of myocardial insulin sensitivity and perfusion in patients with type 2 diabetes.[32] The increased FFA availability in NAFLD may induce a detrimental effect on the creatine phosphate/adenosine triphosphate (PCr/ATP) ratio through oxidative substrate competition or through an impairment of myocardial insulin signaling. Treatment with trimetazidine, a partial FFA-oxidation inhibitor, consistently induced improvement of the LV function and PCr/ATP ratio in patients with heart failure. Of note, in the study of Perseghin and

colleagues,[36] the extrapericardial and intrapericardial fat in NAFLD subjects was inversely correlated with the early/atrial peak filling rate, a parameter of diastolic function. This finding confirms those of previous studies whereby cardiac fat was found to be negatively associated with the cardiac output.[37]

Cardiac Fat, Insulin Resistance, and the Metabolic Syndrome

Experimental and clinical observations suggest both favorable and unfavorable effects of epicardial and perivascular fat.[8,38] Growing evidence suggests that cardiac adiposity may play an important role in the development of an unfavorable cardiovascular risk profile, as epicardial fat could locally modulate the morphology and function of the heart.[7,39] The close anatomic relationship between epicardial adipose tissue and the adjacent myocardium should readily allow local paracrine interactions between these tissues. Although MRI and computed tomography are more reliable,[8] ultrasonography has been often used for the direct assessment of epicardial adipose tissue.[40,41] Epicardial adipose tissue thickness, determined by echo over the free wall of the right ventricle, correlates with visceral abdominal adipose tissue (a CHD risk factor per se), other correlates of CVD such as waist circumference, diastolic blood pressure, plasma insulin, fasting plasma glucose, HDL cholesterol, LDL cholesterol, and adiponectin.[7,40]

Cardiac fat, in particular mediastinal fat, is also associated with increased insulin resistance in subjects without type 2 diabetes[7] but also with the number of factors associated with the MetS and 10-year CHD risk score.[6,39] The same association can be observed in the same subjects if visceral fat is considered, whereas subcutaneous fat does not seem to have a strong association with cardiometabolic risk markers.[6]

Low-Grade Inflammatory State

Emerging evidence also suggests that NAFLD, especially in its necroinflammatory form (NASH), not only is a marker of CVD and cardiac function abnormalities but also might be involved in their pathogenesis, possibly through the systemic release of several pathogenic mediators from the steatotic and inflamed liver (eg, increased CRP, interleukin [IL]-6, tumor necrosis factor α [TNF-α], and other inflammatory cytokines).[34,35] Increased amounts of circulating and intracellular FFA concentration are associated with an increase in the intranuclear and total cellular nuclear factor κB.[42] Soluble forms of the vascular adhesion

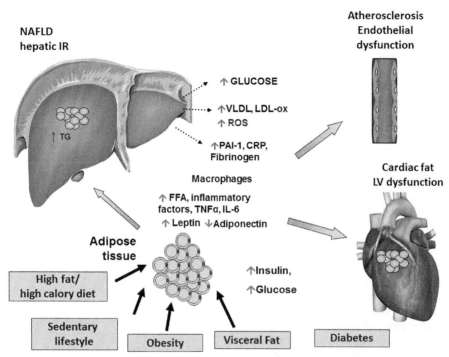

Fig. 2. Interrelationships between abdominal, hepatic, and myocardial steatosis that can explain coronary artery disease in patients with NAFLD. CRP, C-reactive protein; FFA, free fatty acid; IL, interleukin; IR, insulin resistance; LDL-ox, oxidized low-density lipoprotein; LV, left ventricular; NAFLD, nonalcoholic fatty liver disease; ROS, reactive oxygen species; PAI, plasminogen-activator inhibitor; TG, triglyceride; TNF, tumor necrosis factor; VLDL, very low-density lipoprotein.

molecules ICAM-1 and E-selectin are upregulated in patients with higher liver fat content and may participate in endothelial dysfunction.[43] Healthy subjects with NAFLD have increased plasma levels of leptin and E-selectin while adiponectin and resistin are reduced.[36]

Leptin is mainly secreted by subcutaneous adipose tissue, and thus is increased with obesity. It has been suggested the leptin is involved in the accumulation of hepatic triglyceride as a consequence of resistance to leptin action independently of insulin resistance. Several in vitro and in vivo studies have identified a close connection between leptin and liver fibrosis, showing that leptin modulates the biology of different cell types participating in the response to liver injury, such as Kupffer cells, sinusoidal endothelial cells, and myofibroblast-like cells.[44] Leptin is also a potential mediator of cardiac hypertrophy in obesity, possibly by causing an increase in sympathetic vasoconstrictor tone and arterial blood pressure, or through direct stimulation of protein synthesis in cardiomyocytes.[45]

Adiponectin levels are closely correlated with the degree of both peripheral and hepatic insulin sensitivity, although the mechanism of action of action of this adipokine is not completely understood, but is possibly mediated by the activation of PPAR-α and adenosine monophosphate–activated protein kinase (AMPK), which lead to an increase in fatty acid oxidation in muscle and liver, and decreased tissue content of triglycerides. In the liver, adiponectin has a role in the wound-healing process and thus has hepatoprotective and antifibrogenic effects.[44] Adiponectin also exerts a protective effect against the endothelial dysfunction induced by advanced glycation end-products.[46] This process is in part mediated by a decrease in expression of adhesion molecules, and provides evidence of the protective role of adiponectin in the pathogenesis of the vascular complications of obesity/MetS. Low adiponectin levels may impair the ability of the heart to adapt to acute and chronic stress, as suggested from studies of adiponectin deficiency in mice.[19] Epidemiologic studies, however, did not find a relationship between the low adiponectin levels in obese people and the incidence of ischemic heart disease.

A study by Fontana and colleagues[47] in extremely obese subjects undergoing gastric bypass have measured several adipokines in the portal vein and in the radial artery, showing that IL-6 portal concentrations were approximately 50% greater in the portal vein and strongly correlated with CRP produced by the liver. Among the other adipokines, plasma TNF-α, resistin, macrophage chemoattractant protein 1, and adiponectin concentrations were similar in the portal vein and radial artery, while leptin was 20% lower in the portal vein, confirming that this adipokine is mainly released by subcutaneous adipose tissue.

Ectopic Fat Accumulation

Human and animal data have shown that ectopic lipid accumulation is associated with insulin resistance in muscle and liver, and with functional losses in the pancreas and the heart in animal models. Ectopic lipid accumulation can occur because of increased uptake of circulating FFAs due to adipose tissue resistance, increased de novo lipogenesis, and/or reduced FFA oxidation or disposal. Obesity and ectopic fat accumulation are also important risk factors for CVD, and data from animal models suggest a causal relationship between cardiac lipid accumulation, dilated cardiomyopathy and, ultimately, heart failure. Fat in the liver accumulates in proportion to total body fat but is strongly related with visceral fat accumulation,[48] which in turn is associated to increased risk of cardiometabolic disease.[49] It has been postulated that abdominal fat is the marker of dysfunctional adipose tissue, which leads to lipid accumulation in multiple sites such as liver, muscle, heart, and around the vessels (as perivascular fat).[49] Although the mechanisms are still not completely elucidated, it is supposed that visceral fat contributes to the lipotoxic effect of fat accumulation in the organs through the release of cytokines and inflammatory factors (**Fig. 2**).

SUMMARY

The accumulation of triglyceride in the myocardium and around the heart of subjects with fatty liver is significant, and may result from fatty acid overflow to the heart because of a generalized condition of ectopic fat excess. Heart and liver share the peculiarity of first-pass organs into which FFAs drain from visceral fat depots, that is, epicardial and VAT, respectively. Epicardial and visceral fat show similar biochemical properties, including a higher lipolytic rate. Thus hepatic fat content may represent an indicator of a generalized condition of ectopic triglyceride deposition, also involving the cardiac wall; in turn, lipids in the heart wall would be directly responsible for myocardial insulin resistance and energy impairment.

The final effect of lipotoxicity varies according to the target organ: in the heart it translates into an impairment of energetic and mechanical efficiency, whereas in the liver a fibrogenic response is favored

by the abundance of inflammatory cells. Collectively these findings suggest the presence of complex and intertwined interrelationships between NAFLD, myocardial steatosis, and diastolic dysfunction. Further research is needed to elucidate the mechanisms by which NAFLD may contribute to the development of diastolic dysfunction. A reduction in liver fat would seem an attractive target for therapies aimed at preventing the development of abnormal myocardial substrate metabolism and future risk of heart failure.

REFERENCES

1. Falck-Ytter Y, Younossi ZM, Marchesini G, et al. Clinical features and natural history of nonalcoholic steatosis syndromes. Semin Liver Dis 2001;21(1):17–26.
2. de Alwis NM, Day CP. Non-alcoholic fatty liver disease: the mist gradually clears. J Hepatol 2008; 48(Suppl 1):S104–12.
3. Bellentani S, Saccoccio G, Masutti F, et al. Prevalence of and risk factors for hepatic steatosis in Northern Italy. Ann Intern Med 2000;132(2):112–7.
4. Mofrad P, Contos MJ, Haque M, et al. Clinical and histologic spectrum of nonalcoholic fatty liver disease associated with normal ALT values. Hepatology 2003;37(6):1286–92.
5. Ricci C, Longo R, Gioulis E, et al. Noninvasive in vivo quantitative assessment of fat content in human liver. J Hepatol 1997;27(1):108–13.
6. Sironi AM, Petz R, De Marchi D, et al. Impact of increased visceral and cardiac fat on cardiometabolic risk and disease. Diabet Med 2012;29(5): 622–7.
7. Sironi AM, Gastaldelli A, Mari A, et al. Visceral fat in hypertension: influence on insulin resistance and beta-cell function. Hypertension 2004;44(2): 127–33.
8. Sacks HS, Fain JN. Human epicardial adipose tissue: a review. Am Heart J 2007;153(6):907–17.
9. Sironi AM, Sicari R, Folli F, et al. Ectopic fat storage, insulin resistance, and hypertension. Curr Pharm Des 2011;17(28):3074–80.
10. Targher G, Day CP, Bonora E. Risk of cardiovascular disease in patients with nonalcoholic fatty liver disease. N Engl J Med 2010;363(14):1341–50.
11. Ghouri N, Preiss D, Sattar N. Liver enzymes, nonalcoholic fatty liver disease, and incident cardiovascular disease: a narrative review and clinical perspective of prospective data. Hepatology 2010; 52(3):1156–61.
12. Perseghin G. The role of non-alcoholic fatty liver disease in cardiovascular disease. Dig Dis 2010; 28(1):210–3.
13. Gastaldelli A, Kozakova M, Hojlund K, et al. Fatty liver is associated with insulin resistance, risk of coronary heart disease, and early atherosclerosis

in a large European population. Hepatology 2009; 49(5):1537–44.

14. Kozakova M, Palombo C, Paterni M, et al. Fatty liver index, gamma-glutamyltransferase and early carotid plaques. Hepatology 2012;55(5):1406–15.

15. Schindhelm RK, Dekker JM, Nijpels G, et al. Alanine aminotransferase predicts coronary heart disease events: a 10-year follow-up of the Hoorn Study. Atherosclerosis 2007;191(2):391–6.

16. Goessling W, Massaro JM, Vasan RS, et al. Amino-transferase levels and 20-year risk of metabolic syndrome, diabetes, and cardiovascular disease. Gastroenterology 2008;135(6):1935–44.

17. Fraser A, Harris R, Sattar N, et al. Gamma-glutamyl-transferase is associated with incident vascular events independently of alcohol intake: analysis of the British Women's Heart and Health Study and Meta-Analysis. Arterioscler Thromb Vasc Biol 2007; 27(12):2729–35.

18. Paolicchi A, Emdin M, Ghliozeni E, et al. Images in cardiovascular medicine. Human atherosclerotic plaques contain gamma-glutamyl transpeptidase enzyme activity. Circulation 2004;109(11):1440.

19. Paolicchi A, Minotti G, Tonarelli P, et al. Gamma-glutamyl transpeptidase-dependent iron reduction and LDL oxidation—a potential mechanism in atherosclerosis. J Investig Med 1999;47(3):151–60.

20. Targher G, Bertolini L, Padovani R, et al. Relation of nonalcoholic hepatic steatosis to early carotid athero-sclerosis in healthy men: role of visceral fat accumula-tion. Diabetes Care 2004;27(10):2498–500.

21. Targher G, Bertolini L, Padovani R, et al. Prevalence of nonalcoholic fatty liver disease and its association with cardiovascular disease among type 2 diabetic patients. Diabetes Care 2007;30(5):1212–8.

22. Lin YC, Lo HM, Chen JD. Sonographic fatty liver, overweight and ischemic heart disease. World J Gastroenterol 2005;11(31):4838–42.

23. Mirbagheri SA, Rashidi A, Abdi S, et al. Liver: an alarm for the heart? Liver Int 2007;27(7):891–4.

24. Wong VW, Wong GL, Yip GW, et al. Coronary artery disease and cardiovascular outcomes in patients with non-alcoholic fatty liver disease. Gut 2011; 60(12):1721–7.

25. Ding J, Kritchevsky SB, Harris TB, et al. The associ-ation of pericardial fat with calcified coronary pla-que. Obesity (Silver Spring) 2008;16(8):1914–9.

26. Djaberi R, Schuijf JD, van Werkhoven JM, et al. Rela-tion of epicardial adipose tissue to coronary athero-sclerosis. Am J Cardiol 2008;102(12):1602–7.

27. Ekstedt M, Franzen LE, Mathiesen UL, et al. Long-term follow-up of patients with NAFLD and elevated liver enzymes. Hepatology 2006;44(4):865–73.

28. Soderberg C, Stal P, Askling J, et al. Decreased survival of subjects with elevated liver function tests during a 28-year follow-up. Hepatology 2010;51(2): 595–602.

29. Fotbolcu H, Yakar T, Duman D, et al. Impairment of the left ventricular systolic and diastolic function in patients with non-alcoholic fatty liver disease. Cardiol J 2010;17(5):457–63.

30. Perseghin G, Ntali G, De Cobelli F, et al. Abnormal left ventricular energy metabolism in obese men with preserved systolic and diastolic functions is associated with insulin resistance. Diabetes Care 2007;30(6):1520–6.

31. Rijzewijk LJ, Jonker JT, van der Meer RW, et al. Effects of hepatic triglyceride content on myocardial metabolism in type 2 diabetes. J Am Coll Cardiol 2010;56(3):225–33.

32. Lautamaki R, Borra R, Iozzo P, et al. Liver steatosis coexists with myocardial insulin resistance and coro-nary dysfunction in patients with type 2 diabetes. Am J Physiol Endocrinol Metab 2006;291(2):E282–90.

33. Boudina S, Abel ED. Diabetic cardiomyopathy revis-ited. Circulation 2007;115(25):3213–23.

34. Kotronen A, Westerbacka J, Bergholm R, et al. Liver fat in the metabolic syndrome. J Clin Endocrinol Metab 2007;92(9):3490–7.

35. Bugianesi E, McCullough AJ, Marchesini G. Insulin resistance: a metabolic pathway to chronic liver disease. Hepatology 2005;42(5):987–1000.

36. Perseghin G, Lattuada G, De Cobelli F, et al. Increased mediastinal fat and impaired left ventric-ular energy metabolism in young men with newly found fatty liver. Hepatology 2008;47(1):51–8.

37. Kankaanpaa M, Lehto HR, Parkka JP, et al. Myocar-dial triglyceride content and epicardial fat mass in human obesity: relationship to left ventricular func-tion and serum free fatty acid levels. J Clin Endocri-nol Metab 2006;91(11):4689–95.

38. Iacobellis G, Barbaro G. The double role of epicar-dial adipose tissue as pro- and anti-inflammatory organ. Hormone and metabolic research. Horm Metab Res 2008;40(7):442–5.

39. Iacobellis G, Sharma AM. Epicardial adipose tissue as new cardio-metabolic risk marker and potential therapeutic target in the metabolic syndrome. Curr Pharm Des 2007;13(21):2180–4.

40. Iacobellis G, Assael F, Ribaudo MC, et al. Epicardial fat from echocardiography: a new method for visceral adipose tissue prediction. Obes Res 2003; 11(2):304–10.

41. Sicari R, Sironi AM, Petz R, et al. Pericardial rather than epicardial fat is a cardiometabolic risk marker: an MRI vs echo study. J Am Soc Echocardiogr 2011; 24(10):1156–62.

42. Tripathy D, Mohanty P, Dhindsa S, et al. Elevation of free fatty acids induces inflammation and impairs vascular reactivity in healthy subjects. Diabetes 2003;52(12):2882–7.

43. Mullenix PS, Andersen CA, Starnes BW. Athero-sclerosis as inflammation. Ann Vasc Surg 2005; 19(1):130–8.

44. Bertolani C, Marra F. The role of adipokines in liver fibrosis. Pathophysiology 2008;15(2):91–101.

45. Paolisso G, Tagliamonte MR, Galderisi M, et al. Plasma leptin level is associated with myocardial wall thickness in hypertensive insulin-resistant men. Hypertension 1999;34(5):1047–52.

46. Del Turco S, Navarra T, Gastaldelli A, et al. Protective role of adiponectin on endothelial dysfunction induced by AGEs: a clinical and experimental approach. Microvasc Res 2011;82(1):73–6.

47. Fontana L, Eagon JC, Trujillo ME, et al. Visceral fat adipokine secretion is associated with systemic inflammation in obese humans. Diabetes 2007; 56(4):1010–3.

48. Gastaldelli A, Cusi K, Pettiti M, et al. Relationship between hepatic/visceral fat and hepatic insulin resistance in nondiabetic and type 2 diabetic subjects. Gastroenterology 2007;133(2):496–506.

49. Despres JP, Lemieux I. Abdominal obesity and metabolic syndrome. Nature 2006;444(7121):881–7.

Epicardial Steatosis, Insulin Resistance, and Coronary Artery Disease

Peter P. Toth, MD, PhD, FNLA, FCCP[a,b,*]

KEYWORDS

- Adipose tissue • Coronary artery disease • Epicardium • Fatty acid • Inflammation
- Insulin resistance • Metabolic syndrome

KEY POINTS

- Insulin resistance is highly correlated with systemic inflammation and alterations in lipid and lipoprotein metabolism that potentiate visceral organ steatosis and failure.
- Patients with insulin resistance and diabetes mellitus have a dramatic escalation in risk for developing all forms of atherosclerotic disease.
- Increased ectopic fat deposition is associated with insulin resistance. In the setting of insulin resistance, epicardial fat mass and volume expand significantly.
- Insulin-resistant epicardial adipose tissue is dysregulated and is an important source of cytokines and interleukins, that appear to augment risk for developing coronary artery disease and increase risk for cardiovascular events. One possible mechanism for this is that insulin-resistant epicardial fat could shower the adventitial aspect of an epicardial coronary artery with toxic lipids, growth factors, and inflammatory cytokines, thereby promoting intravascular inflammation, intimal injury, and atherogenesis.
- Increased cardiac steatosis also increases risk for reduced coronary flow reserve, endothelial dysfunction, arrhythmogenesis, altered myocardial energy metabolism, and perturbations in contractility.

INTRODUCTION

Insulin resistance (IR) is the accepted primary cause of the metabolic syndrome, a constellation of cardiovascular risk factors that includes abdominal adiposity/obesity, hyperglycemia, elevated blood pressure, and abnormal lipid metabolism (Fig. 1) as manifested by hypertriglyceridemia and low high-density lipoprotein cholesterol (HDL-C).[1] IR is also associated with

- Heightened systemic inflammation
- A prooxidative state
- Hypercoagulability
- Endothelial dysfunction
- Impaired interorgan signaling and functional coordination

The metabolic syndrome and IR increase the risk for cardiovascular disease–related morbidity and mortality and incidental type 2 diabetes mellitus (DM) significantly.[2] There is a rapidly evolving parallel worldwide epidemic of obesity and DM. In 2011, it was estimated that there were 25.8 million patients with DM in the United States, with an estimated 1.9 million new cases annually (http://www.diabetes.org/diabetes-basics/diabetes-statistics). A staggering 79 million people in the

[a] CGH Medical Center, 101 East Miller Road, Sterling, IL 61081, USA; [b] Department of Family and Community Medicine, University of Illinois School of Medicine, Peoria, IL 61605, USA
* CGH Medical Center, 101 East Miller Road, Sterling, IL 61081.
E-mail address: peter.toth@cghmc.com

Heart Failure Clin 8 (2012) 671–678
http://dx.doi.org/10.1016/j.hfc.2012.06.013
1551-7136/12/$ – see front matter © 2012 Elsevier Inc. All rights reserved

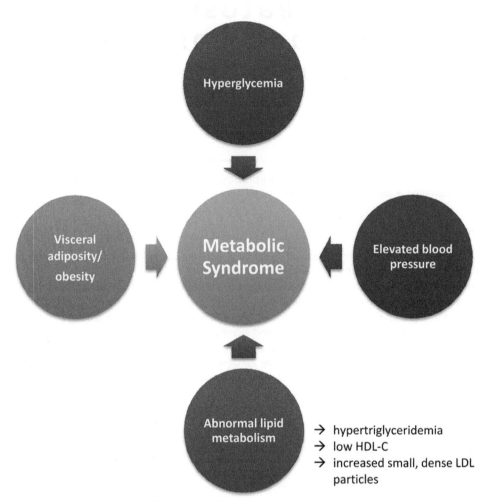

Fig. 1. Metabolic syndrome is a constellation of cardiovascular risk factors that include abdominal adiposity/obesity, hyperglycemia, elevated blood pressure, and abnormal lipid metabolism as manifested by hypertriglyceridemia and low high-density lipoprotein cholesterol (HDL-C). LDL, low-density lipoprotein.

United States are prediabetic. The World Health Organization estimates a global prevalence of DM of approximately 346 million, with all nations as well as all racial and ethnic groups significantly affected (http://www.who.int/mediacentre/factsheets/fs312/en).

Visceral obesity is inversely correlated with insulin sensitivity.[3] Hyperinsulinemia (a surrogate for IR) is highly prevalent in patients with coronary artery disease (CAD).[4] Hyperinsulinemia arises in patients with IR as a compensatory response: the pancreas produces more and more insulin in an effort to promote glucose uptake in systemic tissues that are becoming progressively less responsive to insulin. In patients with IR, lipid and lipoprotein metabolism is severely perturbed. Abnormalities in lipid metabolism give rise to steatosis in multiple organs, including the liver, pancreas, skeletal muscle, and heart. Ectopic steatosis is associated with elevated levels of free fatty acid (FFAs), increased intracellular toxic lipid accumulation and metabolic stress (ie, lipotoxicity), as well as organ dysfunction and failure.[5,6] The pathophysiologic impact of steatosis in the liver, pancreas, and skeletal muscle in patients with IR has been recognized for some time. Evidence is rapidly accumulating to show that epicardial steatosis and expansion of coronary fat pad volume are highly deleterious and associated with increased risk for CAD. Epicardial adipocytes can become insulin resistant and appear to potentiate atherosclerotic disease by continually exposing coronary arteries to increased levels of lipids and inflammatory mediators. This article explores these associations from both biochemical and structural standpoints. Although increased epicardial adiposity is often accompanied by increased intramyocellular lipid deposition, this article focuses solely on changes in epicardial adiposity.

INSULIN RESISTANCE

IR has a complex molecular etiology and is still inadequately understood. In the setting of IR, tissues become progressively less sensitive to the effects of insulin. Under normal circumstances, the binding of insulin to its cell-surface receptor initiates an intracellular signaling cascade that begins with the phosphorylation of tyrosine residues in insulin receptor substrates (IRS)-1 and -2. This in turn activates a series of phosphoinositide-3-kinase–dependent reactions, which promote the nuclear expression of glucose transport (GLUT) proteins that are translocated to the cell surface to promote the uptake of glucose from the extracellular milieu.[7] In patients with IR, visceral adipose tissue becomes dysregulated. Visceral adipocytes (as found in omentum, perimesenteric fat, and perinephric fat) under normal conditions are highly regulated and hydrolyze triglycerides to FFAs and glycerol in response to systemic energy/substrate demands. Insulin serves to inhibit the activity of hormone-sensitive lipase, the enzyme that hydrolyzes triglycerides stored within adipocytes. In insulin-resistant adipocytes, hormone-sensitive lipase remains active and continually allows for the flooding of the portal and systemic circulation with FFAs. As cells take up fatty acid and intracellular FFA levels increase, cells become insulin resistant. The cell undergoes a transition from tyrosine to serine phosphorylation of IRS-1, which alters its ability to initiate the insulin signaling cascade. This process is compounded by the accumulation of toxic intracellular acyl-coenzyme As and diacylglycerol. These changes result in reduced phosphoinositide-3-kinase activity and impaired GLUT expression and translocation.[8]

Adipose tissue is metabolically highly active, and has both endocrine and paracrine signaling capacity. Under normal circumstances adipocytes produce adiponectin, a molecule that sensitizes tissues to the effects of insulin; serum levels of this hormone are inversely correlated with the degree of adiposity.[9] Adipocytes also produce leptin, a hormone that acts on the arcuate nucleus of the hypothalamus to suppress appetite.[10] As adipose tissue volume expands, several changes occur:

- Adiponectin expression decreases
- Leptin increases because patients become leptin resistant with reduced capacity for appetite suppression
- The expression of resistin (an adipocyte-derived hormone that promotes IR) increases[11]
- Inflammatory mediator expression increases ("adipokines," including tumor necrosis factor α [TNF-α], transforming growth factor β, interleukin-1 and interleukin-6, plasminogen activator inhibitor 1, and monocyte chemoattractant protein 1 [MCP-1], among others)[12]

The expression of inflammatory mediators creates a vicious cycle as these molecules potentiate a worsening of IR. The MCP-1 promotes the influx of monocytes into adipose tissue, the liver, and other organs. Monocytes convert to macrophages, which become activated by FFAs and other chemokines.[6] Activated macrophages secrete more inflammatory mediators, and the cycle is propagated and intensified. Adipose tissue that is insulin resistant can thus become an important source of FFAs and a wide variety of inflammatory mediators. Weight loss and increased aerobic activity have been consistently shown to decrease IR,[13,14] reduce hyperglycemia and the severity of dyslipidemia, and regress epicardial steatosis.[15,16]

IR augments cardiovascular risk in numerous other ways. A heralding sign of IR is atherogenic dyslipidemia. In an effort to cope with the massive influx of fatty acid, the liver reassimilates at least some of this fatty acid into triglyceride, which is packaged into very low-density lipoproteins (VLDL) and secreted into the systemic circulation. Because IR is associated with inhibition of lipoprotein lipase, the triglycerides in VLDL particles are not hydrolyzed at a normal rate, and patients become hypertriglyceridemic with impaired clearance of VLDL. As serum triglyceride levels increase, activity of cholesterol ester transfer protein increases and there is increased transfer of triglyceride into HDL and low-density lipoprotein (LDL) particles. This process leads to increased catabolism and clearance of HDL particles and the formation of large numbers of small, dense LDL particles. HDL levels decrease further because of reduced hepatic and adipose tissue biosynthesis of this lipoprotein and decreased release of surface-coat constituents from chylomicrons that can be used to assimilate HDL in serum.[17-19] IR potentiates hyperglycemia secondary to reduced peripheral tissue uptake as well as increased hepatic gluconeogenesis and glycogenolysis. IR also promotes the activation of receptors of advanced glycosylated end products (RAGE). The activation of RAGE is proinflammatory and has been shown to accelerate atherogenesis.[20] Hypertension is caused by endothelial dysfunction, increased central sympathetic outflow of catecholamines, increased production of angiotensin II and vascular expression of the AT1 receptor, increased sodium reabsorption and expansion of intravascular volume, and structural alterations within arterial walls making them less distensible and compliant, among other changes.[21]

EPICARDIAL ADIPOSE TISSUE

Epicardial adipose tissue comprises the fat in between myocardium and the visceral layer of pericardium, and is distinct from pericardial fat, which localizes between the visceral and parietal pericardium.[22] Epicardial fat directly overlies myocardium without a fascial boundary, and is a type of visceral fat that can develop IR. Many articles in the literature refer to the terms epicardial and pericardial interchangeably. The epicardium and myocardium are perfused by the same microcirculation.[22] The epicardial coronary vessels are cushioned along a layer of epicardial fat. Epicardial fat is derived embryologically from brown fat, and several functions have been attributed to it[23,24]:

1. Acts as a readily available source of oxidizable substrate
2. Acts as a buffer against high circulating levels of FFAs by sequestering them, storing them as triglyceride, and reducing toxic exposure
3. Protects the coronary vessels against torsional injury during cardiac contraction and during propagation of the arterial pulse wave
4. Allows for positive remodeling (ectatic expansion in the Glagovian[25] sense) in areas with atherosclerotic lesions/plaque, because adipose tissue is more compliant than adjacent myocardium
5. Houses and protects the intracardiac nervous system (ganglia and ganglionated plexuses)

Several imaging techniques are used to quantitate epicardial fat mass and volume, including echocardiography, computed tomography (CT), and magnetic resonance imaging (MRI).

CORRELATION OF EPICARDIAL FAT WITH IR

The use of multidetector CT imaging has provided important new information about the relationship of epicardial fat to IR and CAD.

Epicardial fat thickness in the atrioventricular groove correlates directly with elevations in blood pressure, hyperglycemia, dyslipidemia, and serum levels of both resistin and high-sensitivity C-reactive protein (hsCRP).[26] Moreover, these investigators showed that as the burden of metabolic syndrome components increased, so did the epicardial fat volume (EFV). Greif and colleagues[27] demonstrated that EFV correlated with low serum levels of adiponectin and HDL-C and increased levels of TNF-α and hsCRP.

In addition to correlations with low HDL-C and hyperglycemia, EFV also shows good correlation with visceral adiposity and waist circumference.[28] Among postmenopausal women, EFV correlates directly with weight, waist circumference, body mass index (BMI), triglycerides, glucose, systolic blood pressure, and use of antihypertensive drugs, and inversely with HDL-C.[29] In the Framingham Heart Study, epicardial fat correlated with low HDL-C, hypertriglyceridemia, hypertension, impaired fasting glucose, DM, and metabolic syndrome after multivariate adjustment.[30] The Framingham investigators further demonstrated that increased epicardial fat is negatively correlated with serum adiponectin and positively correlated with resistin in both men and women.[31] As shown by echocardiography, epicardial fat thickness correlated with waist circumference, diastolic blood pressure, LDL-C, glucose, adiponectin, HDL-C, and fasting insulin levels.[32] Among type I diabetic women with central adiposity, the presence of metabolic syndrome is associated with increased EFV.[33] In prepubertal children, increasing thickness of epicardial fat is associated with BMI, insulin levels, and homeostatic model assessment IR.[34] There is remarkable consistency in the literature showing that defining components of the metabolic syndrome and heightened systemic inflammatory tone correlate with an increasing burden of epicardial fat deposition.

CORRELATION OF EPICARDIAL FAT WITH CAD

It is well established that IR, dyslipidemia, hypertension, hyperglycemia, and inflammation are highly associated with the development of atherosclerotic disease, particularly CAD (**Fig. 2**). Consistent with this is the observation that EFV correlates strongly with coronary calcium burden and coronary atherosclerotic plaques. The Framingham investigators showed that EFV was associated with coronary artery calcification even after adjusting for Framingham risk factors and visceral adiposity (odds ratio 1.21 per 1 standard deviation increase in EFV).[30] In a study by Sarin and colleagues,[35] coronary artery calcium scores tripled once EFV exceeded 100 mL, and more patients with elevated EFV had evidence of nonobstructive or obstructive plaques (46% vs 31%, $P<.05$). EFV correlates with the number of diseased coronary segments, the number of atherosclerotic plaques, and the risk of having noncalcified, calcified, or a mixture of both types of plaque.[27] These investigators also demonstrated that an EFV that exceeds 300 mL is the strongest independent risk factor for CAD (odds ratio 4.1, $P<.05$), with the Framingham risk score, smoking, hypertension, and

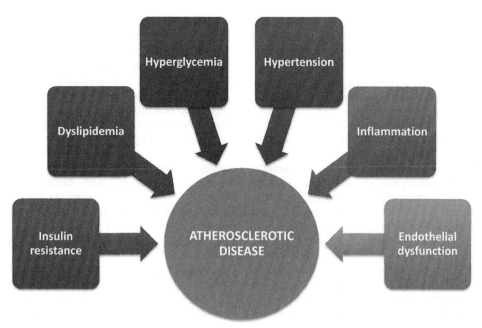

Fig. 2. Several factors are highly associated with the development of atherosclerotic disease, particularly coronary artery disease.

diabetes all having lower odds ratios of 2.8, 1.6, 1.8, and 3.0, respectively.

Other groups have similarly shown that EFV correlates with coronary calcium burden[28] and has a graded relationship with the presence of CAD in women[29] as well as patients with BMI of less than 27 kg/m[2].[36] Among patients with DM, EFV was significantly greater than in nondiabetic patients, and correlated highly and in a graded fashion with coronary calcium score and presence of atherosclerotic plaques that were greater than 50% obstructive.[37] A particularly interesting study of 567 patients with CAD assessing epicardial fat burden with echocardiography showed the following: (1) epicardial fat was thicker in patients with CAD compared with those without CAD (4.0 mm vs 1.5 mm, P<.001); (2) patients with unstable angina had thicker epicardial fat than patients with atypical or stable angina; and (3) an epicardial fat thickness that exceeded 3.0 mm was an independent risk factor for CAD, with an odds ratio of 3.36 (P<.001).[38] In black patients enrolled in the Jackson Heart Study, increased EFV was significantly associated with coronary artery calcium (odds ratio 1.34, P<.004).[39] Carotid intima-media thickness (CIMT) is generally regarded as a validated surrogate for coronary atherosclerosis.[40] In patients with metabolic syndrome infected with the human immunodeficiency virus and receiving highly active antiretroviral therapy, there is a linear relationship between epicardial fat thickness and CIMT.[41]

METABOLIC ALTERATIONS IN THE EPICARDIAL FAT OF PATIENTS WITH IR

IR drives epicardial fat expansion. The metabolism of epicardial fat in patients with metabolic syndrome and IR is active, dysregulated, and abnormal. It is postulated that arterial walls that are showered by lipids and inflammatory mediators undergo recurrent biochemical and histologic injury and are subjected to accelerated atherogenesis.[42,43] Evidence is accruing that epicardial fat in insulin-resistant patients is in fact metabolically abnormal. In the setting of IR and CAD, epicardial fat decreases adiponectin production and increases the biosynthesis of TNF-α and leptin.[44] Fatty acid–binding proteins bind to, and help to solubilize and traffic, long-chain fatty acids within cells. The epicardial adipose tissue of patients with metabolic syndrome massively increases the expression of fatty acid binding protein 4 compared with subjects without metabolic syndrome, which likely reflects a large increase in the need to store and mobilize fatty acids within the epicardium.[45] In patients undergoing cardiac surgery, epicardial adipose tissue has the capacity to increase the production of fibroblast growth factor 21[46] as well as resistin, interleukin-6, and MCP-1.[47]

These data clearly support the hypothesis that epicardial adipose tissue can serve as a source of growth factors and inflammatory mediators.

OTHER CARDIAC ABNORMALITIES ASSOCIATED WITH INCREASED EPICARDIAL ADIPOSITY

Several other manifestations of cardiac disease are associated with increased epicardial adiposity. Among women with chest pain and angiographically normal coronary arteries, increased epicardial fat thickness is associated with reduced coronary flow reserve.[48] Traditional Framingham risk factors in this study were not predictive of microvascular dysfunction. An epicardial fat thickness greater than 0.45 cm had 85% sensitivity and 75% specificity in detecting a coronary flow reserve of less than 2 ($P<.0001$). Consistent with this finding is the observation that there is a negative linear relationship between epicardial fat thickness and flow-mediated dilatation at the brachial artery, suggesting that endothelial dysfunction worsens as epicardial fat thickness increases.[49] In patients with metabolic syndrome, hepatic steatosis, and increased epicardial adiposity, the myocardial phosphorylation potential (a measure of how efficiently adenosine triphosphate can be regenerated by mitochondrial oxidative phosphorylation to meet intramyocellular energy demands) is markedly reduced, despite normal left ventricular morphology as well as normal systolic and diastolic function.[50] Epicardial fat mass is associated with decreased left ventricular circumferential shortening and reduced regional systolic function[51] and, as it expands and increases in mass, increases the workload of cardiac pumping activity.[23] Patients with metabolic syndrome and increased epicardial fat thickness have blunted recovery of heart rate after a maximal graded exercise stress test.[52] Of interest, epicardial fat thickness of 5.5 mm or more correlates with blunting of heart-rate recovery with 84% sensitivity and 52% specificity. Finally, increased epicardial fat has been proposed to increase predisposition to atrial arrhythmias.[53] Increased epicardial fat is associated with increased fatty infiltration of the left atrium and pulmonary vein. Lin and colleagues[53] suggest that the combination of these 2 fatty infiltrative phenomena is associated with an increase in ectopic foci, automaticity, triggered activity, and electrical and structural remodeling.

SUMMARY

IR increases visceral organ steatosis caused by abnormalities in lipid trafficking and metabolism.

Expansion of epicardial fat thickness, volume, and mass are associated with all components of the metabolic syndrome. Epicardial fat can become insulin resistant and a potent source of lipids, adipokines that regulate insulin sensitivity, inflammatory mediators, and growth factors. Increased epicardial adiposity is associated with coronary atherosclerosis, endothelial dysfunction, reduced coronary flow reserve, impaired intramyocellular energy metabolism, and other cardiac abnormalities. Epicardial adiposity is a clinically significant structural and functional adverse sequela of IR. Epicardial adiposity constitutes an important focus of continued research, and may emerge as a target of therapy in patients with metabolic syndrome and/or DM.

REFERENCES

1. Executive Summary of The Third Report of The National Cholesterol Education Program (NCEP) expert panel on detection, evaluation, and treatment of high blood cholesterol in adults (adult treatment panel III). JAMA 2001;285(19):2486–97.
2. Lakka HM, Laaksonen DE, Lakka TA, et al. The metabolic syndrome and total and cardiovascular disease mortality in middle-aged men. JAMA 2002;288(21):2709–16.
3. Fujimoto WY, Abbate SL, Kahn SE, et al. The visceral adiposity syndrome in Japanese-American men. Obes Res 1994;2(4):364–71.
4. Lamarche B, Tchernof A, Mauriege P, et al. Fasting insulin and apolipoprotein B levels and low-density lipoprotein particle size as risk factors for ischemic heart disease. JAMA 1998;279(24):1955–61.
5. Oresic M. Systems biology strategy to study lipotoxicity and the metabolic syndrome. Biochim Biophys Acta 2010;1801(3):235–9.
6. Virtue S, Vidal-Puig A. Adipose tissue expandability, lipotoxicity and the metabolic syndrome—an allostatic perspective. Biochim Biophys Acta 2010;1801(3):338–49.
7. Leto D, Saltiel AR. Regulation of glucose transport by insulin: traffic control of GLUT4. Nat Rev Mol Cell Biol 2012;13(6):383–96.
8. Erion DM, Shulman GI. Diacylglycerol-mediated insulin resistance. Nat Med 2010;16(4):400–2.
9. Ukkola O, Santaniemi M. Adiponectin: a link between excess adiposity and associated comorbidities? J Mol Med (Berl) 2002;80(11):696–702.
10. Myers MG, Cowley MA, Munzberg H. Mechanisms of leptin action and leptin resistance. Annu Rev Physiol 2008;70:537–56.
11. Steppan CM, Bailey ST, Bhat S, et al. The hormone resistin links obesity to diabetes. Nature 2001;409(6818):307–12.

12. Kahn SE, Hull RL, Utzschneider KM. Mechanisms linking obesity to insulin resistance and type 2 diabetes. Nature 2006;444(7121):840–6.

13. Franssila-Kallunki A, Rissanen A, Ekstrand A, et al. Effects of weight loss on substrate oxidation, energy expenditure, and insulin sensitivity in obese individuals. Am J Clin Nutr 1992;55(2):356–61.

14. DeFronzo RA, Sherwin RS, Kraemer N. Effect of physical training on insulin action in obesity. Diabetes 1987;36(12):1379–85.

15. Kim MK, Tomita T, Kim MJ, et al. Aerobic exercise training reduces epicardial fat in obese men. J Appl Physiol 2009;106(1):5–11.

16. Bosy-Westphal A, Kossel E, Goele K, et al. Association of pericardial fat with liver fat and insulin sensitivity after diet-induced weight loss in overweight women. Obesity (Silver Spring) 2010; 18(11):2111–7.

17. Zhang Y, McGillicuddy FC, Hinkle CC, et al. Adipocyte modulation of high-density lipoprotein cholesterol. Circulation 2010;121(11):1347–55.

18. Toth PP. Reverse cholesterol transport: high-density lipoprotein's magnificent mile. Curr Atheroscler Rep 2003;5(5):386–93.

19. Toth PP. Adiponectin and high-density lipoprotein: a metabolic association through thick and thin. Eur Heart J 2005;26(16):1579–81.

20. Naka Y, Bucciarelli LG, Wendt T, et al. RAGE axis: animal models and novel insights into the vascular complications of diabetes. Arterioscler Thromb Vasc Biol 2004;24(8):1342–9.

21. Toth PP. Pleiotropic effects of angiotensin receptor blockers: addressing comorbidities by optimizing hypertension therapy. J Clin Hypertens (Greenwich) 2011;13(1):42–51.

22. Iacobellis G. Epicardial and pericardial fat: close, but very different. Obesity (Silver Spring) 2009; 17(4):625 [author reply: 626–27].

23. Iacobellis G, Sharma AM. Epicardial adipose tissue as new cardio-metabolic risk marker and potential therapeutic target in the metabolic syndrome. Curr Pharm Des 2007;13(21):2180–4.

24. Rabkin SW. Epicardial fat: properties, function and relationship to obesity. Obes Rev 2007;8(3): 253–61.

25. Glagov S, Bassiouny HS, Giddens DP, et al. Pathobiology of plaque modeling and complication. Surg Clin North Am 1995;75(4):545–56.

26. Wang TD, Lee WJ, Shih FY, et al. Relations of epicardial adipose tissue measured by multidetector computed tomography to components of the metabolic syndrome are region-specific and independent of anthropometric indexes and intraabdominal visceral fat. J Clin Endocrinol Metab 2009;94(2): 662–9.

27. Greif M, Becker A, von Ziegler F, et al. Pericardial adipose tissue determined by dual source CT is a risk factor for coronary atherosclerosis. Arterioscler Thromb Vasc Biol 2009;29(5):781–6.

28. Dey D, Wong ND, Tamarappoo B, et al. Computer-aided non-contrast CT-based quantification of pericardial and thoracic fat and their associations with coronary calcium and metabolic syndrome. Atherosclerosis 2010;209(1):136–41.

29. de Vos AM, Prokop M, Roos CJ, et al. Peri-coronary epicardial adipose tissue is related to cardiovascular risk factors and coronary artery calcification in post-menopausal women. Eur Heart J 2008; 29(6):777–83.

30. Rosito GA, Massaro JM, Hoffmann U, et al. Pericardial fat, visceral abdominal fat, cardiovascular disease risk factors, and vascular calcification in a community-based sample: the Framingham Heart Study. Circulation 2008;117(5):605–13.

31. Jain SH, Massaro JM, Hoffmann U, et al. Cross-sectional associations between abdominal and thoracic adipose tissue compartments and adiponectin and resistin in the Framingham Heart Study. Diabetes Care 2009;32(5):903–8.

32. Iacobellis G, Ribaudo MC, Assael F, et al. Echocardiographic epicardial adipose tissue is related to anthropometric and clinical parameters of metabolic syndrome: a new indicator of cardiovascular risk. J Clin Endocrinol Metab 2003;88(11):5163–8.

33. Momesso DP, Bussade I, Epifanio MA, et al. Increased epicardial adipose tissue in type 1 diabetes is associated with central obesity and metabolic syndrome. Diabetes Res Clin Pract 2011;91(1):47–53.

34. Hizli S, Ozdemir O, Abaci A, et al. Relation of subepicardial adipose tissue thickness and clinical and metabolic parameters in obese prepubertal children. Pediatric Diabetes 2010;11(8):556–62.

35. Sarin S, Wenger C, Marwaha A, et al. Clinical significance of epicardial fat measured using cardiac multislice computed tomography. Am J Cardiol 2008;102(6):767–71.

36. Park JS, Ahn SG, Hwang JW, et al. Impact of body mass index on the relationship of epicardial adipose tissue to metabolic syndrome and coronary artery disease in an Asian population. Cardiovasc Diabetol 2010;9:29.

37. Wang CP, Hsu HL, Hung WC, et al. Increased epicardial adipose tissue (EAT) volume in type 2 diabetes mellitus and association with metabolic syndrome and severity of coronary atherosclerosis. Clin Endocrinol 2009;70(6):876–82.

38. Ahn SG, Lim HS, Joe DY, et al. Relationship of epicardial adipose tissue by echocardiography to coronary artery disease. Heart 2008;94(3):e7.

39. Liu J, Fox CS, Hickson D, et al. Pericardial adipose tissue, atherosclerosis, and cardiovascular disease risk factors: the Jackson heart study. Diabetes Care 2010;33(7):1635–9.

40. Crouse JR 3rd, Raichlen JS, Riley WA, et al. Effect of rosuvastatin on progression of carotid intima-media

thickness in low-risk individuals with subclinical atherosclerosis: the METEOR Trial. JAMA 2007; 297(12):1344–53.

41. Iacobellis G, Sharma AM, Pellicelli AM, et al. Epicardial adipose tissue is related to carotid intima-media thickness and visceral adiposity in HIV-infected patients with highly active antiretroviral therapy-associated metabolic syndrome. Curr HIV Res 2007;5(2):275–9.

42. Shimabukuro M. Cardiac adiposity and global cardiometabolic risk: new concept and clinical implication. Circ J 2009;73(1):27–34.

43. Iacobellis G, Willens HJ. Echocardiographic epicardial fat: a review of research and clinical applications. J Am Soc Echocardiogr 2009;22(12):1311–9 [quiz: 1417–8].

44. Gormez S, Demirkan A, Atalar F, et al. Adipose tissue gene expression of adiponectin, tumor necrosis factor-alpha and leptin in metabolic syndrome patients with coronary artery disease. Intern Med 2011;50(8):805–10.

45. Vural B, Atalar F, Ciftci C, et al. Presence of fatty-acid-binding protein 4 expression in human epicardial adipose tissue in metabolic syndrome. Cardiovasc Pathol 2008;17(6):392–8.

46. Kotulak T, Drapalova J, Kopecky P, et al. Increased circulating and epicardial adipose tissue mRNA expression of fibroblast growth factor-21 after cardiac surgery: possible role in postoperative inflammatory response and insulin resistance. Physiol Res 2011; 60(5):757–67.

47. Kremen J, Dolinkova M, Krajickova J, et al. Increased subcutaneous and epicardial adipose tissue production of proinflammatory cytokines in cardiac surgery patients: possible role in postoperative insulin resistance. J Clin Endocrinol Metab 2006; 91(11):4620–7.

48. Sade LE, Eroglu S, Bozbas H, et al. Relation between epicardial fat thickness and coronary flow reserve in women with chest pain and angiographically normal coronary arteries. Atherosclerosis 2009;204(2):580–5.

49. Aydin H, Toprak A, Deyneli O, et al. Epicardial fat tissue thickness correlates with endothelial dysfunction and other cardiovascular risk factors in patients with metabolic syndrome. Metab Syndr Relat Disord 2010;8(3):229–34.

50. Perseghin G, Lattuada G, De Cobelli F, et al. Increased mediastinal fat and impaired left ventricular energy metabolism in young men with newly found fatty liver. Hepatology 2008;47(1):51–8.

51. Sironi AM, Pingitore A, Ghione S, et al. Early hypertension is associated with reduced regional cardiac function, insulin resistance, epicardial, and visceral fat. Hypertension 2008;51(2):282–8.

52. Sengul C, Duman D. The association of epicardial fat thickness with blunted heart rate recovery in patients with metabolic syndrome. Tohoku J Exp Med 2011;224(4):257–62.

53. Lin YK, Chen YJ, Chen SA. Potential atrial arrhythmogenicity of adipocytes: implications for the genesis of atrial fibrillation. Med Hypotheses 2010; 74(6):1026–9.

Index

Note: Page numbers of article titles are in **boldface** type.

Heart Failure Clin 8 (2012) 679–683
http://dx.doi.org/10.1016/S1551-7136(12)00082-7
1551-7136/12/$ – see front matter © 2012 Elsevier Inc. All rights reserved.

heartfailure.theclinics.com

United States Postal Service
Statement of Ownership, Management, and Circulation
(All Periodicals Publications Except Requestor Publications)

1. Publication Title	2. Publication Number	3. Filing Date
Heart Failure Clinics	0 2 5 - 0 5 5	9/14/12

4. Issue Frequency	5. Number of Issues Published Annually	6. Annual Subscription Price
Jan, Apr, July, Oct	4	$224.00

7. Complete Mailing Address of Known Office of Publication (*Not printer*) (*Street, city, county, state, and ZIP+4®*)

Elsevier Inc.
360 Park Avenue South
New York, NY 10010-1710

Contact Person
Stephen R. Bushing
Telephone (*Include area code*)
215-239-3688

8. Complete Mailing Address of Headquarters or General Business Office of Publisher (*Not printer*)

Elsevier Inc., 360 Park Avenue South, New York, NY 10010-1710

9. Full Names and Complete Mailing Addresses of Publisher, Editor, and Managing Editor (*Do not leave blank*)

Publisher (*Name and complete mailing address*)

Kim Murphy, Elsevier, Inc., 1600 John F. Kennedy Blvd. Suite 1800, Philadelphia, PA 19103-2899

Editor (*Name and complete mailing address*)

Barbara Cohen-Kligerman, Elsevier, Inc., 1600 John F. Kennedy Blvd. Suite 1800, Philadelphia, PA 19103-2899

Managing Editor (*Name and complete mailing address*)

Barbara Cohen-Kligerman, Elsevier, Inc., 1600 John F. Kennedy Blvd. Suite 1800, Philadelphia, PA 19103-2899

10. Owner (*Do not leave blank. If the publication is owned by a corporation, give the name and address of the corporation immediately followed by the names and addresses of all stockholders owning or holding 1 percent or more of the total amount of stock. If not owned by a corporation, give the names and addresses of the individual owners. If owned by a partnership or other unincorporated firm, give its name and address as well as those of each individual owner. If the publication is published by a nonprofit organization, give its name and address.*)

Full Name	Complete Mailing Address
Wholly owned subsidiary of	1600 John F. Kennedy Blvd., Ste. 1800
Reed/Elsevier, US holdings	Philadelphia, PA 19103-2899

11. Known Bondholders, Mortgagees, and Other Security Holders Owning or Holding 1 Percent or More of Total Amount of Bonds, Mortgages, or Other Securities. If none, check box ☐ None

Full Name	Complete Mailing Address
N/A	

12. Tax Status (*For completion by nonprofit organizations authorized to mail at nonprofit rates*) (*Check one*)
The purpose, function, and nonprofit status of this organization and the exempt status for federal income tax purposes:
☐ Has Not Changed During Preceding 12 Months
☐ Has Changed During Preceding 12 Months (*Publisher must submit explanation of change with this statement*)

PS Form 3526, September 2007 (Page 1 of 3 (Instructions Page 3)) PSN 7530-01-000-9931 PRIVACY NOTICE: See our Privacy policy in www.usps.com

---

13. Publication Title	14. Issue Date for Circulation Data Below
Heart Failure Clinics	July 2012

15. Extent and Nature of Circulation			Average No. Copies Each Issue During Preceding 12 Months	No. Copies of Single Issue Published Nearest to Filing Date
a. Total Number of Copies (*Net press run*)			231	195
b. Paid Circulation (By Mail and Outside the Mail)	(1)	Mailed Outside-County Paid Subscriptions Stated on PS Form 3541. (*Include paid distribution above nominal rate, advertiser's proof copies, and exchange copies*)	66	65
	(2)	Mailed In-County Paid Subscriptions Stated on PS Form 3541 (*Include paid distribution above nominal rate, advertiser's proof copies, and exchange copies*)		
	(3)	Paid Distribution Outside the Mails Including Sales Through Dealers and Carriers, Street Vendors, Counter Sales, and Other Paid Distribution Outside USPS®	16	17
	(4)	Paid Distribution by Other Classes Mailed Through the USPS (e.g. First-Class Mail®)		
c. Total Paid Distribution (*Sum of 15b (1), (2), (3), and (4)*)		►	82	82
d. Free or Nominal Rate Distribution (By Mail and Outside the Mail)	(1)	Free or Nominal Rate Outside-County Copies Included on PS Form 3541	62	57
	(2)	Free or Nominal Rate In-County Copies Included on PS Form 3541		
	(3)	Free or Nominal Rate Copies Mailed at Other Classes Through the USPS (e.g. First-Class Mail)		
	(4)	Free or Nominal Rate Distribution Outside the Mail (Carriers or other means)		
e. Total Free or Nominal Rate Distribution (*Sum of 15d (1), (2), (3) and (4)*)		►	62	57
f. Total Distribution (*Sum of 15c and 15e*)		►	144	139
g. Copies not Distributed (See instructions to publishers #4 (page #3))		►	87	56
h. Total (*Sum of 15f and g*)		►	231	195
i. Percent Paid (15c divided by 15f times 100)			56.94%	58.99%

16. Publication of Statement of Ownership

If the publication is a general publication, publication of this statement is required. Will be printed ☐ Publication not required
in the October 2012 issue of this publication.

17. Signature and Title of Editor, Publisher, Business Manager, or Owner

Stephen R. Bushing

Stephen R. Bushing – Inventory/Distribution Coordinator

Date
September 14, 2012

I certify that all information furnished on this form is true and complete. I understand that anyone who furnishes false or misleading information on this form or who omits material or information requested on the form may be subject to criminal sanctions (including fines and imprisonment) and/or civil sanctions (including civil penalties).

PS Form 3526, September 2007 (Page 2 of 3)

Moving?

Make sure your subscription moves with you!

To notify us of your new address, find your **Clinics Account Number** (located on your mailing label above your name), and contact customer service at:

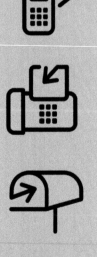

Email: journalscustomerservice-usa@elsevier.com

800-654-2452 (subscribers in the U.S. & Canada)
314-447-8871 (subscribers outside of the U.S. & Canada)

Fax number: 314-447-8029

Elsevier Health Sciences Division
Subscription Customer Service
3251 Riverport Lane
Maryland Heights, MO 63043